Thieme

# Colloid Cysts of the Third Ventricle

## Natural History, Decision-Making, and Operative Management

**Peter Nakaji, MD**
Professor and Chair
Department of Neurosurgery
University of Arizona College of Medicine
Phoenix, Arizona, USA

**Thomas L. Beaumont, MD, PhD**
Assistant Professor
Department of Neurological Surgery
University of California, San Diego
La Jolla, California, USA

**Ralph G. Dacey, Jr., MD, FACS, FRCSI (Hon)**
Professor and Former Chairman
Department of Neurosurgery
Washington University School of Medicine
St. Louis, Missouri, USA

295 Illustrations

Thieme
New York • Stuttgart • Delhi • Rio de Janeiro

**Library of Congress Cataloging-in-Publication Data** is available from the publisher.

**Important note:** Medicine is an ever-changing science undergoing continual development. Research and clinical experience are continually expanding our knowledge, in particular our knowledge of proper treatment and drug therapy. Insofar as this book mentions any dosage or application, readers may rest assured that the authors, editors, and publishers have made every effort to ensure that such references are in accordance with **the state of knowledge at the time of production of the book.**

Nevertheless, this does not involve, imply, or express any guarantee or responsibility on the part of the publishers in respect to any dosage instructions and forms of applications stated in the book. **Every user is requested to examine carefully** the manufacturers' leaflets accompanying each drug and to check, if necessary, in consultation with a physician or specialist, whether the dosage schedules mentioned therein or the contraindications stated by the manufacturers differ from the statements made in the present book. Such examination is particularly important with drugs that are either rarely used or have been newly released on the market. Every dosage schedule or every form of application used is entirely at the user's own risk and responsibility. The authors and publishers request every user to report to the publishers any discrepancies or inaccuracies noticed. If errors in this work are found after publication, errata will be posted at www.thieme.com on the product description page.

Some of the product names, patents, and registered designs referred to in this book are in fact registered trademarks or proprietary names even though specific reference to this fact is not always made in the text. Therefore, the appearance of a name without designation as proprietary is not to be construed as a representation by the publisher that it is in the public domain.

Thieme addresses people of all gender identities equally. We encourage our authors to use gender-neutral or gender-equal expressions wherever the context allows.



Thieme Publishers New York
333 Seventh Avenue, 18th Floor
New York, NY 10001, USA
www.thieme.com
+ 1 800 782 3488, customerservice@thieme.com

Cover design: © Thieme
Cover image source: © Thieme/Illustration by Matthew Holt, Medical Illustrator
Typesetting by TNQ Tech Private Limited, India

Printed in India by Replika Press Pvt. Ltd. 5 4 3 2 1

MIX
Paper | Supporting responsible forestry
FSC™ C016779
www.fsc.org

DOI: 10.1055/b000000352

ISBN: 978-1-68420-156-3

Also available as an e-book:
eISBN (PDF): 978-1-68420-157-0
eISBN (epub): 978-1-63853-680-2

# Contents

# Videos

# Foreword

It is easy to write a foreword for a topic which holds a great deal of personal interest. I have my own preference with colloid cysts, which is a small midline transcallosal exposure without the use of rigid retraction allowing complete visualization with extrication of the entire cyst. However, there are many neurosurgeons of equal aptitude, whose convictions on how to treat these enigmatic lesions are different from mine, and what this book beautifully provides is a rational review from master practitioners of their personal preferences, allowing the readers a choice of well-reasoned and thoughtful options to form their own preference of treatment.

There are few conditions that provoke more consternation and controversy among neurosurgeons than the colloid cyst. The sudden coma and death for which the colloid cyst is justly infamous for has left many neurosurgeons to ponder on how best to manage these patients. At the same time, the surgical risk, especially of forniceal damage with the risk of antegrade memory loss, is not insignificant in a mostly asymptomatic group of patients who may harbor these lesions for decades. Thus, the decision on whether to intervene in an asymptomatic patient remains difficult. Unfortunately, there has been a lack of long-term, reliable, natural history data to help with solid evidence-based decision-making.

Should the decision to operate be made, various treatment options are available, including cerebrospinal fluid diversion, stereotactic drainage, transcortical or transcallosal microsurgery, and endoscopic removal, leaving ample room for debate as to which is the "best" solution for any specific patient.

The present volume embodies the efforts of three editors who represent a cross-section of career stages. My contemporary and friend Ralph Dacey had a distinguished career practicing microneurosurgery including a long and distinguished service as Chair at Washington University, St. Louis. My former fellow and colleague Peter Nakaji is in the early years of his own service as Chair at the University of Arizona College of Medicine in Phoenix, where he performs complex microsurgery and minimally invasive and endoscopic surgery. Their colleague Thomas Beaumont is in the early middle part of his career at the University of California San Diego, where he also practices both cranial microsurgery and neuroendoscopy. The author list includes an honor roll of acknowledged experts in neurosurgery in general and on colloid cysts in particular, both from North America and from around the globe.

This volume contains much that will interest the student of neurosurgery at any phase, from residency to those in established practice. The clear presentation and insightful illustrations enrich a fundamentally useful tome.

I hope you will find it as thought-provoking and informative to read as I did. Fundamentally, this book is about bringing together what is known and what is controversial, providing ample fodder for vigorous debate. With the knowledge gleaned from these pages we can provide up-to-date thoughtful options to our patients with colloid cysts and their families.

Recommended with enthusiasm, enjoy!

*Robert Spetzler, MD, PhD*
*Emeritus President and CEO*
*Department of Neurosurgery*
*Barrow Neurological Institute*
*Phoenix, Arizona, USA*

# Preface

Why write a book about colloid cysts of the third ventricle? The truth is, I have been fascinated by the colloid cyst of the third ventricle since I first became aware of the pathology as a resident. There are a few clinical scenarios that neurosurgeons learn early in their residencies to treat with special respect: cauda equina, aneurysmal rupture, uncal herniation, and ventricular obstruction from a colloid cyst of the third ventricle. Of these, the colloid cyst is singular in the particularly insidious way that a completely intact patient with a benign disease, indeed just a cell layer thick, can go from talking with a headache to irretrievably comatose. In the clinic, one teeters between having every patient with a colloid cyst to go to the emergency department immediately and the observation that there are plenty of people who have a known cyst who have remained asymptomatic and with stable imaging for years. Colloid cysts are more similar to one another than many other pathologies: there is a constancy to the pathology in that most are simple cysts with a consistent location. Yet in this book, we will see that there is a great deal of nuance in presentation and situation (and somewhat in form and anatomy as well). We have all seen a great diversity of contrasting patient stories: those with headaches and a moderately small cyst (say, 7 mm) without any hydrocephalus; patients who neglected their cysts and come in years later with precipitous decline; those who come with no symptoms but have enlarged ventricles, or just one enlarged ventricle; those with giant cysts and very thin fornices, and already with memory decline; and those who have headaches and a known cyst who just want temporizing management—in one case motivated by the patient being at the peak of his career who was not willing to risk any loss in memory. These circumstances make what otherwise may seem like binary issues (small vs. large, hydrocephalus vs. no hydrocephalus, pressure headaches vs. asymptomatic) more complex. Nonetheless, there are some "classic" presentations that are more common. The finding of an incidental colloid cyst, identified on imaging for some other reason, is one of the classic quandaries, especially when headaches are mild, and the ventricles are small. A second group is the patient, often also without enlarged ventricles (or very mildly so), who presents a long history of headaches and is found to have a cyst in the 7- to 9-mm range, who feels compelled to go to the ER for a scan every time he or she has a bad headache (which may or may not be of the "pressure" or Valsalva-associated variety), in case this is "the time." Like the patient with the unruptured aneurysm who presents to the office who really could (but probably won't soon) deteriorate suddenly, counselling the odds is fine unless it is indeed *that time*. And who can say? This is the obverse of the whole psychology of buying lottery tickets: after all, sooner or later, it has to be someone.

I think of three patients in particular, out of many. In the first sobering case, the patient presented to the Emergency Department at an outside hospital with a severe headache, much out of keeping with her prior headaches, and who deteriorated within hours to completely comatose. By the time she received an external ventricular drain at our hospital (also only hours) she had suffered irrecoverable injury. The second is a medical provider who had a small colloid cyst diagnosed without ventriculomegaly after a mild biking accident as a young man. He decided on conservative management with serial imaging, but as many young people might do, stopped following up after a number of years. When he developed severe headache and nausea and vomiting, a case of flu was suspected—he forgot about the cyst and did not associate it with the symptoms anymore, and his fiancée was unaware of the diagnosis. Fortunately, due to the astuteness of an emergency room doctor he received a prompt CT scan which demonstrated profound ventriculomegaly, and an on-call neurosurgeon placed an external ventricular drain in time. He underwent successful endoscopic removal with an excellent outcome. The third patient was a military fighter pilot who stepped out of his aircraft with sudden vertigo after performing high-G maneuvers and was found to have a colloid cyst with hydrocephalus. Successful endoscopic removal eventually returned him to combat duty.

Neurosurgery is a hard profession whose stakes are often high. This is certainly true in the case of the colloid cyst. Gathering our collective wisdom and especially our best sense of how we should manage this pathology is a great cause. We are delighted that so many of our colleagues have come together to try to define the summation of our knowledge on this subject. Advances in neurosurgical technique, both endoscopic and microsurgical, have created options for patients that sometimes leave the "best" approach in any given case very much a subject of debate. Our goal in this volume is to present the background information and context related colloid cysts necessary to interpret the variety of treatments and approaches that the assembled experts herein detail. As Dr. Spetzler notes in his Foreword, for many aspects of this subject, expert opinion is as close to authority as we can come. In this case, at least we can endorse that the quality of the expert opinion is excellent.

We hope that you will find much in this book which will help you and your patients with colloid cyst to get the best care currently available and that it will also stimulate the thought processes of new colleagues who ultimately will advance the field to the benefit of all, and foremost, to our patients.

Enjoy!

**Peter Nakaji, MD**

# Contributors

**Thiago Albonette-Felicio, MD**
Neurosurgeon
Department of Neuroscience
University of Uninassau
Vilhena, Rondônia, Brazil

**Thomas L. Beaumont, MD, PhD**
Assistant Professor
Department of Neurological Surgery
University of California, San Diego
La Jolla, California, USA

**Alan R. Cohen, MD, FACS, FAAP, FAANS**
Chief of Pediatric Neurosurgery;
Carson-Spiro Professor of Pediatric Neurosurgery;
Director, Pediatric Neurosurgery Fellowship
The Charlotte R. Bloomberg Children's Center;
Professor of Neurosurgery, Oncology, and Pediatrics
The Johns Hopkins University School of Medicine
Baltimore, Maryland, USA

**Ralph G. Dacey, Jr., MD, FACS, FRCSI (Hon)**
Professor and Former Chairman
Department of Neurosurgery
Washington University School of Medicine
St. Louis, Missouri, USA

**Sonika Dahiya, MD**
Associate Professor
Department of Pathology & Immunology
Washington University School of Medicine
St. Louis, Missouri, USA

**Arthur Day, MD**
Professor
Department of Neurosurgery
University of Texas Health Science Center at Houston
Houston, Texas, USA

**Jonathan Engh, MD**
Neurosurgeon
Lexington Brain and Spine Institute
West Columbia, South Carolina, USA

**Andre Felix Gentil, MD, PhD**
Neurosurgeon
Department of Neurosurgery
Hospital Israelita Albert Einstein
São Paulo, São Paulo, Brazil

**Gaurav Gupta, MD, FAANS, FACS**
Associate Professor
Department of Neurosurgery
Rutgers Robert Wood Johnson Medical School
New Brunswick, New Jersey, USA

**Costas Hadjipanayis, MD, PhD**
Professor and Executive Vice-Chairman
Department of Neurological Surgery
University of Pittsburgh Medical Center
Pittsburgh, Pennsylvania, USA

**Simon Hanft, MD, FAANS**
Associate Professor
Department of Neurosurgery
Westchester Medical Center, New York Medical College
Valhalla, New York, USA

**Douglas A. Hardesty, MD**
Associate Professor
Department of Neurosurgery
Creighton University
Omaha, Nebraska, USA

**Albert Isaacs, MD, PhD, FRCSC FAANS**
Assistant Professor
Department of Neuroscience
Nationwide Children's Hospital
Columbus, Ohio, USA

**Roland Jabre, MD**
Clinical Assistant Professor
Department of Surgery
Division of Neurosurgery
University of Montreal
Montreal, Quebec, Canada

**Nikita Lakomkin, MD**
Resident
Department of Neurologic Surgery
Mayo Clinic
Rochester, Minnesota, USA

**David Limbrick, MD, PhD**
T.S. Park Chair in Neurosurgery;
Professor of Neurological Surgery and Pediatrics;
Neurosurgeon-in-Chief
St. Louis Children's Hospital
Washington University School of Medicine
St. Louis, Missouri, USA

**Islas-Aguilar Mario Alberto, MD**
Chair
Department of Neurosurgery
Hospital Central Dr. Ignacio Morones Prieto
San Luis Potosi, SLP, Mexico

**Sascha Marx, MD**
Resident
Department of Neurosurgery
University Medicine Greifswald
Sauerbruchstr, Greifswald, Germany

**Michael W. McDermott, MD, FAANS**
Chief Medical Executive
Department of Neurological Surgery
Miami Neuroscience Institute
Baptist Health South Florida
Miami, Florida, USA

**Sean D. McEvoy, MD**
Assistant Professor
Department of Neurological Surgery
Washington University School of Medicine
St. Louis, Missouri, USA

**Peter Nakaji, MD**
Professor and Chair
Department of Neurosurgery
University of Arizona College of Medicine
Phoenix, Arizona, USA

**Anil Nanda, MD, MPH, FACS**
Professor
Department of Neurosurgery
Rutgers Robert Wood Johnson Medical School
New Brunswick, New Jersey, USA

**Vinayak Narayan, MD, FACS, FRCS (Ed)**
Clinical Assistant Professor
Department of Neurological Surgery
University of Pittsburgh
UPMC Neurological Institute
Harrisburg, Pennsylvania, USA

**David M. Panczykowski, MD**
Neurosurgeon
Department of Neurosurgery
The University of Texas Health Science Center at Houston
Houston, Texas, USA

**Daniel M. Prevedello, MD**
Professor
Department of Neurological Surgery;
Director
Minimally Invasive Cranial Surgery Program;
Director
Skull Base and Pituitary Surgery Program;
The Ohio State University
Columbus, Ohio, USA

**Eduardo Carvalhal Ribas, MD, PhD**
Privat-Docent Professor
Neurosurgeon
Department of Neurosurgery
Hospital Israelita Albert Einstein
São Paulo, São Paulo, Brazil

**Guilherme Carvalhal Ribas, MD, PhD**
Privat-Docent Professor
Neurosurgeon
Department of Neurosurgery
Hospital Israelita Albert Einstein
São Paulo, São Paulo, Brazil

**Keith M. Rich, MD**
Professor
Department of Neurosurgery
Washington University
St. Louis, Missouri, USA

**Roberto Rodriguez Rubio, MD**
Associate Professor
Department of Neurological Surgery
University of California, San Francisco
San Francisco, California, USA

**Henry W. S. Schroeder, MD, PhD**
Professor and Chairman
Department of Neurosurgery
University Medicine Greifswald
Greifswald, Mecklenburg-Vorpommern, Germany

**Robert Spetzler, MD, PhD**
Emeritus President and CEO
Department of Neurosurgery
Barrow Neurological Institute
Phoenix, Arizona, USA

**Jaime Gerardo Torres-Corzo, MD**
Chair
Department of Neurosurgery
Hospital Central Dr. Ignacio Morones Prieto
San Luis Potosi, SLP, Mexico

**Franz J. Wippold II, MD, FACR**
Emeritus Professor of Radiology;
Former Chief of Neuroradiology
Department of Radiology
Mallinckrodt Institute of Radiology
Washington University School of Medicine
Chesterfield, Missouri, USA

**Jacob S. Young, MD**
Resident
Department of Neurological Surgery
University of California
San Francisco, California, USA

**Hussein A. Zeineddine, MD**
Resident
Department of Neurosurgery
University of Texas Health Science Center at Houston
Houston, Texas, USA

# The History of Surgery for Colloid Cysts

*Alan R. Cohen and Ralph G. Dacey*

## Introduction

Colloid cysts are small, slow-growing, histologically benign lesions occurring at the anterior aspect of the third ventricle. They are rare, comprising between 0.5 and 1% of all brain tumors,[1,2,3,4] with an estimated annual incidence of 3.2 per million,[5] although it has been suggested that they are being recognized with increased frequency due to advances in neuroimaging.[6,7,8,9,10] Despite their rarity, these cysts have long presented a challenge to the neurosurgeon tasked with their removal because of their location in the center of the brain, adjacent to critical neurovascular structures at the foramina of Monro. Here we trace the evolution of surgery for colloid cysts from craniotomy to microsurgery to stereotactic approaches up to the early neuroendoscopic experience. More recent microsurgical and endoscopic techniques will be covered in subsequent chapters.

## Background

Colloid cysts are generally spherical in shape and are composed of a capsule of variable thickness lined by columnar epithelium with a gelatinous center of variable viscocity.[11] They are usually located at the anterior superior aspect of the third ventricle and can cause noncommunicating hydrocephalus by unilateral or bilateral obstruction at the foramina of Monro. The clinical presentation of colloid cysts is broad and ranges from an incidental finding on imaging studies to sudden death from increased intracranial pressure.

The natural history of colloid cysts remains incompletely understood. In 1989, Camacho and colleagues retrospectively reviewed 84 patients with colloid cysts at the Mayo Clinic.[7] Of these, 24 patients, most of whom had normal-sized ventricles, were managed nonoperatively and none required surgery over an average follow-up interval of 19 months. A decade later, Pollock and Huston expanded on this series, studying 68 patients in whom colloid cysts were found incidentally, including the 24 cases previously reported by Camacho et al, and concluded that this cohort can be managed safely with observation and serial neuroimaging.[12] Over a 10-year period, only two patients undergoing surveillance imaging showed progression, one with cyst growth and one with hydrocephalus. They concluded that patients with asymptomatic colloid cysts could be followed safely with observation and serial neuroimaging. No patient in this series experienced sudden death.

In 2016, Beaumont and colleagues at Washington University retrospectively reviewed the natural history of 163 patients with colloid cysts treated at their institution over two decades.[13] Half of the colloid cysts were identified incidentally, and 58% of these incidental colloid cysts were followed with surveillance neuroimaging, with a mean follow-up of 5.1 years. No patient with an incidentally discovered colloid cyst went on to develop acute hydrocephalus or neurological deterioration in the absence of antecedent trauma. Risk factors for symptomatic lesions were younger age (<65 years), headache at presentation, larger cyst diameter (≥7 mm), hyperintensity on FLAIR MRI, and cyst location in a third ventricle risk zone (either anteriorly adjacent to the foramina of Monro or posteriorly adjacent to the aqueduct of Sylvius).

The "classical history" of colloid cysts presenting with paroxysmal headache associated with changes in head position is actually rare.[2,14,15,16] This reflects the fact that these lesions are relatively sessile and do not move significantly in the absence of trauma or procedures, such as lumbar puncture, that alter cerebrospinal fluid (CSF) dynamics. The most common presenting complaints of patients with symptomatic colloid cysts are related to hydrocephalus: headache, nausea, vomiting, blurred vision, diplopia, dizziness, syncope, ataxia, and cognitive decline.[13] Other presentations include progressive dementia and gait disturbance with urinary ataxia without headache or papilledema.[2,15,17] Seizures are a recognized but infrequent presentation of colloid cysts. Incidental colloid cysts often come to light during a workup for trauma.

Colloid cysts can present with hydrocephalus due to symptomatic obstruction of the foramina of Monro. A feared consequence of colloid cysts is sudden neurological deterioration and death.[2,3,5,7,15,16,18,19,20,21,22,23] A colloid cyst headache can be misinterpreted as migraine, and sudden deterioration and death from acute obstructive noncommunicating hydrocephalus is one of the more dramatic presentations in neurosurgery. Although sudden neurological deterioration and death remains a concern in the era of modern neuroimaging, it is uncommon in patients presenting without preceding symptoms.[12,13]

## History

The first description of a colloid cyst was by Wallman in 1858 as a postmortem finding in a man with ataxia and incontinence. A lipoma of the choroid plexus was also identified.[24] But it was Walter Dandy of Johns Hopkins who performed the first colloid cyst surgery and who pioneered both the transcallosal and the transcortical approaches that are still in use today (▶ Fig. 1).[25]

The first localization and surgical resection of a colloid cyst was performed by Dandy in 1921.[25,26] His patient was a 24-year-old woman who complained of headaches for 10 years. She had bilateral papilledema measuring 6 diopters, a right lateral rectus palsy, and a left ptosis (▶ Fig. 2).

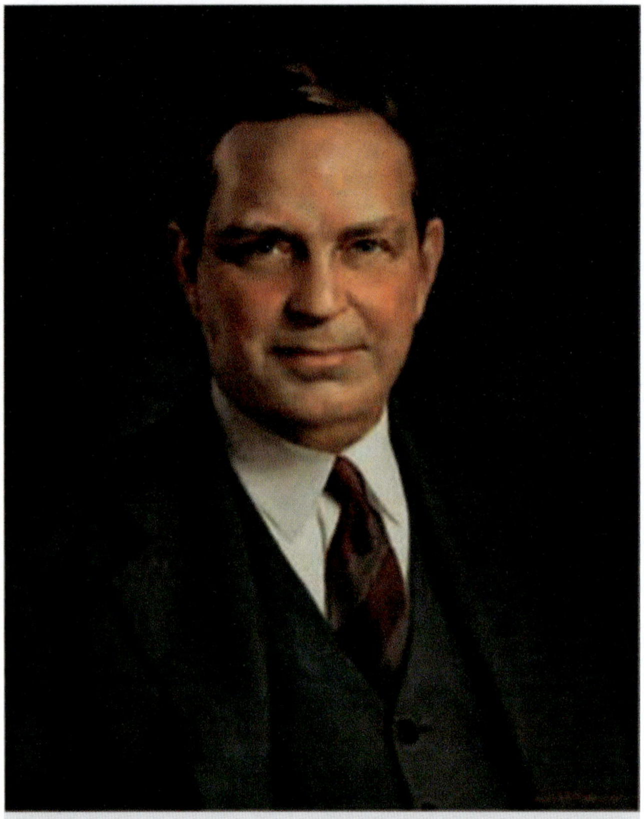

**Fig. 1** Walter Edward Dandy. (Reproduced with permission from the Chesney Archives of Johns Hopkins Medicine, Nursing, and Public Health.)

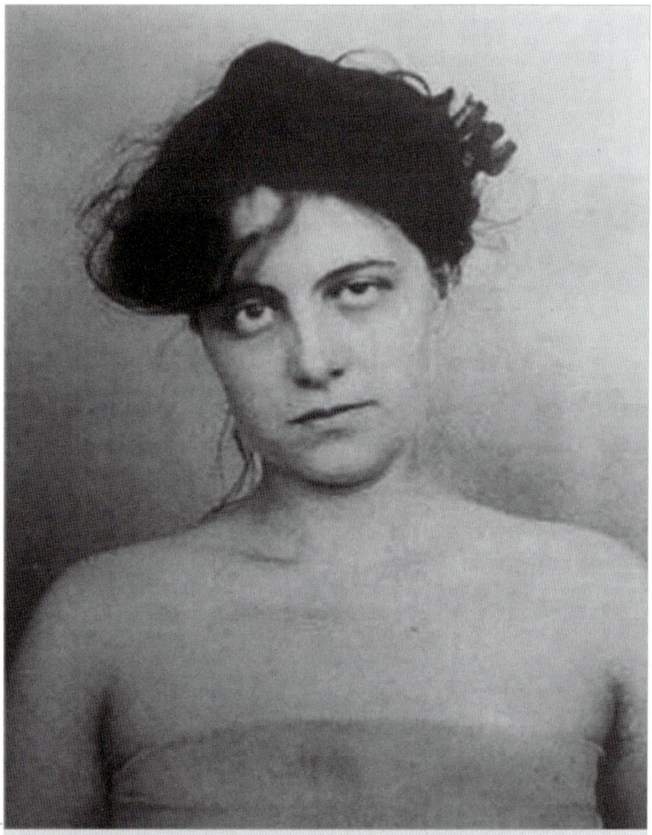

**Fig. 2** In a landmark operation, this 24-year-old woman underwent surgical resection of a third ventricular colloid cyst by Walter Dandy in 1921. This was the first time a colloid cyst was successfully diagnosed, localized, and removed. (Reproduced from Benign Tumors in the Third Ventricle of the Brain: Diagnosis and Treatment. By Walter E. Dandy, M.D., Adjunct Professor of Surgery, the Johns Hopkins University. Cloth. Price, $5. Pp. 171, with 120 illustrations. Springfield & Baltimore: Charles C. Thomas, 1933.)

Localization of the tumor to the third ventricle was performed by air ventriculography (▶ Fig. 3). Sequential injection of air into each dilated lateral ventricle failed to fill the third ventricle, which was occupied by the tumor, or the contralateral ventricle, because the septum pellucidum was intact. Dandy operated on October 18, 1921 under ether anesthesia. He turned a large bone flap on the right side, tapped the lateral ventricle, and used a posterior interhemispheric transcallosal approach. This included division of a long 5 to 6 cm portion of the corpus callosum and sectioning of one of the fornices to facilitate the exposure (▶ Fig. 4). He was able to remove the 1-cm diameter colloid cyst, although the patient had a stormy postoperative course, with high fevers from a large gluteal abscess that was caused by a burn from an overheated water bottle. She developed a "marked mental disturbance" with disorientation, short-term memory loss, and confabulation that Dandy and a psychiatric consultant attributed to her prolonged fever. She also had a hemiparesis that was caused by an injury to the internal capsule during the operation when, in Dandy's words, "at one time the operator had lost his bearings." Ultimately the patient's mental status and hemiparesis improved markedly. She was discharged 2.5 months after the surgery (▶ Fig. 5) and she remained well at Dandy's follow-up examination 10.5 years later.

Dandy subsequently developed the frontal transcortical transventricular approach and used it on October 11, 1930 to remove a colloid cyst from an 11-year-old girl who had presented with headaches for 8 months (▶ Fig. 6). He exposed the cyst by sectioning the fornix at the anterior foramen of Monro and then opened the cyst capsule and drained the contents, which included a small hard concretion. There was a large vein stuck to the cyst capsule that Dandy had to coagulate, clip, and divide in order to get the cyst out. The child had a smooth postoperative course and was discharged from the hospital after 3 weeks (▶ Fig. 7) and remained well at a follow-up of 1.5 years.

Between 1921 and 1932, Dandy removed colloid cysts from five patients, with one perioperative death.[25] All patients presented with headache. In two patients he noted that the severity of the headache varied with changes in posture. In each case the tumor was localized with air ventriculography. Dandy used the posterior transcallosal approach in three patients and the anterior transcortical transventricular approach in two. He was successful in removing the colloid cyst from all the patients. The single

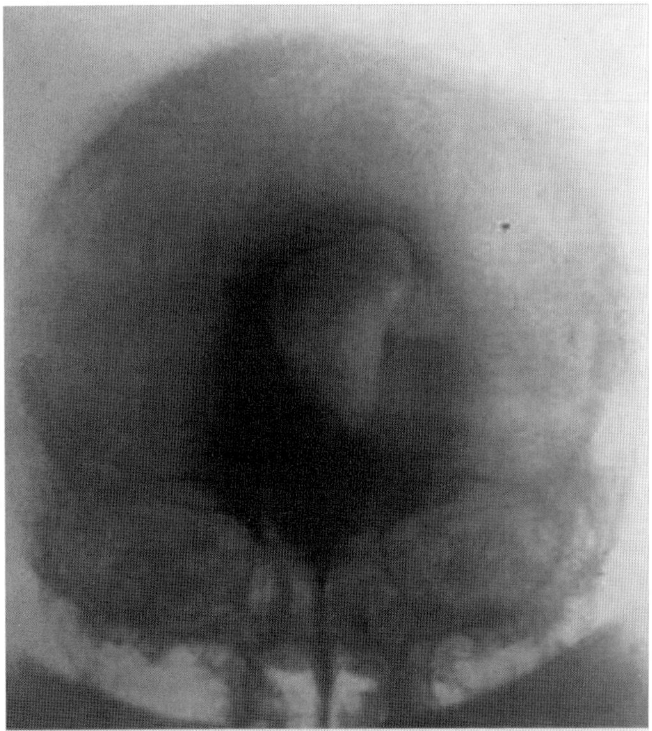

Fig. 3 Dandy localized the tumor using air ventriculography, a technique that he had pioneered. (Reproduced from Benign Tumors in the Third Ventricle of the Brain: Diagnosis and Treatment. By Walter E. Dandy, M.D., Adjunct Professor of Surgery, the Johns Hopkins University. Cloth. Price, $5. Pp. 171, with 120 illustrations. Springfield & Baltimore: Charles C. Thomas, 1933.)

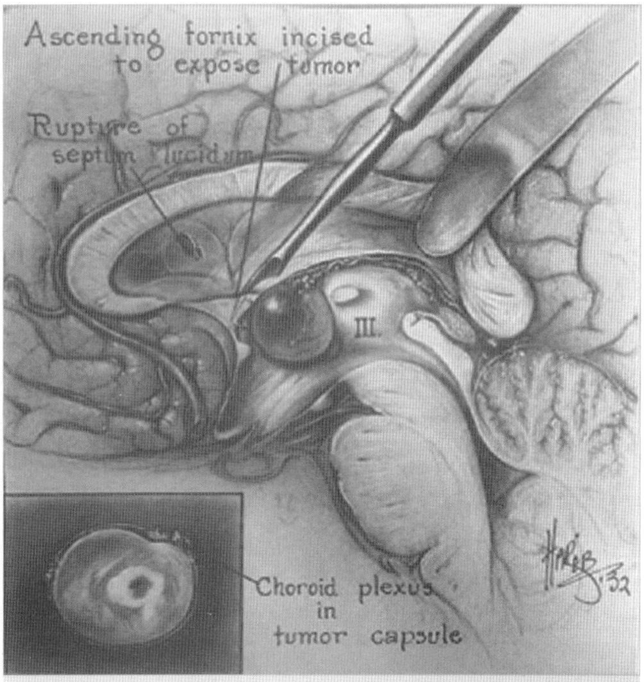


Fig. 4 Dandy removed the tumor using a posterior interhemispheric transcallosal approach. (Reproduced from Benign Tumors in the Third Ventricle of the Brain: Diagnosis and Treatment. By Walter E. Dandy, M.D., Adjunct Professor of Surgery, the Johns Hopkins University. Cloth. Price, $5. Pp. 171, with 120 illustrations. Springfield & Baltimore: Charles C. Thomas, 1933.)

death was from occlusion of the aqueduct of Sylvius that occurred in a 42-year-old woman, 1 month following transcortical transventricular cyst resection.

In 1951, Wylie McKissock of the National Hospital, Queen Square, London reported using the transcortical transventricular approach to remove colloid cysts in 21 patients, with 6 deaths.[27] Of the 15 patients who survived the surgery, 11 were symptom-free postoperatively.

The anterior interhemispheric transcallosal approach was introduced by James Greenwood at the Methodist Hospital in Houston, Texas in 1949.[28] This was a modification of Dandy's earlier posterior transcallosal operation. Greenwood was able to demonstrate the feasibility of this approach, although both patients undergoing this surgery had a poor outcome. In 1964, Cassinari and Bernasconi in Milan, Italy used the transcallosal approach for tumors in the anterior third ventricle.[29] In 1966, Thomas Milhorat and Maitland Baldwin, working at the NIH, reported using the transcallosal microdissection in experimental animals to expose structures deep in the cerebral midline, describing it as safe, simple, and delicate.[30] In 1969, George Ehni of the Baylor College of Medicine created a movie demonstrating the efficacy of the transcallosal approach for removing brain tumors.[31] He later published his experience with 52 transcallosal procedures and emphasized the benefits of this approach over the transcortical route.[32]

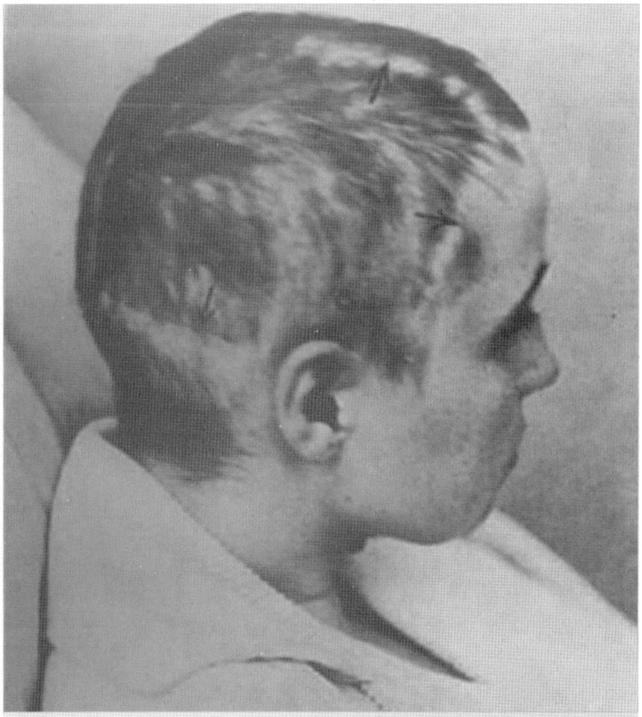

Fig. 5 Dandy's first colloid cyst patient at the time of discharge from the hospital, 2.5 months after the operation. (Reproduced from Benign Tumors in the Third Ventricle of the Brain: Diagnosis and Treatment. By Walter E. Dandy, M.D., Adjunct Professor of Surgery, the Johns Hopkins University. Cloth. Price, $5. Pp. 171, with 120 illustrations. Springfield & Baltimore: Charles C. Thomas, 1933.)

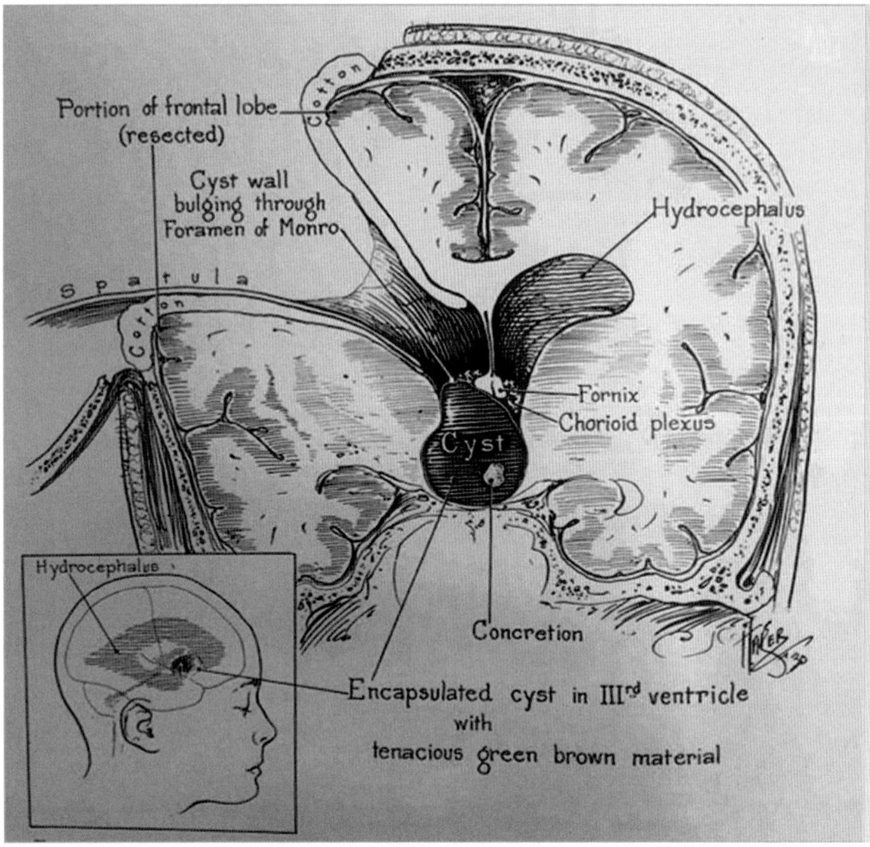


**Fig. 6** Dandy's third colloid cyst removal. The patient was an 11-year-old girl. For this case, Dandy used the frontal transcortical transventricular corridor, another approach he developed. (Reproduced from Benign Tumors in the Third Ventricle of the Brain: Diagnosis and Treatment. By Walter E. Dandy, M.D., Adjunct Professor of Surgery, the Johns Hopkins University. Cloth. Price, $5. Pp. 171, with 120 illustrations. Springfield & Baltimore: Charles C. Thomas, 1933.)

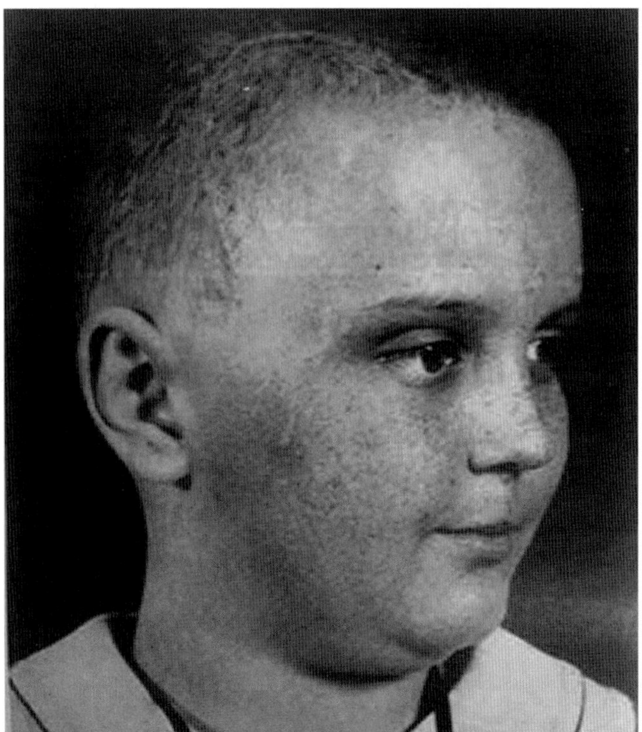

**Fig. 7** The patient 3 weeks after Dandy's successful transcortical transventricular colloid cyst resection. (Reproduced from Benign Tumors in the Third Ventricle of the Brain: Diagnosis and Treatment. By Walter E. Dandy, M.D., Adjunct Professor of Surgery, the Johns Hopkins University. Cloth. Price, $5. Pp. 171, with 120 illustrations. Springfield & Baltimore: Charles C. Thomas, 1933.)

In 1973, Donlin Long and Shelly Chou reported a favorable experience using the anterior transcallosal corridor to remove six craniopharyngiomas located primarily in the third ventricle.[33]

It was William Shucart and Bennett Stein who popularized the transcallosal approach to the anterior ventricular system, reporting their experience with 25 patients in 1978, 6 of whom had third ventricular colloid cysts.[31] In 2017, Alexander Konovalov and colleagues at the Burdenko Neurosurgery Institute in Moscow described their experience treating a large series of 377 patients with colloid cysts. They used the transcallosal corridor almost exclusively with total cyst removal in 96% of cases and a low complication rate.[34]

Currently, the two conventional craniotomies for the microsurgical resection of third ventricular colloid cysts remain the anterior transcortical transventricular approach and the anterior interhemispheric transcallosal approach, each of which was originally pioneered by Dandy.

Over the years, surgeons have searched for less invasive alternatives for approaching the elusive third ventricular colloid cyst. In 1975, Gutierrez-Lara and colleagues treated five patients by introducing a catheter into the third ventricular cyst using external skull landmarks and ventriculography.[35] They punctured the cyst, aspirated its contents, and converted the catheter to a ventriculoatrial shunt with satisfactory results and no morbidity or mortality.

The work of Gutierrez-Lara paved the way for the novel technique of stereotactic cyst aspiration. In 1978,

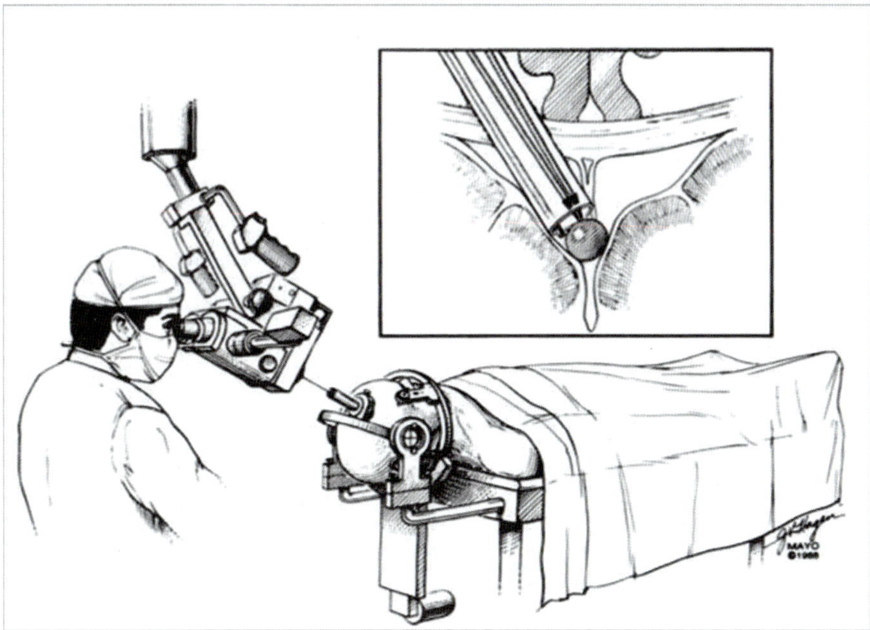

**Fig. 8** Stereotaxic microsurgical laser craniotomy performed through a cylindrical tube. (Reproduced with permission from Abernathey CD, et al. Treatment of colloid cysts of the third ventricle by stereotaxic microsurgical laser craniotomy. J Neurosurgery 1989;70:535–539. An Open Access or Creative Commons publishing model conveys no rights to use this material in any format without written permission from the JNS Publishing Group.)

Bosch et al reported successful treatment of four patients at the Karolinska Hospital by CT-guided stereotactic cyst aspiration.[36] Other investigators have reported generally favorable short-term outcomes for stereotactic aspiration of colloid cysts, despite technical limitations of the procedure.[37,38,39,40,41]

In 1989, Chad Abernathey et al at the Mayo Clinic combined stereotaxy with a transcortical approach for colloid cysts by microsurgical laser craniotomy through a 2-cm diameter cylindrical tube (▶ Fig. 8).[42] They reported good results with no mortality and minimal morbidity over an average follow-up duration of 19 months and offered the technique as a viable alternative to transcallosal craniotomy. Kondziolka and Lunsford treated 20 patients with colloid cysts using a limited craniotomy, small corticectomy, and stereotactically guided trajectory to the foramen of Monro.[43] They achieved total or near-total resection in all cases with an excellent outcome in all over a mean follow-up of 4.3 years. Extracranial ventricular shunting has been used infrequently to treat patients with colloid cysts and although some successes have been reported, shunting is generally considered the least satisfactory method of treatment.[7]

## Complications of Craniotomy and Stereotactic Approaches

Microsurgical craniotomy, either via the transcortical or transcallosal route, and stereotactic surgery to approach these benign deep-seated lesions is not without risk.

Craniotomy carries risks of hydrocephalus, seizures, subdural hygromas, venous infarction, and cerebral swelling. Camacho et al reported complications in 10 of 36 patients undergoing colloid cyst resection via the transcortical transventricular route.[7] Antunes et al noted 4 deaths and 7 complications in 23 patients undergoing colloid cyst resection using this technique.[6] Fritsch used the transcortical transventricular approach in 18 patients with no deaths and no major morbidities, although 1 patient had a generalized seizure 2 years after surgery, 4 had a transient "organic mental syndrome," and 6 required ventriculoperitoneal shunt placement.[44] Morita and Kelly identified 10 complications in 30 patients undergoing resection of third ventricular tumors using a computer-assisted volumetric stereotactic approach, including short-term memory loss, hydrocephalus, subdural hygroma, and the syndrome of inappropriate antidiuretic hormone.[45]

Although the transcallosal corridor eliminates cortical disruption, it can result in injury to thrombosis of the superior sagittal sinus, venous infarction from division of bridging veins, disconnection syndrome, injury to the pericallosal arteries, injury to the fornices, and subdural effusions. In their series, Shucart and Stein noted a postoperative hemiparesis from venous infarction in one of six patients with colloid cyst and mutism in one of two patients with a craniopharyngioma.[31] In 1979, Jeeves et al in Adelaide, South Australia used the transcallosal route to remove a third ventricular colloid cyst in two patients.[46] Each patient developed a disturbance of short-term memory, presumably related to division of the forniceal pillars to facilitate exposure, and one of them required placement of a ventriculoatrial shunt. Hall and Lunsford used the transcallosal approach in eight patients with third ventricular colloid cysts and noted venous infarction with hemiparesis in two, *Serratia marscescens* meningitis in one, and hydrocephalus requiring ventricular shunting in one.[37] In 1996, Hernesniemi and Leivo of Finland reported a good functional outcome in 31 patients undergoing transcallosal resection of colloid cysts with several postoperative complications.[5] One patient suffered a memory deficit, one sustained a hemorrhagic venous infarction, one developed a chronic subdural hematoma, one had meningitis and a brain abscess with hemiparesis, and one had a superficial wound infection.

The initial enthusiasm for stereotactic surgery for colloid cysts has been tempered by treatment failure in several cases. Stereotactic needle puncture can lead to neural or vascular injury if the procedure is not visualized. Other failures have been attributed to the thick, viscous, semi-solid nature of some colloid cysts resulting in incomplete aspiration or to deflection of small, pedunculated cysts away from the stereotactic needle.[5] Kondziolka and Lunsford retrospectively identified two factors on preoperative CT predicting failure of stereotactic aspiration: small cyst size (≤1.0 mL volume) and hyperdense cyst appearance, correlating with increased cyst viscocity.[5] El Khoury and colleagues have correlated the MR finding of a low signal on T2-weighted fast spin echo sequences with increased cyst viscosity in 19 patients.[5] These cysts proved more difficult to remove using neuroendoscopic techniques.

Simple stereotactic cyst aspiration can be associated with a high recurrence rate if the cyst wall remains. Mathiesen and colleagues at the Karolinska Institute found a high recurrence rate in 16 patients with colloid cysts treated by stereotactic aspiration.[3] Eight of the aspirations were performed using ventriculoscopic guidance. Reoperation was required in 13 of the 16 patients, which included a second aspiration in 6, 2 further aspirations in 2, microsurgical resection in 5, and ventricular shunt insertion in 3. Late recurrences were common, with 7 of the 16 patients developing a recurrence 8 or more years after cyst aspiration. The authors emphasized the need for long-term follow-up. Complications included coma from transtentorial herniation in four patients. Three patients had headaches, temporary memory deficit, mild personality change postoperatively, and one patient suffered unilateral arm pain feltto be from thalamic injury.

## Neuroendoscopic Management

Endoscopic surgery was introduced as a balanced middle ground between open microsurgery and stereotactic aspiration. The endoscope allows the operator to work under direct vision in the CSF-filled ventricular cavity with minimal disruption of the cortex. The cyst capsule can be opened sharply or with a fiberoptic laser and the cyst contents, even if viscous or semi-solid, can be emptied. The cyst wall can be reduced, and significant amounts of the wall can be removed. In some cases, the colloid cyst can be removed en bloc.

The first endoscopic treatment of colloid cysts was described in 1983 by Powell et al working at the Frenchay Hospital in Bristol, UK.[48] They were able to successfully aspirate five of six colloid cysts using a rigid endoscope and coagulate the cyst capsule with diathermy. Included in their five successes were two patients in whom the cyst was aspirated endoscopically but the surgeon nevertheless chose to proceed with craniotomy to resect the cyst wall.

In 1988, Auer et al attempted to resect a third ventricular colloid cyst endoscopically using an Nd YAG laser. They were able to shrink the cyst but could not open the cyst wall; so the procedure was converted to a transcortical transventricular craniotomy for cyst removal.[49] In 1991, Eiras Ajuria and Alberdi Viñas in Zargosa, Spain described successful endoscopic management of eight patients with varied brain lesions including one colloid cyst of the third ventricle.[50] Merienne and colleagues in Paris, France reported using an endoscope with stereotactic guidance and an Nd YAG laser to treat two patients with colloid cysts in 1992.[51]

In 1992, Cohen and Shucart removed two colloid cysts and decompressed a third endoscopically using neuronavigation and placing the burr hole more anteriorly and laterally than the standard precoronal mid-pupillary line site to maximize exposure of the face of the cyst in the foramen of Monro (▶ Fig. 9).[52] Subsequently, in 1998 Abdou and Cohen reported their experience with endoscopic treatment of colloid cysts in 13 patients, with a near-total resection in 10 over a mean follow-up duration of 4 years and no mortality (▶ Fig. 10).[53] The use of frameless stereotactic image guidance permitted a more anterior and lateral placement of the burr hole, which provided an optimal view of the cyst at the foramen of Monro (▶ Fig. 11).[53] Three patients required ventricular shunt placement, although in one of the three hydrocephalus developed despite complete removal of the cyst. Philippe Decq et al in Creteil, France operated on 15 patients with colloid cysts endoscopically using stereotactic guidance, perforating the cyst wall with a needle, aspirating the cyst contents, and coagulating the cyst capsule.[54] The procedure was successful in 12 of the 15 cases with a mean duration of follow-up of 15 months, with no mortality or major morbidity. One patient had an asymptomatic recurrence after 1 year.

Lewis and coworkers reported on seven patients who underwent endoscopic resection of colloid cysts, none of whom required conversion to open craniotomy.[22] They compared this cohort to eight patients operated on by transcallosal microsurgery and found that the endoscopic group had a shorter operative time, shorter hospitalization, lower perioperative complication rate, and earlier return to work. Caemaert et al in Ghent, Belgium described endoscopic treatment of six patients with colloid cysts and hydrocephalus, with three total and three subtotal resections.[55] The hydrocephalus was successfully treated in all patients and nopatient required ventricular shunting. Other investigators have considered the endoscope the first line of treatment for colloid cysts with the understanding that in select cases the procedure may need to be converted to microsurgical craniotomy.[56,57,58,59]

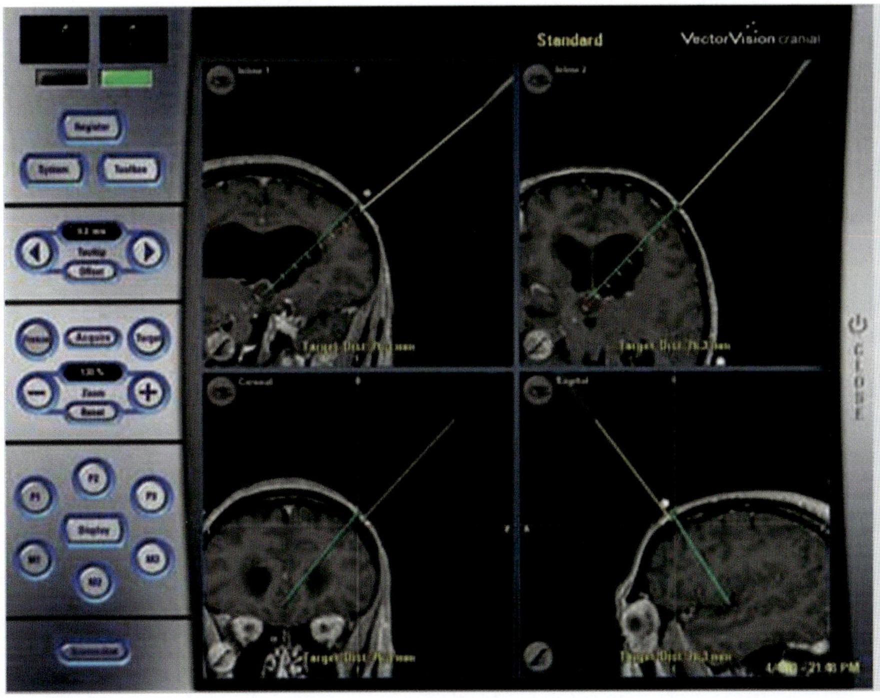


**Fig. 9** Frameless stereotactic guidance permits precise calculation of a trajectory for endoscopic colloid cyst resection. (Reproduced with permission from Alan R. Cohen.)

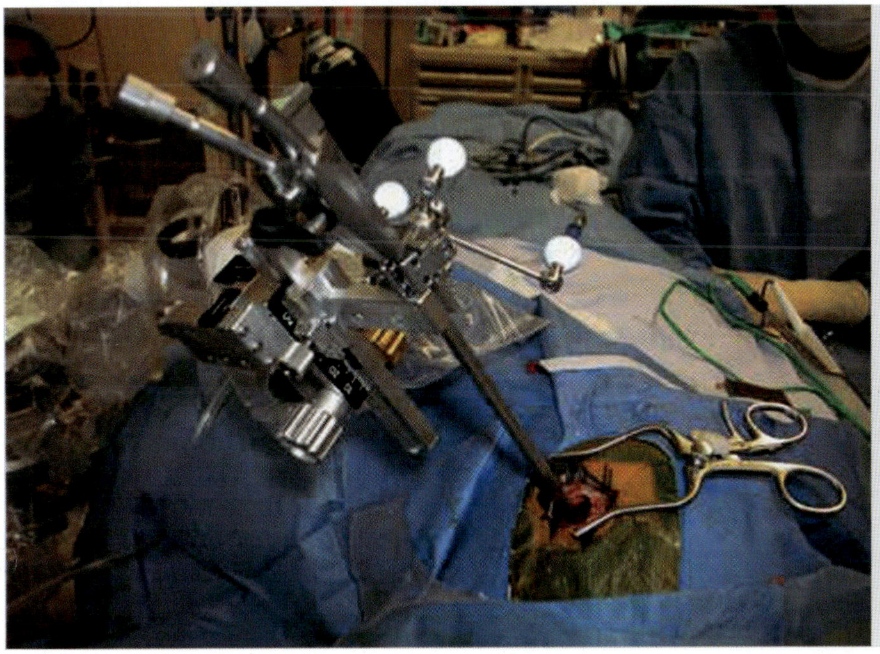

**Fig. 10** An endoscope holder can be useful. This device has a nitrogen-powered pneumatic arm along with a micromanipulator that allows small incremental movements. (Reproduced with permission from Alan R. Cohen.)

## Complications of Neuroendoscopic Approaches

Multiple investigators have described a generally favorable experience with the endoscopic management of colloid cysts.[52,53,60,61,62,63,64,65,66,67,68,69,70,71] As is the case for stereotactic cyst resection, the duration of follow-up for endoscopic cases has been relatively short, and the question is whether these results will be durable in the long run. Complications of endoscopic colloid cyst surgery are similar to those of stereotactic approaches: neurovascular injury including short-term memory dysfunction from forniceal injury, infection, low grade headache, and fever from aseptic ventriculitis and hydrocephalus.[3,52,55,72,73,74] Transient postoperative depression in consciousness with normal intracranial pressure has been reported and ascribed, possibly, to extensive irrigation with normal saline leading to a depletion of calcium and potassium ions that could disturb neural transmission.[55]

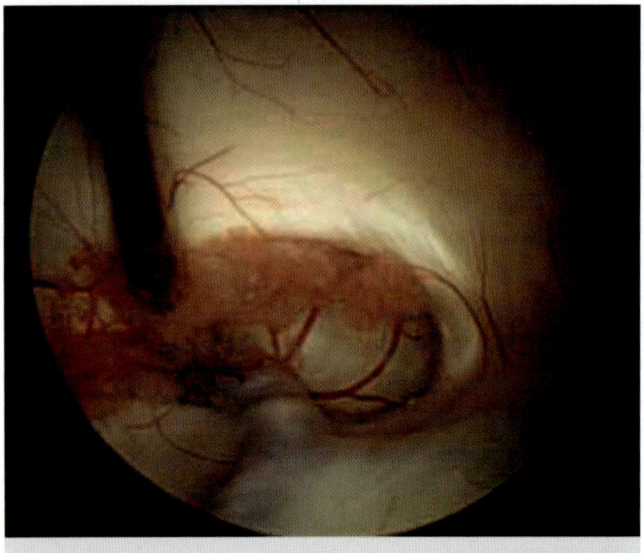

**Fig. 11** Endoscopic view of a colloid cyst obstructing the right foramen of Monro, with overlying choroid plexus. The septal vein can be seen coursing vertically. Placing the burr hole more anteriorly and laterally with neuronavigation permits a face-on view of the cyst filling the foramen. (Reproduced with permission from Alan R. Cohen.)

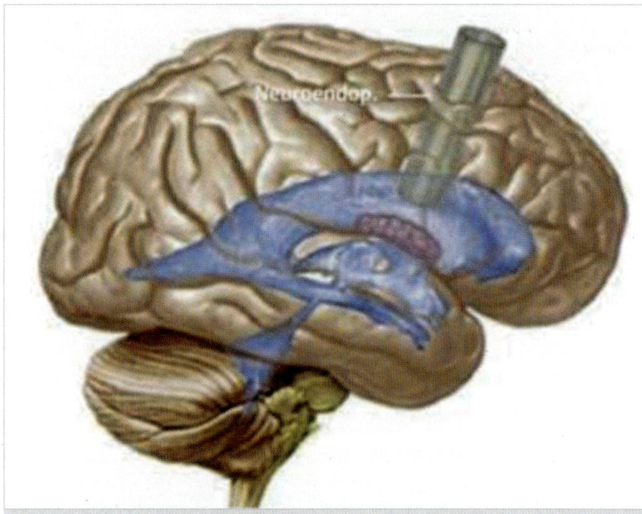

**Fig. 12** Endoscopic port surgery through a transparent cylinder (neuroendoport) to permit bimanual dissection. (From Engh JA. Stereotactically guided endoscopic port surgery for intraventricular tumor and colloid cyst resection. Operative Neurosurgery 2010;67:198–205.)

## Future Surgical Advances

Microsurgical transcallosal or transcortical resection remains the workhorse technique for resection of the challenging colloid cysts of the third ventricle. Endoscopic approaches combined with stereotactic guidance have proven to be a safe minimally invasive alternative to craniotomy. Long-term follow-up is essential to assess for recurrence, which may occur years after the initial resection. The growing experience with neuroendoscopic surgery along with technical advances in optics and illumination will likely lead to better clinical outcomes.

Improvement in equipment has enabled some investigators to perform endoscopic colloid cyst resections using a dual instrument technique.[75,76] Transtubular "endoport" surgery has been performed as a middle ground between endoscopy and microsurgery, enabling the operator to use bimanual techniques through small corticotomies under endoscopic guidance.[77,78,79] This is an expansion of the original stereotactic tubular endoscopy introduced by Kelly et al at the Mayo Clinic. Jho and Alfieri developed a clever technique of operating through a narrow transparent rollable vinyl tube.[80] Engh and colleagues modified this as an 11.5-mm transparent figure conduit (Endoport) which they deployed under stereotactic guidance, with successful gross total resection of 31 of 32 colloid cysts (▶ Fig. 12).[77] Transtubular surgery can be carried out under "exoscopic" guidance. Here the exoscope is situated outside the skull to serve as a high-definition video telescope. These exoscopes can provide excellent illumination and magnification with wide-field two- or three-dimensional exposure that may lead to effective results for colloid cyst resection. The current challenge in managing colloid cysts is to find minimally invasive approaches that are safe, effective, and durable.

## References


[1] Batnitzky S, Sarwar M, Leeds NE, Schechter MM, Azar-Kia B. Colloid cysts of the third ventricle. Radiology. 1974; 112(2):327–341

[2] Little JR, MacCarty CS. Colloid cysts of the third ventricle. J Neurosurg. 1974; 40(2):230–235

[3] Mathiesen T, Grane P, Lindquist C, von Holst H. High recurrence rate following aspiration of colloid cysts in the third ventricle. J Neurosurg. 1993; 78 (5):748–752

[4] Cohen AR, Perneczky A. Endoscopy and the management of third ventricular lesions. In: Apuzzo MLJ, ed. Surgery of the Third Ventricle. 2nd ed. Baltimore, MD: Williams and Wilkins; 1998:869–936

[5] Hernesniemi J, Leivo S. Management outcome in third ventricular colloid cysts in a defined population: a series of 40 patients treated mainly by transcallosal microsurgery. Surg Neurol. 1996; 45(1):2–14

[6] Antunes JL, Louis KM, Ganti SR. Colloid cysts of the third ventricle. Neurosurgery. 1980; 7(5):450–455

[7] Camacho A, Abernathey CD, Kelly PJ, Laws ER, Jr. Colloid cysts: experience with the management of 84 cases since the introduction of computed tomography. Neurosurgery. 1989; 24(5):693–700

[8] Bullard DE, Osborne D, Cook WA, Jr. Colloid cyst of the third ventricle presenting as a ring-enhancing lesion on computed tomography. Neurosurgery. 1982; 11(6):790–791

[9] Ganti SR, Antunes JL, Louis KM, Hilal SK. Computed tomography in the diagnosis of colloid cysts of the third ventricle. Radiology. 1981; 138(2):385–391

[10] Zilkha A. Computed tomography of colloid cysts of the third ventricle. Clin Radiol. 1981; 32(4):397–401

[11] Burger P, Shcheithauer B, Vogel F. Surgical Pathology of the Nervous System and Its Coverings. New York: Churchill Livingstone; 1991

[12] Pollock BE, Huston J, III. Natural history of asymptomatic colloid cysts of the third ventricle. J Neurosurg. 1999; 91(3):364–369

[13] Beaumont TL, Limbrick DD, Jr, Rich KM, Wippold FJ, II, Dacey RG, Jr. Natural history of colloid cysts of the third ventricle. J Neurosurg. 2016; 125(6):1420–1430

[14] Bull JWD, Sutton D. The diagnosis of paraphysial cysts. Brain. 1949; 72:487–516

[15] Kelly R. Colloid cysts of the third ventricle; analysis of twenty-nine cases. Brain. 1951; 74(1):23–65

[16] Yenermen MH, Bowerman CI, Haymaker W. Colloid cyst of the third ventricle; a clinical study of 54 cases in the light of previous publications. Acta Neuroveg (Wien). 1958; 17(3–4):211–277

[17] Riddoch G. Progressive dementia, without headache or changes in the optic discs, due to tumors of the third ventricle. Brain. 1936; 59:225–233

[18] Cairns H, Mosberg WH, Jr. Colloid cyst of the third ventricle. Surg Gynecol Obstet. 1951; 92(5):545–570

[19] Demirci S, Dogan KH, Erkol Z, Gulmen MK. Sudden death due to a colloid cyst of the third ventricle: report of three cases with a special sign at autopsy. Forensic Sci Int. 2009; 189(1–3):e33–e36

[20] Aronica PA, Ahdab-Barmada M, Rozin L, Wecht CH. Sudden death in an adolescent boy due to a colloid cyst of the third ventricle. Am J Forensic Med Pathol. 1998; 19(2):119–122

[21] Büttner A, Winkler PA, Eisenmenger W, Weis S. Colloid cysts of the third ventricle with fatal outcome: a report of two cases and review of the literature. Int J Legal Med. 1997; 110(5):260–266

[22] Lewis AI, Crone KR, Taha J, van Loveren HR, Yeh HS, Tew JM, Jr. Surgical resection of third ventricle colloid cysts. Preliminary results comparing transcallosal microsurgery with endoscopy. J Neurosurg. 1994; 81(2): 174–178

[23] Macdonald RL, Humphreys RP, Rutka JT, Kestle JR. Colloid cysts in children. Pediatr Neurosurg. 1994; 20(3):169–177

[24] Wallman H. Eine colloidcyste im dritten Hirnventrkl und eine lipom im plexus choroides. Virchows Arch. 1858; 11:385–388

[25] Dandy WE. Benign Tumors of the Third Ventricle of the Brain. Diagnosis and Treatment. Springfield, Illinois: Charles C. Thomas; 1933

[26] Dandy WE. Diagnosis localization and removal of tumors of the third ventricle. Bull Johns Hopkins Hosp. 1922; 33:188–189

[27] McKissock W. The surgical treatment of colloid cyst of the third ventricle; a report based upon twenty-one personal cases. Brain. 1951; 74(1):1–9

[28] Greenwood J, Jr. Paraphysial cysts of the third ventricle; with report of eight cases. J Neurosurg. 1949; 6(2):153–159

[29] Cassinari V, Bernasconi V. Tumori della parte anteriore del terzo ventricolo. Acta Neurochir (Wien). 1964; 11:236–271

[30] Milhorat TH, Baldwin M. A technique for surgical exposure of the cerebral midline: experimental transcallosal microdissection. J Neurosurg. 1966; 24(3): 687–691

[31] Shucart WA, Stein BM. Transcallosal approach to the anterior ventricular system. Neurosurgery. 1978; 3(3):339–343

[32] Ehni G. Interhemispheric and percallosal (transcallosal) approach to the cingulate gyri, intraventricular shunt tubes, and certain deeply placed brain lesions. Neurosurgery. 1984; 14(1):99–110

[33] Long DM, Chou SN. Transcallosal removal of cranio-pharyngiomas within the third ventricle. J Neurosurg. 1973; 39(5):563–567

[34] Konovalov AN, Pitskhelauri DI, Shkarubo M, Buklina SB, Poddubskaya AA, Kolycheva M. Microsurgical treatment of colloid cysts of the third ventricle. World Neurosurg. 2017; 105:678–688

[35] Gutierrez-Lara F, Patiño R, Hakim S. Treatment of tumors of the third ventricle: a new and simple technique. Surg Neurol. 1975; 3(6):323–325

[36] Bosch DA, Rähn T, Backlund EO. Treatment of colloid cysts of the third ventricle by stereotactic aspiration. Surg Neurol. 1978; 9(1):15–18

[37] Hall WA, Lunsford LD. Changing concepts in the treatment of colloid cysts. An 11-year experience in the CT era. J Neurosurg. 1987; 66(2):186–191

[38] Kondziolka D, Lunsford LD. Stereotactic management of colloid cysts: factors predicting success. J Neurosurg. 1991; 75(1):45–51

[39] Mohadjer M, Teshmar E, Mundinger F. CT-stereotaxic drainage of colloid cysts in the foramen of Monro and the third ventricle. J Neurosurg. 1987; 67(2):220–223

[40] Musolino A, Fosse S, Munari C, Daumas-Duport C, Chodkiewicz JP. Diagnosis and treatment of colloid cysts of the third ventricle by stereotactic drainage. Report on eleven cases. Surg Neurol. 1989; 32(4):294–299

[41] Rivas JJ, Lobato RD. CT-assisted stereotaxic aspiration of colloid cysts of the third ventricle. J Neurosurg. 1985; 62(2):238–242

[42] Abernathey CD, Davis DH, Kelly PJ. Treatment of colloid cysts of the third ventricle by stereotaxic microsurgical laser craniotomy. J Neurosurg. 1989; 70(4): 525–529

[43] Kondziolka D, Lunsford LD. Microsurgical resection of colloid cysts using a stereotactic transventricular approach. Surg Neurol. 1996; 46(5):485–490, discussion 490–492

[44] Fritsch H. Colloid cysts—a review including 19 own cases. Neurosurg Rev. 1988; 11(2):159–166

[45] Morita A, Kelly PJ. Resection of intraventricular tumors via a computer-assisted volumetric stereotactic approach. Neurosurgery. 1993; 32(6):920–926, discussion 926–927

[46] Jeeves MA, Simpson DA, Geffen G. Functional consequences of the transcallosal removal of intraventricular tumours. J Neurol Neurosurg Psychiatry. 1979; 42 (2):134–142

[47] El Khoury C, Brugières P, Decq P, et al. Colloid cysts of the third ventricle: are MR imaging patterns predictive of difficulty with percutaneous treatment? AJNR Am J Neuroradiol. 2000; 21(3):489–492

[48] Powell MP, Torrens MJ, Thomson JL, Horgan JG. Isodense colloid cysts of the third ventricle: a diagnostic and therapeutic problem resolved by ventriculoscopy. Neurosurgery. 1983; 13(3):234–237

[49] Auer LM, Holzer P, Ascher PW, Heppner F. Endoscopic neurosurgery. Acta Neurochir (Wien). 1988; 90(1–2):1–14

[50] Eiras Ajuria J, Alberdi Viñas J. [Endoscopic treatment of intracranial lesions. Apropos of 8 cases] Neurochirurgie. 1991; 37(4):278–283

[51] Merienne L, Leriche B, Roux FX, Devaux B. [Use of Nd-YAG laser in intracranial endoscopy. An initial experience in stereotaxy] Neurochirurgie. 1992; 38(4): 245–247

[52] Cohen AR, Shucart WA. Ventriculoscopic management of colloid cysts of the third ventricle. In: Manwaring K, Crone KR, eds. Neuroendoscopy. New York: Mary Ann Liebert; 1992:109–117

[53] Abdou MS, Cohen AR. Endoscopic treatment of colloid cysts of the third ventricle. Technical note and review of the literature. J Neurosurg. 1998; 89 (6):1062–1068

[54] Decq P, Le Guerinel C, Brugières P, et al. Endoscopic management of colloid cysts. Neurosurgery. 1998; 42(6):1288–1294, discussion 1294–1296

[55] Caemaert J, Abdullah J, Calliauw L. Endoscopic diagnosis and treatment of para- and intra-ventricular cystic lesions. Acta Neurochir Suppl (Wien). 1994; 61:69–75

[56] Horn EM, Feiz-Erfan I, Bristol RE, et al. Treatment options for third ventricular colloid cysts: comparison of open microsurgical versus endoscopic resection. Neurosurgery. 2007; 60(4):613–618, discussion 618–620

[57] Gaab MR. Colloid cysts: endoscopic or microsurgical resection? World Neurosurg. 2014; 82(6):1017–1019

[58] Sheikh AB, Mendelson ZS, Liu JK. Endoscopic versus microsurgical resection of colloid cysts: a systematic review and meta-analysis of 1,278 patients. World Neurosurg. 2014; 82(6):1187–1197

[59] Osorio JA, Clark AJ, Safaee M, et al. Intraoperative conversion from endoscopic to open transcortical-transventricular removal of colloid cysts as a salvage procedure. Cureus. 2015; 7(2):e247

[60] Apuzzo ML, Chandrasoma PT, Zelman V, Giannotta SL, Weiss MH. Computed tomographic guidance stereotaxis in the management of lesions of the third ventricular region. Neurosurgery. 1984; 15(4):502–508

[61] Heikkinen ER. Stereotactic neurosurgery: new aspects of an old method. Ann Clin Res. 1986; 18 Suppl 47:73–83

[62] Cohen AR. Images in clinical medicine. Colloid cyst of the third ventricle. N Engl J Med. 1995; 332(19):1267

[63] Grunert P, Perneczky A, Resch K. Endoscopic procedures through the foramen interventriculare of Monro under stereotactical conditions. Minim Invasive Neurosurg. 1994; 37(1):2–8

[64] Deinsberger W, Böker DK, Bothe HW, Samii M. Stereotactic endoscopic treatment of colloid cysts of the third ventricle. Acta Neurochir (Wien). 1994; 131 (3–4):260–264

[65] Grotenuis A. Manual of Endoscopic Procedures in Neurosurgery. Nijmegen: Machaon; 1995

[66] Hellwig D, Bauer BL. Minimally invasive neurosurgery by means of ultrathin endoscopes. Acta Neurochir Suppl (Wien). 1992; 54:63–68

[67] Teo C. Complete endoscopic removal of colloid cysts: issues of safety and efficacy. Neurosurg Focus. 1999; 6(4):E11

[68] Margetis K, Christos PJ, Souweidane M. Endoscopic resection of incidental colloid cysts. J Neurosurg. 2014; 120(6):1259–1267

[69] El-Ghandour NM. Endoscopic treatment of third ventricular colloid cysts: a review including ten personal cases. Neurosurg Rev. 2009; 32(4):395–402

[70] Schroeder HW, Gaab MR. Endoscopic resection of colloid cysts. Neurosurgery. 2002; 51(6):1441–1444, discussion 1444–1445

[71] Vazhayil V, Sadashiva N, Nayak N, Prabhuraj AR, Shukla D, Somanna S. Surgical management of colloid cysts in children: experience at a tertiary care center. Childs Nerv Syst. 2018; 34(6):1215–1220

[72] Cohen AR. Ventriculoscopic surgery. Clin Neurosurg. 1994; 41:546–562

[73] Chowdhry SA, Cohen AR. Intraventricular neuroendoscopy: complication avoidance and management. World Neurosurg. 2013; 79(2) Suppl:15.e1–15.e10

[74] Caemaert J, Abdullah J. Endoscopic management of colloid cysts. In: Cohen AR, ed. Technique in Neurosurgery. Hagerstown, MD: Lippincott-Raven; 1995:185–200

[75] Wilson DA, Fusco DJ, Wait SD, Nakaji P. Endoscopic resection of colloid cysts: use of a dual-instrument technique and an anterolateral approach. World Neurosurg. 2013; 80(5):576–583

[76] Bergsneider M. Complete microsurgical resection of colloid cysts with a dual-port endoscopic technique. Neurosurgery. 2007; 60(2) Suppl 1: ONS33–ONS42, discussion ONS42–ONS43

[77] Engh JA, Lunsford LD, Amin DV, et al. Stereotactically guided endoscopic port surgery for intraventricular tumor and colloid cyst resection. Neurosurgery. 2010; 67(3) Suppl Operative:ons198–ons204, discussion ons204–ons205

[78] Ajlan AM, Kalani MA, Harsh GR. Endoscopic transtubular resection of a colloid cyst. Neurosciences (Riyadh). 2014; 19(1):43–46

[79] Cohen-Gadol AA. Minitubular transcortical microsurgical approach for gross total resection of third ventricular colloid cysts: technique and assessment. World Neurosurg. 2013; 79(1):207.e7–207.e10

[80] Jho HD, Alfieri A. Endoscopic removal of third ventricular tumors: a technical note. Minim Invasive Neurosurg. 2002; 45(2):114–119

# Part I

## Development, Anatomy, and Neuroimaging



I

# 1 Developmental Origins of the Cerebral Ventricular System and Colloid Cysts

*Albert Isaacs, Sonika Dahiya, Sean D. McEvoy, Keith M. Rich, and David Limbrick*

**Abstract**
Colloid cysts are rare, benign brain tumors, predominantly located in the third ventricle and constitute less than 3% of all benign intracranial tumors. Although they can occur in various brain regions, the vast majority are found within the third ventricle. The genetic basis of colloid cysts remains largely undefined, although there have been reports of occasional familial instances. The etiology of colloid cysts has been a subject of debate, with theories suggesting both neuroectodermal and enterogenous origins. This chapter focuses on the embryological origins of colloid cysts within the context of nervous system development, emphasizing the anatomy around the third ventricle to understand their primary embryological sources. The development of the human ventricular system, from the closure of the neural tube to the formation of the ventricular system, underpins the understanding of colloid cyst pathophysiology. The chapter explores the differentiation of the choroid plexus and ependymal cells, shedding light on the complexities of the ventricular system and its association with colloid cyst formation. An anatomical and histopathological examination attributes the origins of colloid cysts to abnormal embryonic foldings that trap endodermal elements, suggesting that these cysts likely originate from detached embryonic diencephalic vesicular recesses or remnants of the paraphysis cerebri. This insight provides a comprehensive understanding of colloid cyst development and its clinical implications, highlighting the significance of embryological perspectives in diagnosing and managing these tumors.

*Keywords:* development, embryology, paraphysis, colloid cyst, cerebral ventricle, ependyma, neural tube

## 1.1 Background

Colloid cysts are slow-growing developmental lesions that constitute approximately 0.2 to 3% of all benign brain tumors.[1,2,3,4,5,6] Although they have been identified in many regions of the brain including the fourth ventricle,[7,8] parenchyma,[9] sella,[10] and within the leaflets of the septum pellucidum,[6,11,12,13,14] approximately 99% of identified colloid cysts are located within the third ventricle[15] (▶ Fig. 1.1). The role of genetics in colloid cysts development has not been characterized; however, rare familial clusters have been documented.[16,17,18,19,20] Since colloid cysts were first reported in 1858,[21] there has been considerable debate on their pathophysiology and embryological origins.[22] Indeed, several studies have implicated structures within the vicinity of the third ventricle, including the paraphysis cerebri,[23,24] velum interpositum,[11,22] ependyma, and choroid plexus neuroepithelium,[23,25] as potential embryological origins. Other studies have suggested an enterogenous origin (e.g., respiratory epithelium[26,27,28]).

The objective of this chapter is to describe the current thinking regarding the embryological basis of colloid cysts, particularly in the context of the development of the nervous system. A close examination of the anatomical structures within the vicinity of the third ventricle will provide the background to understand the embryological origins of the vast majority of colloid cysts.

## 1.2 Neurodevelopment and the Cerebral Ventricles

Human development originates from three primitive embryonic layers, namely, ectoderm, mesoderm, and endoderm, which are formed through purposeful cell movement and organization following fertilization.[29] During neurulation, around 2 weeks of embryonic development, the neural plate thickens and invaginates into a neural groove along its midline, which then fuses into a rostro-caudal neural tube.[29,30] The neural tube momentarily remains in communication with the surrounding environment via its rostral (anterior) and caudal (posterior) neuropores, until they both eventually close off to form the closed ventricular system[29] (▶ Fig. 1.2). The closed anterior neuropore can later be identified as the ***lamina terminalis*** in the developed brain.

During neurulation, the anterior and posterior neuropores close to isolate the ventricular system from its embryonic environment. Formation of the five-vesicle complex structure and differential expansion of regions around the neural tube flexures along with the neural canal create the cerebral ventricles.

Around week 3, the rostral end of the neural tube undergoes rapid morphogenetic movement and expansions to develop three symmetric primary swellings: the prosencephalon (forebrain), mesencephalon (midbrain), and rhombencephalon (hindbrain). The three-vesicle stage is facilitated by symmetric folding of the neural tube rostrally along its lateral axis to form two flexures: the cephalic flexure which develops between the prosencephalon and mesencephalon, and cervical flexure which divides the rhombencephalon and the spinal cord.[29] Due to significantly restricted morphogenesis at the cephalic flexure in relation to the rest of the prosencephalon, two distinct structures develop: the telencephalon rostrally and the diencephalon caudally. At approximately 6 weeks, the pontine flexure develops to demarcate the rhombencephalon into myelencephalon and metencephalon. Thus, by week 7, the three primary vesicles have developed into five secondary vesicles,[29] which are (from rostral to caudal): telencephalon (*future cerebral hemispheres*), diencephalon (*future thalami, hypothalamic and optic cups*) mesencephalon (*future midbrain*), metencephalon (*future pons and cerebellum*), and myelencephalon (*future medulla oblongata*)[29] (▶ Fig. 1.2).

Development of the ventricular system is a fascinating and clinically important topic in its own right and is integral to understanding the complexities of ventricular-associated pathologies such as colloid cysts. In the developed human brain, the ventricular system comprises of two lateral (telencephalic) ventricles that connect through the foramen of Monro to the third (diencephalic) ventricle, which in turn connects to the fourth

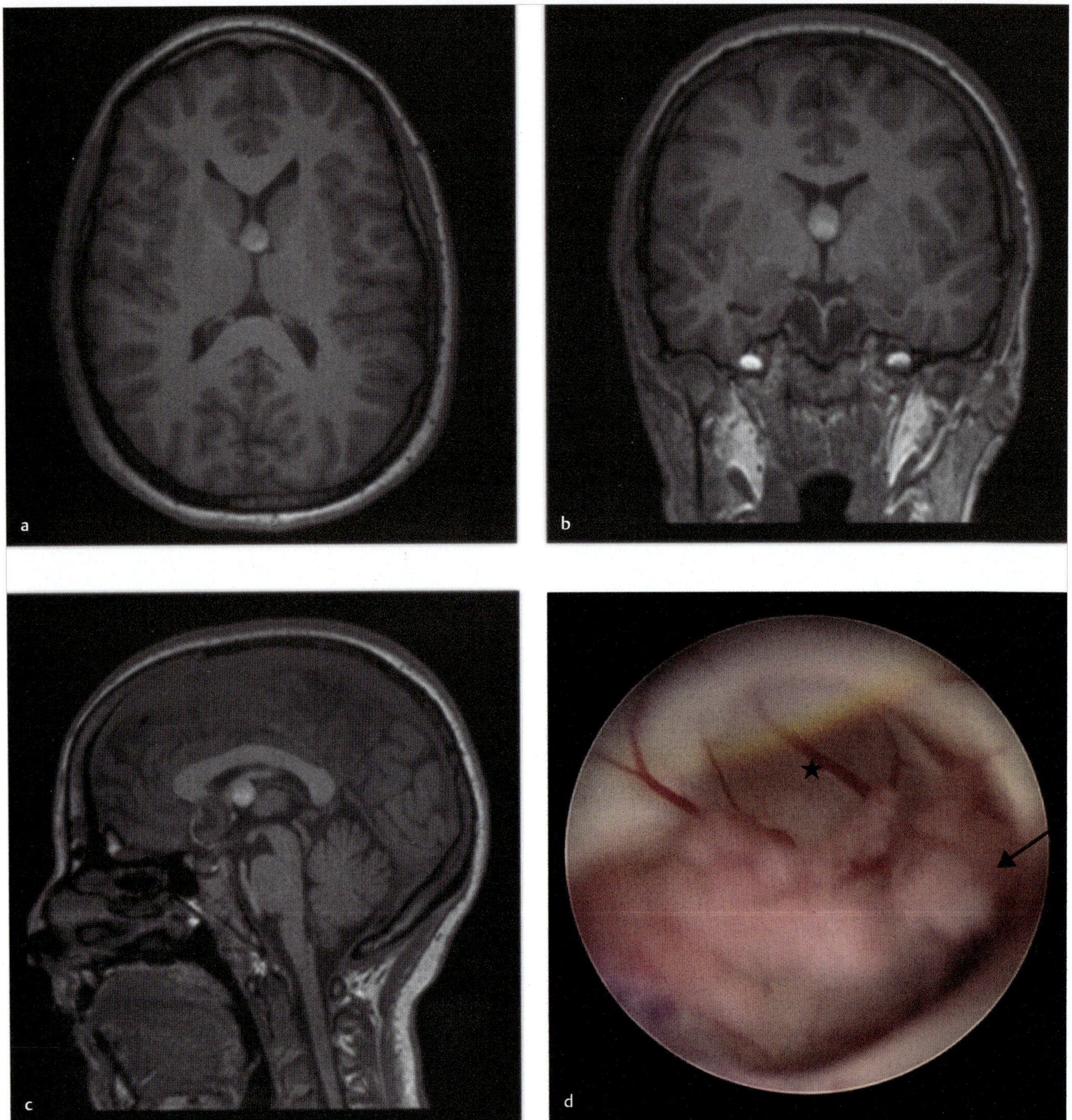

**Fig. 1.1** Case presentation. Representative axial **(a)**, coronal **(b)**, and sagittal **(c)** T1-weighted (T1W) magnetic resonance imaging (MRI) images of a 21-year-old female demonstrating a colloid cyst located at the roof of the third ventricle that appears to obstruct the foramina of Monro, but without features of hydrocephalus. An endoscopic view **(d)** showing the cyst (★) with a vascularized smooth glistening wall draped by choroid plexus (*arrow*) as in the foramen of Monro.

(rhombencephalic) ventricle via the cerebral aqueduct. Although the ventricular system is continuous with the central canal of the spinal cord during development, and potentially thereafter, it communicates with the subarachnoid space through the foramen of Magendie and foramina of Lushka at the level of the pons.

Embryonic ventricular development is heralded by closure of the anterior and posterior neuropores, which are connected midline by a cerebrospinal fluid (CSF)-filled lumen lined by ependymal cells—the neural canal (▶ Fig. 1.2). Development of the three-dimensional ventricular structure from the primitive neural tube configuration is mediated by complex mechanisms of morphogenesis, which include both physical forces and interactions that occur concurrently with neural tube expansion. Physical forces are created through osmotic absorption of water

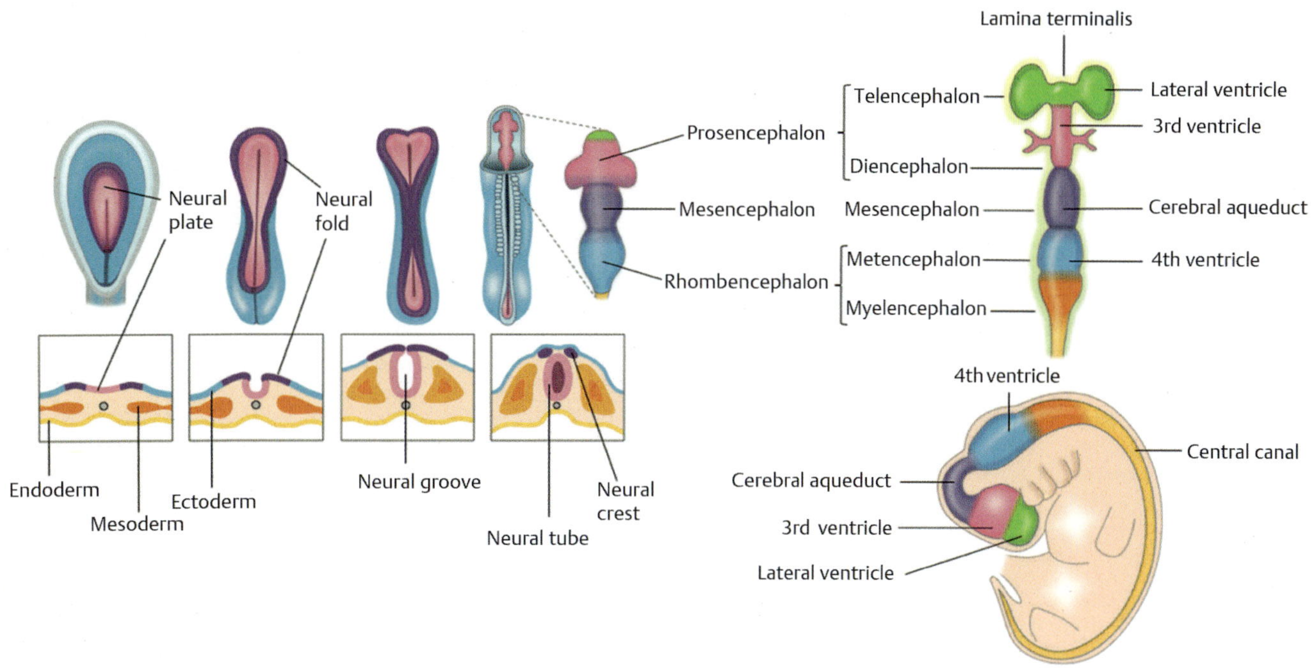


**Fig. 1.2** Embryological origins of ventricular development.

by cells lining the primitive ventricles and by secretion of fluid into the ventricular cavity by the choroid plexus (see below for details of choroid plexus development). The segment of the neural canal that spans the telencephalon develops into the *lateral ventricles* (▶ Fig. 1.2). The lateral ventricles maintain a large, inflated shape due to massive CSF production by the choroid plexus in those regions. The C-shaped configuration of the lateral ventricles occurs as a result of ventromedial expansion of the ganglionic eminence bilaterally.[29] The lateral ventricles and the fornices are separated later around weeks 10 to 12[31] into left and right by a thin membranous bridge, the *septum pellucidum*. The septum pellucidum develops inextricably with the corpus callosum and anterior and hippocampal commissures from the basal medial portion of the *lamina terminalis* known as the commissural plate[31,32,33] (▶ Fig. 1.3). During week 6 of gestation, the *foramen of Monro* is formed from the anterior enlargement of the initial slit-like communication between the diencephalon and bilateral telencephalon vesicles (▶ Fig. 1.2). The *velum interpositum* on the other hand derives from duplication of the pia–arachnoid layer that overlies the roof of the diencephalon and superior walls of the telencephalon, as they undergo a U-shaped infolding (▶ Fig. 1.3). While the cavity in the diencephalon forms the *third ventricle*, the *cerebral aqueduct* forms from the remnant of the neural canal at the level of the mesencephalon (▶ Fig. 1.2). The fourth ventricle develops from splaying of the pontine flexure (▶ Fig. 1.2). Unlike the fourth ventricle which enlarges during formation of the rostral neural tube structures, the cerebral aqueduct is relatively large during early embryological stages, but later narrows. The remainder of the neural canal stretches inferiorly as the central canal of the spinal cord.

### 1.2.1 Ependyma Development

During neurodevelopment, progenitor stem cell proliferation occurs in the ventricular zone, an area immediately *adjacent* to the ventricles. The stem cells either migrate via radial glial cells to differentiate into neurons of the cerebral cortex or supporting glial structures, which include ependymal cells that form the ventricular CSF–brain barrier.[34] During neurulation, the ventricular zone spans the entire neural tube, but as the brain matures it is replaced by the ependymal layer and limited portions of the stem cells are largely limited to specific areas of the subventricular zone. These stem cells retain restorative and repair capabilities, for example, regenerating neurons of the olfactory bulb and dentate gyrus via the rostral migratory stream.[35,36] Histologically, the ependyma contains multiciliated cuboidal cells with cilia that, among other purposes, may facilitate the movement of CSF through the ventricular system.

### 1.2.2 Choroid Plexus Development

As development of the neural tube progresses, a shallow sulcus limitans at the caudal end demarcates the roof and alar plates from the floor and basal plates. Further differentiation of non-neural tissues at the roof plate forms the highly vascularized choroid plexus that are found within each cerebral ventricle.[37] After neural tube closure, the choroid plexus in the fourth ventricle appear first, which is followed by those of the lateral ventricles synchronously, and then lastly in the third ventricle.[38] Despite their distinct appearance, the choroid plexuses in the lateral ventricles from the choroid fissures merge at the exit levels of foramina of Monro, and fuse with the third ventricle plexus to form a continuous choroid plexus structure.[38,39,40] The many functions of the choroid plexus have been extensively described in the literature and include CSF secretion,[38,41] solute transport,[42] and immune system regulation.[43] Histologically, the choroid plexus comprises of a network of connective tissues and fenestrated capillaries, surrounded by cuboidal epithelial cells that are held together by tight and adherens junctions to form the blood–CSF barrier.

## 1.2.3 Development of Colloid Cysts

Given the intimate anatomical proximity of the sellar region to the third ventricle, the differential diagnoses of colloid cysts may include other cystic lesions that originate in the vicinity, such as Rathke's cleft cysts and cystic craniopharyngiomas.[44] Rathke's cleft cysts develop between the lobes of the pituitary as cystic remnants of the craniopharyngeal duct, while craniopharyngiomas are considered neoplastic transformation of ectodermal-derived epithelial cell remnants of the craniopharyngeal duct and Rathke's pouch.[45,46] Although the embryological origins of Rathke's cleft cysts and craniopharyngiomas are considered by many to be distinct from colloid cysts, it has been hypothesized that the presence of some endodermal features that are common to colloid cysts and Rathke's cleft cysts suggests they may be embryologically related.[47]

### Third Ventricle Anatomy

Majority of colloid cysts originate from structures around the roof of the third ventricle. The third ventricle is defined by the foramen of Monro, lamina terminalis, columns of the fornix, and the anterior commissure, while the posterior border is defined by the cerebral aqueduct and the suprapineal recess[48] (▶ Fig. 1.3). The two lateral walls are defined by the left and right diencephalon, which comprises of the thalami, interthalamic adhesion, hypothalami, paraventricular nuclei, and subthalami. The floor extends from the optic chiasm anteriorly to the orifice of the cerebral aqueduct posteriorly with intermediary structures such as the infundibular recess, tuber cinereum, mamillary bodies, posterior perforated substance, and tegmentum[48] (▶ Fig. 1.3).

The roof of the third ventricle, where majority of colloid cysts are located, is defined superiorly to inferiorly by five layers. The first layer, the superior layer, is formed by the fornix. The next two layers, the tela choroidea layers, are characterized by a bundle of choroid plexus around the choroidal fissures that attaches to the choroid plexus of the third ventricle. The fourth layer, velum interpositum, is a vascular layer that contains the internal cerebral and medial posterior choroidal arteries. The fifth layer is the choroid plexus layer (▶ Fig. 1.3).

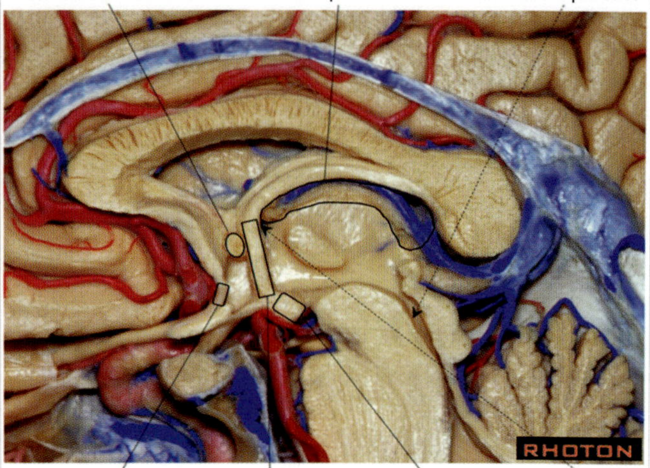


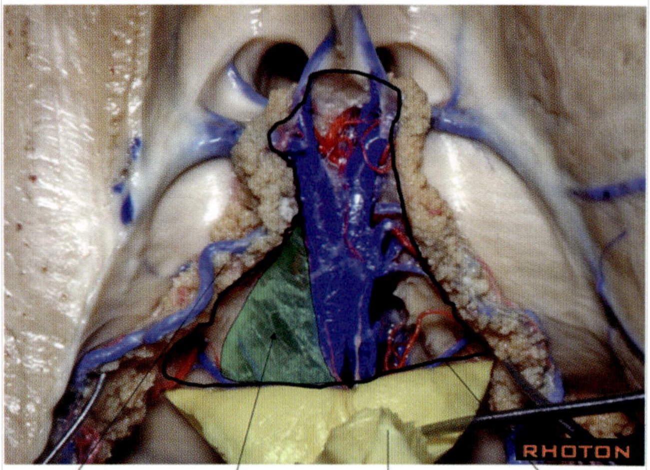


**Fig. 1.3** Borders and roof of the third ventricle. *Top:* Sagittal view of third ventricular anatomy demonstrating the anterior border demarcated by the lamina terminalis, anterior commissure, and column of fornix, and posterior border demarcated by the cerebral aqueduct and suprapineal recess. The velum interpositum is seen at the roof. *Bottom:* A superior view of the roof of the third ventricle demonstrating structures that form its five layers; layer 1 (fornix) has been reflected to reveal layers 2 and 3 (telea) and the demarcated layer 4 (velum interpositum). The choroid plexus is labelled to depict layer 5 (choroid plexus layer). (Used with permission from the Rhoton Collection, American Association of Neurological Surgeons [AANS]/Neurosurgical Research and Education Foundation [NREF].)

### Histopathology of Colloid Cysts

On gross pathology, colloid cysts are typically spherical to ovoid in shape with a smooth, partially translucent cyst wall (▶ Fig. 1.1). Their contents are highly variable and can range from clear, semi-viscous fluid to gelatinous or even rock solid[49,50,51] (▶ Fig. 1.4). Histological analyses of explanted colloid cysts demonstrate a fibrous collagenous outer layer.[52] Piloid gliosis with Rosenthal material may also be seen in the cyst wall bed, as can sometimes adhered choroid plexus tissue (▶ Fig. 1.4). The lining epithelium is variable, albeit often well-differentiated and mature, and may contain columnar to cuboidal epithelium with or without a pseudostratified appearance with mucin secretory organelles[52,53] (▶ Fig. 1.4). It is possible that the secretory activity of mucin organelles is partly responsible for the slow enlargement of colloid cysts,[54] as symptomatic colloid cysts, which tend be larger than nonsymptomatic ones, and often demonstrate a T2-weighted (T2W) signal indicative of relatively higher mucinous content. However, the osmotic effects of intracystic mucin-laden electrolytes[55] such as sodium, calcium, and magnesium that may draw fluid into the cyst cannot be discounted. Majority

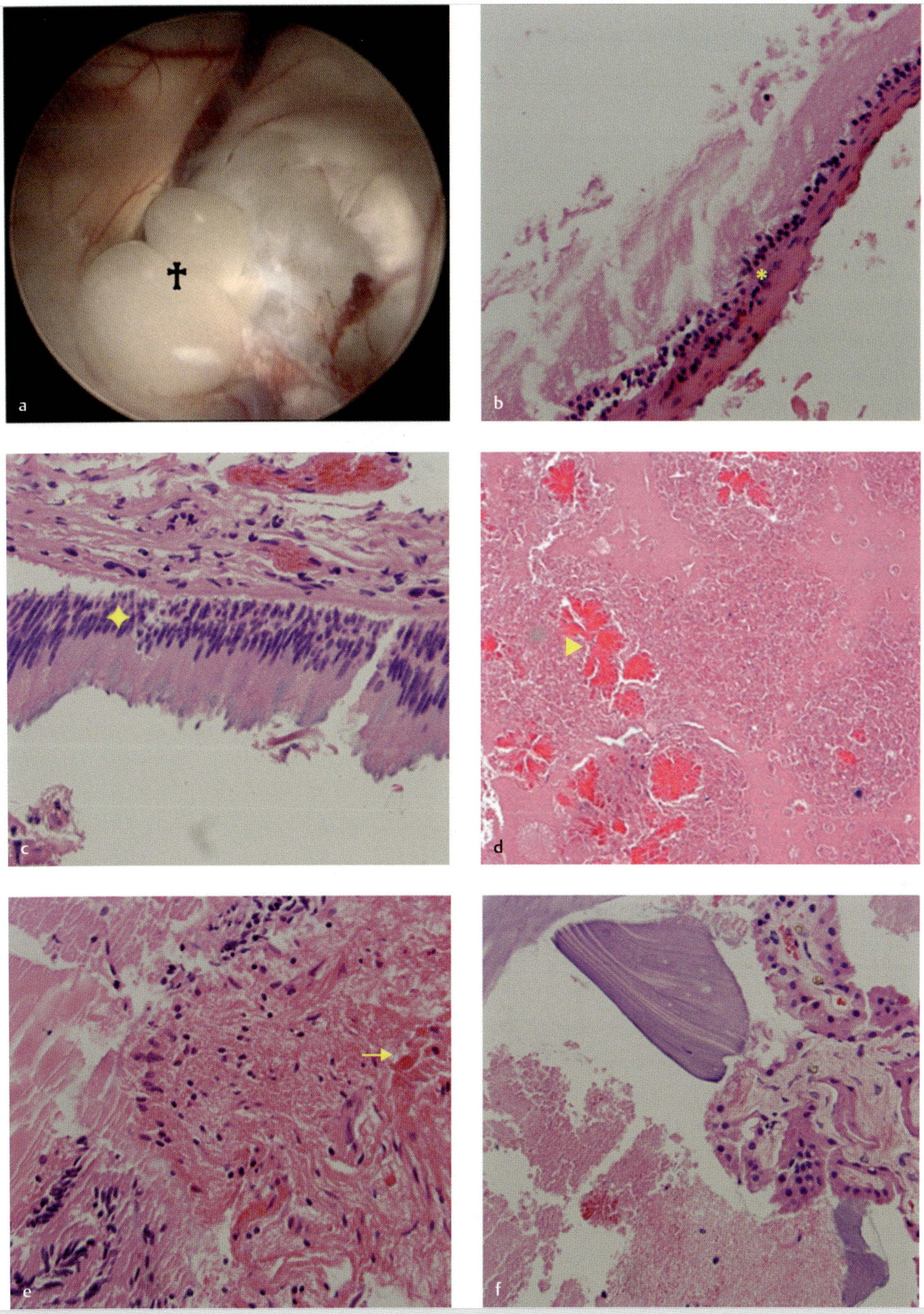

**Fig. 1.4** Representative pathological and histological features a colloid cyst. Intraoperative endoscopic image of a colloid cyst **(a)** showing extruded gelatinous cyst contents following surgical opening of the cyst wall. The H&E stained images of an explanted colloid cyst demonstrating a thin fibrous layer and simple cuboidal to columnar epithelium (**b**, ❊) to pseudostratified mucinous epithelium (**c**, ✦) from two different examples. Often the predominant pathology material is composed of acellular proteinaceous material, that is, cyst contents **(d)**, which can sometimes form small aggregates resembling crystalloids (*arrowhead*). Piloid gliosis with Rosenthal material (*arrow*) may also be seen in the cyst wall bed **(e)**, and sometimes adhered choroid plexus tissue also **(f)**.

of colloid cysts also contain cilia and basal bodies or mucin (resembling bronchogenic epithelium)[26,28,49,52,56]; however, variants that lack cilia have been reported.[26,28] Commonly, fragments of normal choroid plexus may be found attached to the cyst (▶ Fig. 1.4). Rarely, intralesional hemorrhage due to colloid cyst apoplexy[57,58] may be identified.

To correlate colloid cysts with potential structures of their origin, several stains and antibodies have been employed on explanted colloid cysts to better characterize their microstructure, some of which have been outlined in ▶ Table 1.1.

**Table 1.1** Histological stains and antibodies that have been used to characterize the cellular microstructure of colloid cysts

| Stain/Antibody | Result |
|---|---|
| Epithelial membrane antigen | Positive[52,59,60] |
| Keratin | Positive[52,59] |
| PAS | Positive[6,52,61] |
| S100 | Positive[52] |
| Trichrome | Positive[52,62] |
| Cytokeratin (CAM 5.2) | Positive[63] |
| GFAP | Negative[52] |
| Monoclonal antibody HNK-1 | Negative[59] |
| Leukocyte antigen | Negative[52,59] |
| Neurofilament | Negative[52] |
| Silver | Negative[52] |
| Enolase | Inconsistent[52,59] |
| Vimentin | Inconsistent[52] |

Abbreviations: GFAP, glial fibrillary acidic protein; PAS, periodic acid-Schiff stain.

## Paraphyseal Origin of Colloid Cysts

Sjövall first described the etiology of colloid cysts as remnants of nondegenerated paraphysis,[24] an embryonic structure that develops from the neuroectodermal paraphyseal arch,[23] which is anatomically located at the border of the diencephalon and the telencephalon in the developing embryo[23,24] (▶ Fig. 1.2). In later development, the paraphyseal arch defines the roof of the third ventricle.[23,24] The paraphysis starts around week 7 of embryonic development, at approximately 15- to 17-mm embryonic crown–rump (CR) length, as a solid bud that projects from the paraphyseal arch.[23] The bud then forms one or more lumens, which subsequently develop into vesicles (▶ Fig. 1.5). Typically, there is significant variation in the rates and patterns of differentiation of the vesicles. However, as the embryo develops further, the principal vesicular anlagen, the most developed midline paraphyseal vesicle, persists near the roof of the third ventricle, while the remaining vesicles regress.[23] Complete degeneration of all vesicular rudiments is normally observed by 3.5 months of gestation at approximately 100-mm CR length.[23] However, occasionally one or more vesicular remnants fail to regress, which may later develop into a colloid cyst. McLean postulated that it is the weight of the paraphyseal cysts that projects it downward into the third ventricle from the velum interpositum.[64] It remains unclear whether one or a coalescing of two or more persistent vesicular rudiments develop into a colloid cyst. Nevertheless, given their anatomical location, embryological development, and histological features that are for the most part similar to that of colloid cysts, the paraphysis has been hypothesized as the precursor to colloid cysts for many decades.[8,13,23,24,52,65,66,67,68]

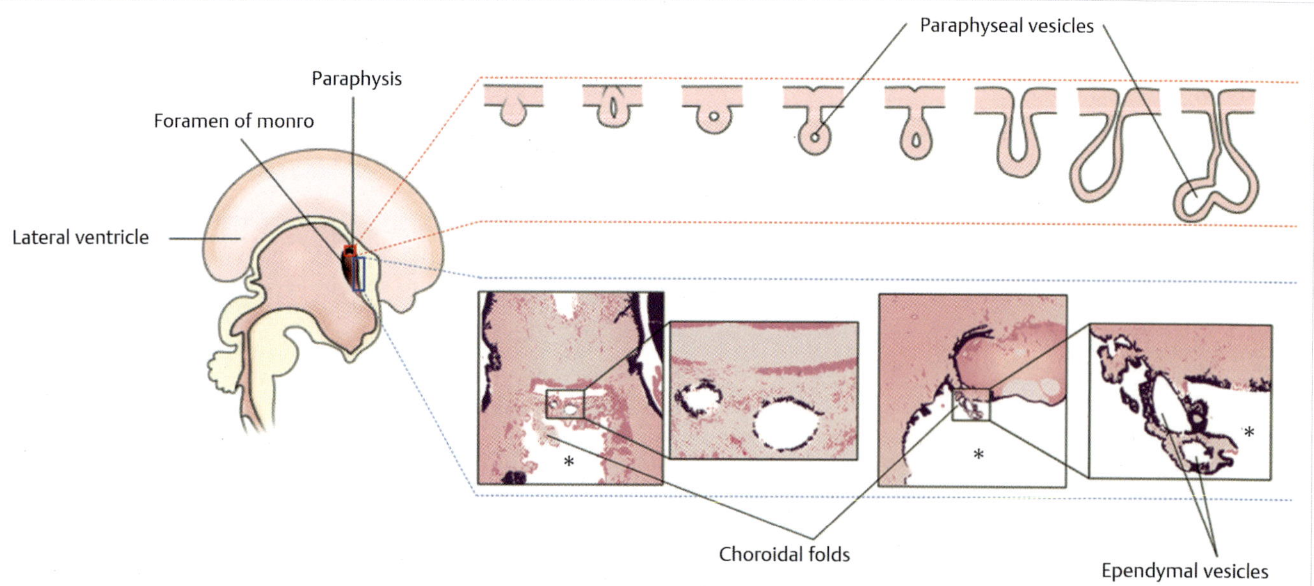


**Fig. 1.5** Schematic representation of colloid cyst development demonstrating paraphyseal and ependymal origins of a third ventricle colloid cyst, as described by Kappers.[23] A solid paraphyseal bud develops from the paraphyseal bud around embryonic week 7. The bud then develops a lumen, and several vesicles may form. A vesicular anlage that fails to regress gets incorporated into a choroidal fold. An ependymal recess may also detach as a closed vesicle and get incorporated into a choroidal fold. A choroidal fold containing paraphyseal or ependymal vesicular anlage may hang from the superior aspect of the third ventricle (*) as a colloid cyst.

### Ependymal Origin of Colloid Cysts

Although the paraphysis is arguably one of the most likely referenced etiologies for third ventricle colloid cysts,[8,13,23,24,52,65,66,67,68] it is important to note that there are several findings that do not fit this narrative. For example, a paraphyseal origin does not explain posteriorly located third ventricle colloid cysts,[52,69] let alone those that are found in the fourth ventricle[7,8] or at extraventricular sites.[6,9,10,11,12,13,14] In addition, majority of explanted colloid cysts demonstrate histological features of cilia while the paraphysis is noncilliated,[22,23] although Ho and Garcia[26] and Macaulay et al[28] both reported a mixed population of ciliated and nonciliated cells in their respective cohorts of explanted colloid cysts.[26,28]

Considering the shortfalls of the hypothesis of paraphysis-based pathophysiology, Kappers[23] suggested that colloid cysts arise from recesses that develop in the ependyma of the diencephalic postvelar arch, which then detach as closed vesicles surrounded by connective tissues of the velum interpositum[24] (▶ Fig. 1.5). However, based on reports of paraphyseal rudiments found to be buried within choroidal folds of patients with colloid cysts,[25] Kappers suggested the paraphysis is plausible, yet an uncommon, precursor of colloid cysts.[23] However, a distinction can be made in that cysts with cilia are more likely to be of ependymal origin, whereas those that lack cilia may be of paraphyseal origin.[23] Kappers's proposed mechanisms of third ventricle colloid cyst development[23] is perhaps the most comprehensive pathophysiological perspective to date.[22] For one, it considers the intricate anatomic relationships between diencephalic–telencephalic junctional structures such as the third ventricle, foramina of Monro, ependymal layer, and choroid plexus to propose the development of colloid cysts.[23] Second, in addition to recognizing the paraphysis as a potential origin of colloid cysts,[24] Kappers's ependymal origin helps reconcile presence of cilia in colloid cysts, which the paraphysis theory was unable to address.[22,23] From an anatomical perspective, both of the paraphyseal and ependymal derived colloid cysts[23] appear to originate from Zone I of Beaumont et al's three-zone stratification of the third ventricle into colloid cyst risk zones.[48] Zone I, defined as the region of the third ventricle anterior to a line tangential to the mamillary body and the massa intermedia, is also associated with nearly all colloid cysts that present with pre-aqueductal hydrocephalus.[48]

## 1.3 Conclusion

Majority of colloid cysts are consistently located in the anterior roof of the third ventricle, near foramen of Monroe, and are thought to originate from abnormal folding of the primitive neuroectoderm resulting in trapping of endodermal elements within velum interpositum in the course of the later stages of primary neurulation. Although there have been several theories on the embryological basis of colloid cysts, a unifying hypothesis is that majority of the lesions arise from detached and degenerated embryonic diencephalic vesicular recesses, while some may develop from remnants of the paraphysis cerebri.

## References

[1] Batnitzky S, Sarwar M, Leeds NE, Schechter MM, Azar-Kia B. Colloid cysts of the third ventricle. Radiology. 1974; 112(2):327–341

[2] Gemperlein J. Paraphyseal cysts of the third ventricle. Report of two cases in infants. J Neuropathol Exp Neurol. 1960; 19(1):133–134

[3] Antunes JL, Louis KM, Ganti SR. Colloid cysts of the third ventricle. Neurosurgery. 1980; 7(5):450–455

[4] Mohadjer M, Teshmar E, Mundinger F. CT-stereotaxic drainage of colloid cysts in the foramen of Monro and the third ventricle. J Neurosurg. 1987; 67(2): 220–223

[5] Pollock BE, Schreiner SA, Huston J, III. A theory on the natural history of colloid cysts of the third ventricle. Neurosurgery. 2000; 46(5):1077–1081, discussion 1081–1083

[6] Turillazzi E, Bello S, Neri M, Riezzo I, Fineschi V. Colloid cyst of the third ventricle, hypothalamus, and heart: a dangerous link for sudden death. Diagn Pathol. 2012; 7:144

[7] Kchir N, Haouet S, Chatti S, et al. Colloid cyst of the fourth ventricle. Apropos of a case. Arch Anat Cytol Pathol. 1992; 40(1–2):36–38

[8] Parkinson D, Childe AE. Colloid cyst of the fourth ventricle; report of a case of two colloid cysts of the fourth ventricle. J Neurosurg. 1952; 9(4): 404–409

[9] Campbell DA, Varma TRK. An extraventricular colloid cyst: case report. Br J Neurosurg. 1991; 5(5):519–522

[10] Sener RN, Jinkins JR. CT of intrasellar colloid cyst. J Comput Assist Tomogr. 1991; 15(4):671–672

[11] Demirci S, Dogan KH, Erkol Z, Gulmen MK. Sudden death due to a colloid cyst of the third ventricle: report of three cases with a special sign at autopsy. Forensic Sci Int. 2009; 189(1–3):e33–e36

[12] Boogaarts HD, Decq P, Grotenhuis JA, et al. Long-term results of the neuroendoscopic management of colloid cysts of the third ventricle: a series of 90 cases. Neurosurgery. 2011; 68(1):179–187

[13] Ciric I, Zivin I. Neuroepithelial (colloid) cysts of the septum pellucidum. J Neurosurg. 1975; 43(1):69–73

[14] Hingwala DR, Sanghvi DA, Shenoy AS, Dange NN, Goel AH. Colloid cyst of the velum interpositum: a common lesion at an uncommon site. Surg Neurol. 2009; 72(2):182–184

[15] McKISSOCK W. The surgical treatment of colloid cyst of the third ventricle; a report based upon twenty-one personal cases. Brain. 1951; 74(1):1–9

[16] Partington MW, Bookalil AJ. Familial colloid cysts of the third ventricle. Clin Genet. 2004; 66(5):473–475

[17] Joshi SM, Gnanalingham KK, Mohaghegh P, Wilson A, Elsmore A. A case of familial third ventricular colloid cyst. Emerg Med J. 2005; 22(12):909–910

[18] Nader-Sepahi A, Hamlyn PJ. Familial colloid cysts of the third ventricle: case report. Neurosurgery. 2000; 46(3):751–753

[19] Socin HV, Born J, Wallemacq C, Betea D, Legros JJ, Beckers A. Familial colloid cyst of the third ventricle: neuroendocrinological follow-up and review of the literature. Clin Neurol Neurosurg. 2002; 104(4):367–370

[20] Stoodley MA, Nguyen TP, Robbins P. Familial fatal and near-fatal third ventricle colloid cysts. Aust N Z J Surg. 1999; 69(10):733–736

[21] Wallman H. Colloid cyst in the third ventricle and lipoma in the plexus chorioideus. Virchows Arch. 1858; 14:385–388

[22] Laidlaw J, Kaye AH. Colloid cysts. In: Kaye AH, Laws ER, Jr, eds. Brain Tumors. Churchill Livingstone; 2012:849–863

[23] Kappers JA. The development of the paraphysis cerebri in man with comments on its relationship to the intercolumnar tubercle and its significance for the origin of cystic tumors in the third ventricle. J Comp Neurol. 1955; 102(2): 425–509

[24] Sjövall E. über eine Ependymzyste embryonalen Charakters im dritten Hirnventrikel mit tödlichem Ausgang. Beitr Pathol Anat. 1909; 47:248–269

[25] Stookey B. Intermittent obstruction of the foramen of Monro by neuroepithelial cysts of the third ventricle. Symptoms, diagnosis and treatment. Bull Neurol Inst NY.. 1934; 3:446–500

[26] Ho KL, Garcia JH. Colloid cysts of the third ventricle: ultrastructural features are compatible with endodermal derivation. Acta Neuropathol. 1992; 83(6): 605–612

[27] Lach B, Scheithauer BW. Colloid cyst of the third ventricle: a comparative ultrastructural study of neuraxis cysts and choroid plexus epithelium. Ultrastruct Pathol. 1992; 16(3):331–349

[28] Macaulay RJB, Felix I, Jay V, Becker LE. Histological and ultrastructural analysis of six colloid cysts in children. Acta Neuropathol. 1997; 93(3):271–276

[29] Carpenter EM. Development of brain ventricles and choroid plexus. In: Neman J, Chen TC, eds. The Choroid Plexus and Cerebrospinal Fluid: Emerging Roles in CNS Development, Maintenance, and Disease Progression. Academic Press; 2015:15–27
[30] Smith JL, Schoenwolf GC. Neurulation: coming to closure. Trends Neurosci. 1997; 20(11):510–517
[31] Loeser JD, Alvord EC, Jr. Agenesis of the corpus callosum. Brain. 1968; 91(3): 553–570
[32] Sarwar M. The septum pellucidum: normal and abnormal. AJNR Am J Neuroradiol. 1989; 10(5):989–1005
[33] Loeser JD, Alvord EC, Jr. Clinicopathological correlations in agenesis of the corpus callosum. Neurology. 1968; 18(8):745–756
[34] Rowitch DH, Kriegstein AR. Developmental genetics of vertebrate glial-cell specification. Nature. 2010; 468(7321):214–222
[35] Wang C, Liu F, Liu Y-Y, et al. Identification and characterization of neuroblasts in the subventricular zone and rostral migratory stream of the adult human brain. Cell Res. 2011; 21(11):1534–1550
[36] Sanai N, Nguyen T, Ihrie RA, et al. Corridors of migrating neurons in the human brain and their decline during infancy. Nature. 2011; 478(7369):382–386
[37] Lun MP, Monuki ES, Lehtinen MK. Development and functions of the choroid plexus-cerebrospinal fluid system. Nat Rev Neurosci. 2015; 16(8):445–457
[38] Lun MP, Johnson MB, Broadbelt KG, et al. Spatially heterogeneous choroid plexus transcriptomes encode positional identity and contribute to regional CSF production. J Neurosci. 2015; 35(12):4903–4916
[39] Lehtinen MK, Walsh CA. Neurogenesis at the brain-cerebrospinal fluid interface. Annu Rev Cell Dev Biol. 2011; 27:653–679
[40] Shechter R, Miller O, Yovel G, et al. Recruitment of beneficial M2 macrophages to injured spinal cord is orchestrated by remote brain choroid plexus. Immunity. 2013; 38(3):555–569
[41] Doetsch F, Caillé I, Lim DA, García-Verdugo JM, Alvarez-Buylla A. Subventricular zone astrocytes are neural stem cells in the adult mammalian brain. Cell. 1999; 97(6):703–716
[42] Redzic ZB, Preston JE, Duncan JA, Chodobski A, Szmydynger-Chodobska J. The choroid plexus-cerebrospinal fluid system: from development to aging. Curr Top Dev Biol. 2005; 71:1–52
[43] Hébert JM, Mishina Y, McConnell SK. BMP signaling is required locally to pattern the dorsal telencephalic midline. Neuron. 2002; 35(6):1029–1041
[44] Bender B, Honegger JB, Beschorner R, Ernemann U, Horger M. MR imaging findings in colloid cysts of the sellar region: comparison with colloid cysts of the third ventricle and Rathke's cleft cysts. Acad Radiol. 2013; 20(11):1457–1465
[45] Eisenberg HM, Sarwar M, Schochet S, Jr. Symptomatic Rathke's cleft cyst. Case report. J Neurosurg. 1976; 45(5):585–588
[46] Fager CA, Carter H. Intrasellar epithelial cysts. J Neurosurg. 1966; 24(1):77–81
[47] Graziani N, Dufour H, Figarella-Branger D, Donnet A, Bouillot P, Grisoli F. Do the suprasellar neurenteric cyst, the Rathke cleft cyst and the colloid cyst constitute a same entity? Acta Neurochir (Wien). 1995; 133(3–4):174–180
[48] Beaumont TL, Limbrick DD, Jr, Rich KM, Wippold FJ, II, Dacey RG, Jr. Natural history of colloid cysts of the third ventricle. J Neurosurg. 2016; 125(6): 1420–1430
[49] Ganti SR, Antunes JL, Louis KM, Hilal SK. Computed tomography in the diagnosis of colloid cysts of the third ventricle. Radiology. 1981; 138(2):385–391
[50] Symon L, Pell M. The transcortical approach. In: Advances and Technical Standards in Neurosurgery. Vol. 17. Springer; 1990:122–133
[51] Yasargil MG, Sarioglu AC, Adamson TE. The interhemispheric-transcallosal approach. In: Advances and Technical Standards in Neurosurgery. Vol. 17. Springer; 1990:133–143
[52] Kondziolka D, Bilbao JM. An immunohistochemical study of neuroepithelial (colloid) cysts. J Neurosurg. 1989; 71(1):91–97
[53] Mosberg WH, Jr, Blackwood W. Mucus-secreting cells in colloid cysts of the third ventricle. J Neuropathol Exp Neurol. 1954; 13(3):417–426
[54] Pollock BE, Huston J, III. Natural history of asymptomatic colloid cysts of the third ventricle. J Neurosurg. 1999; 91(3):364–369
[55] Donaldson JO, Simon RH. Radiodense ions within a third ventricular colloid cyst. Arch Neurol. 1980; 37(4):246
[56] Ferrand B, Pecker J, Javalet A, et al. Colloid cysts of the 3rd ventricle. Anatomo-pathological and pathogenic study. Ann Anat Pathol (Paris). 1971; 16(4):429–450
[57] Mathiesen T, Grane P, Lindgren L, Lindquist C. Third ventricle colloid cysts: a consecutive 12-year series. J Neurosurg. 1997; 86(1):5–12
[58] Godano U, Ferrai R, Meleddu V, Bellinzona M. Hemorrhagic colloid cyst with sudden coma. Minim Invasive Neurosurg. 2010; 53(5–6):273–274
[59] Miettinen M, Clark R, Virtanen I. Intermediate filament proteins in choroid plexus and ependyma and their tumors. Am J Pathol. 1986; 123(2):231–240
[60] Perentes E, Rubinstein LJ. Recent applications of immunoperoxidase histochemistry in human neuro-oncology. An update. Arch Pathol Lab Med. 1987; 111(9):796–812
[61] Armao D, Castillo M, Chen H, Kwock L. Colloid cyst of the third ventricle: imaging-pathologic correlation. AJNR Am J Neuroradiol. 2000; 21(8): 1470–1477
[62] Mackenzie IR, Gilbert JJ. Cysts of the neuraxis of endodermal origin. J Neurol Neurosurg Psychiatry. 1991; 54(7):572–575
[63] Scaravilli F, Lidov H, Spalton DJ, Symon L. Neuroenteric cyst of the optic nerve: case report with immunohistochemical study. J Neurol Neurosurg Psychiatry. 1992; 55(12):1197–1199
[64] McLean AJ. Paraphysial cysts. Arch Neuro Psychiatr. 1936; 36(3):485–513
[65] Palacios E, Azar-Kia B, Shannon M, Messina AV. Neuroepithelial (colloid) cysts. Pathogenesis and unusual features. AJR Am J Roentgenol. 1976; 126 (1):56–62
[66] Bailey P. Morphology of the roof plate of the forebrain and the lateral choroid plexuses in the human embryo. J Comp Neurol. 1916; 26(1):79–120
[67] Little JR, MacCarty CS. Colloid cysts of the third ventricle. J Neurosurg. 1974; 40(2):230–235
[68] Shuangshoti S, Roberts MP, Netsky MG. Neuroepithelial (colloid) cysts: pathogenesis and relation to choroid plexus and ependyma. Arch Pathol. 1965; 80: 214–224
[69] Shuangshoti S, Netsky MG. Neuroepithelial (colloid) cysts of the nervous system: further observations on pathogenesis, location, incidence, and histochemistry. Neurology. 1966; 16(9):887

# 2 Anatomy of the Third Ventricle

*Eduardo Carvalhal Ribas, Andre Felix Gentil, and Guilherme Carvalhal Ribas*

**Abstract**

The third ventricle is a single cavity, located deep inside the brain, between both thalami. It can be approached by neurosurgeons, microsurgically or endoscopically, to address lesions at this region or perform CSF diversion procedures. Detailed anatomical understanding of this cavity and nearby structures is fundamental to obtain safe and accurate surgeries at this region.

*Keywords:* neuroanatomy, third ventricle, CSF, thalami, hypothalamus, fornix

## 2.1 Introduction

The third ventricle is a single cavity located in the center of the brain, between the thalami.[1,2] It receives cerebrospinal fluid (CSF) from the lateral ventricles through both foramina of Monro, located next to each other at the anterior part of its roof, and drains into the fourth ventricle through the aqueduct of Sylvius, with the opening of the aqueduct located in the posterior part of the third ventricle floor. Some CSF is also produced within the third ventricle by two small strains of choroid plexus located along the roof.

It is usually a narrow and funnel-shaped space, but the presence of hydrocephalus and CSF accumulation can dilate its walls and confer a more globous appearance. In approximately two-third of brains, this cavity is traversed by a connection of the upper one-half surfaces of both thalami, named massa intermedia.[2]

The third ventricle has six distinct anatomic boundaries: two lateral walls, an anterior and a posterior wall, a roof, and a floor.

## 2.2 Lateral Walls

The lateral walls of the third ventricle are constituted by the mesial aspect of both thalami, with both interventricular foramina of Monro located next to each other at the most anterior and superior aspect of this ventricular cavity (▶ Fig. 2.1, ▶ Fig. 2.2, ▶ Fig. 2.3).

On each side, the shallow hypothalamic sulcus extends from the foramen of Monro toward the orifice of the aqueduct, separating the thalamus from the ipsilateral hypothalamus. The hypothalamus extends basally between both thalami; hence, these three surfaces form a U-shaped configuration. The lateral arms of the "U" correspond to the lateral walls of the third ventricle, with the upper two-third constituted by the thalamus and the lower third by the hypothalamus. The bottom of the "U" is constituted by the hypothalamus and corresponds to the floor of the third ventricle.

The superior limit of each lateral wall is demarcated by the stria medullaris thalami which runs along the superomedial border of each thalamus, from the foramen of Monro to the habenular commissure, a structure that connects both habenulae, which are small eminences located on the dorsomedial surfaces of both the thalami, superior to the posterior commissure.

## 2.3 Anterior Wall

The anterior wall of the third ventricle is formed by the lamina terminalis, which is a thin membrane that stretches from the anterior commissure (superiorly and posteriorly) to the optic chiasm (inferiorly and anteriorly) that forms a prominence at the anterior margin of the floor.[2] The small recess between the lamina terminalis and the optic chiasm is named the optic

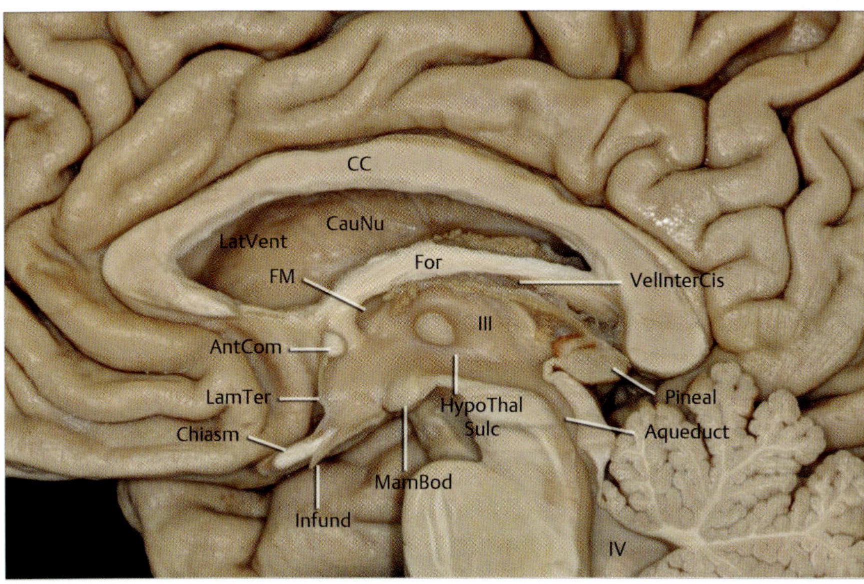


**Fig. 2.1** Sagittal view of the third ventricle. Its anterior wall is mainly formed by the lamina terminalis, stretching from the anterior commissure to the optic chiasm; its roof extends from the foramen of Monro to the habenular commissure and has the velum interpositum cistern, a space between two layers of tela choroidea; its posterior wall extends from the suprapineal recess to the opening of the aqueduct, having the pineal gland at the center; and its floor extends from the optic chiasm to the opening of the aqueduct, divided into an anterior hypothalamic part (inferior to the hypothalamic sulcus) and a posterior mesencephalic part by the mammillary bodies. (Anatomical dissections performed by Eduardo Carvalhal Ribas, MD.)

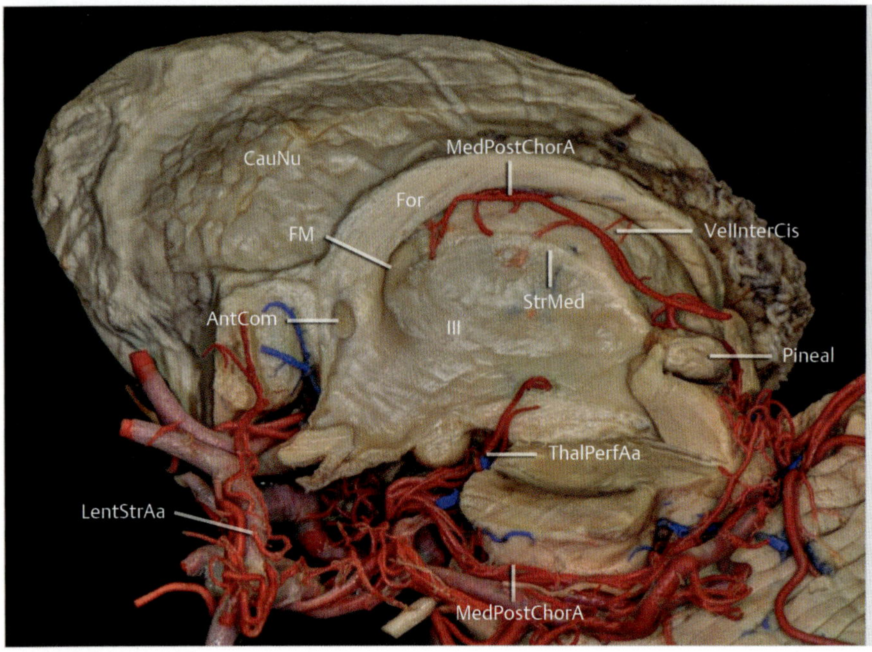


**Fig. 2.2** Arteries related to the third ventricle. The third ventricle can be seen in this sagittal view after removing all cerebral lobes and the left central core; the arteries were perfused with red silicone. The lenticulostriate arteries arise from the M1 segment of the middle cerebral artery and enter the anterior perforated substance (not related to the third ventricle). The thalamoperforating arteries arise from the basilar artery tip and proximal segments of the posterior cerebral artery and enter the inferior aspect of the third ventricle at the posterior perforated substance. The lateral and medial posterior choroidal arteries also arise from the proximal segments of the posterior cerebral artery; the former enters the lateral ventricle, and the latter has first a posterior trajectory around the midbrain, then upward to the pineal region, and finally anteriorly to enter the velum interpositum cistern. (Anatomical dissections performed by Eduardo Carvalhal Ribas, MD.)

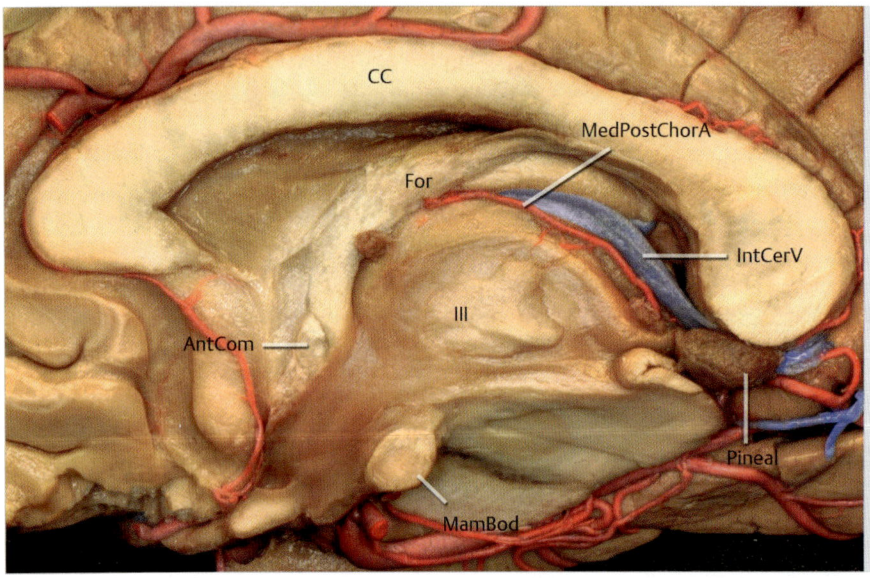


**Fig. 2.3** Internal cerebral vein. The third ventricle is seen in this sagittal view, with the arteries and veins perfused with red and blue silicone, respectively. The internal cerebral vein is formed by the junction of the anterior septal vein and the thalamostriate vein and can be found at the velum interpositum cistern. It exits this cistern posteriorly, over the pineal gland, and joins the basal vein of Rosenthal to form the great vein of Galen. The medial posterior choroidal arteries are also present inside the velum interpositum cistern. (Anatomical dissections performed by Eduardo Carvalhal Ribas, MD.)

recess. While the superior third of the lamina terminalis is hidden posterior to the rostrum of the corpus callosum, the lower two-third lies within the lamina terminalis cistern, which harbors the anterior communicating artery.

## 2.4 Posterior Wall

The posterior wall extends from the suprapineal recess, located superiorly to the habenular commissure, to the opening of the aqueduct, and includes, from superior to inferior, the suprapineal recess, the habenular commissure, the pineal gland, the pineal recess, and the posterior commissure, which is the upper aspect of the opening of the aqueduct.

The pineal gland is found in the quadrigeminal cistern, already outside the third ventricle, and is attached to the posterior wall by a double stalk that projects superiorly to the habenular commissure and inferiorly to the posterior commissure. The pineal recess is anterior to the pineal gland and constitutes an extension of the third ventricle cavity between the upper and lower attachments of the pineal gland.

There is also a small posterior extension of the third ventricle located above the habenular commissure referred to as the suprapineal recess.

## 2.5 Floor

The floor of the third ventricle extends from the optic chiasm to the orifice of the aqueduct of Sylvius that has the posterior commissure as its superior margin and the mesencephalic tegmentum as its inferior margin. The floor can be divided into an anterior hypothalamic part and a posterior mesencephalic part. The anterior part is composed, from anterior to posterior, by the optic chiasm, the infundibulum, the tuber cinereum, and the mammillary bodies, while the posterior part corresponds to the roof of the interpeduncular fossa and is formed by the mesencephalic tegmentum. The infundibulum is continuous with the pituitary stalk and connects the hypothalamus to the posterior lobe of the pituitary gland (neurohypophysis) through the supraoptico-paraventriculo-hypophyseal tract, which transports colloid droplets containing oxytocin and vasopressin hormones.[3]

When the floor is seen from above and from inside the ventricle, the infundibular recess can be easily identified between the optic chiasm prominence and the infundibulum, and the mammillary bodies appear as two prominences posterior to the infundibular recess. An endoscopic third ventriculostomy should be performed by opening the thin and commonly translucent area between the infundibular recess and the mammillary bodies, corresponding to the tuber cinereum. The procedure is then completed by opening of the underlying Liliequist membrane, hence communicating the third ventricle with the prepontine cistern, meanwhile taking particular care of the basilar artery. Posterior to the mammillary bodies, the floor of the third ventricle has a concave and smooth surface, marked by the triangular-shaped opening of the aqueduct more posteriorly.

When seen from outside within the encephalon base, the floor of the third ventricle is located just posterior to the optic chiasm and between the optic tracts and cerebral peduncles, with the roof of the interpeduncular fossa corresponding to the anterior aspect of the mesencephalic part of the third ventricle floor. While the anterior perforated substance spreads along the basal areas anteriorly to both optic tracts, the posterior perforated substance spreads along all the inferior aspect of the third ventricle floor.

## 2.6 Roof

The roof of the third ventricle extends from the foramina of Monro to the habenular commissure, and is formed by four layers of structures: the superior layer comprised of the fornices, then layers consisting of the superior and the inferior tela choroidea, with the space between these two thin membranes corresponding to the velum interpositum cistern.

The superior neural layer is anteriorly constituted by both the bodies of the fornices which run juxtaposed. While the upper sheet of tela choroidea is in intimate contact with the inferior borders of both the fornices, the lower sheet of tela choroidea is attached to both the stria medullaris that run along the superomedial thalamic borders.

The velum interpositum cistern in between the tela choroidea layers ends anteriorly at the level of both foramina of Monro and opens posteriorly into the quadrigeminal or pineal cistern. It harbors the medial posterior choroidal arteries and the internal cerebral veins within its small trabeculae.

The internal cerebral veins are formed by the junction of the anterior septal vein and the thalamostriate vein, which usually happens close to the entry point into the velum interpositum cistern as they pass underneath the fornix through the choroidal fissure, next to the foramen of Monro. The internal cerebral veins exit the velum interpositum cistern posteriorly, over the pineal gland, and join the basal vein of Rosenthal to form the great vein of Galen.

Two small strands of choroid plexus project downward from the lower sheet of tela choroidea into the third ventricle along both sides of the midline. Each of these choroid plexus strands is continuous along its pedicle with the choroid plexus of the ipsilateral lateral ventricle through the choroidal fissure, which defines the lateral aspect of the third ventricle roof.

Understanding the anatomy of the roof of the third ventricle is paramount to perform a safe and precise transchoroidal approach (▶ Fig. 2.4). The choroid plexus is identified after opening the body of the lateral ventricle. It is attached to the choroidal fissure, which is the natural cleft between the thalamus and the fornix. This attachment is made by two taenias that stretch from the choroid plexus: the taenia fornicis to the fornix and the taenia choroidea to thalamus. These taenias are the continuation of the ependyma that covers the internal surface of the ventricular cavity. Either taenia can be opened to approach the choroidal fissure. However, the more lateral taenia choroidea is closely related to the small veins that drain the superior surface of the thalamus, and the thalamostriate vein will stop the surgeon from opening the choroidal fissure further anteriorly since this approach is done laterally to both internal cerebral veins (subchoroidal approach). Crossing the taenia fornicis is an ideal route by making an incision between the fornix medially and the choroid plexus laterally through the choroidal fissure to access the velum interpositum cistern (transchoroidal approach). At this level, the ipsilateral internal cerebral vein is identified first, and the contralateral vein is seen further medially. Between both the veins the inferior tela choroidea is opened and the third ventricle is approached through its roof. The anterior septal vein can be sacrificed if it is necessary to access the anterior part of the third ventricle.[4] Conceptually, both the subchoroidal and the transchoroidal are done through the choroidal fissure and are trans-velum approaches, differing only in the choroidal fissure side of entrance.

See ▶ Table 2.1 for brain structures related to the third ventricle and ▶ Fig. 2.5 for understanding this region's anatomy through endoscopic views.

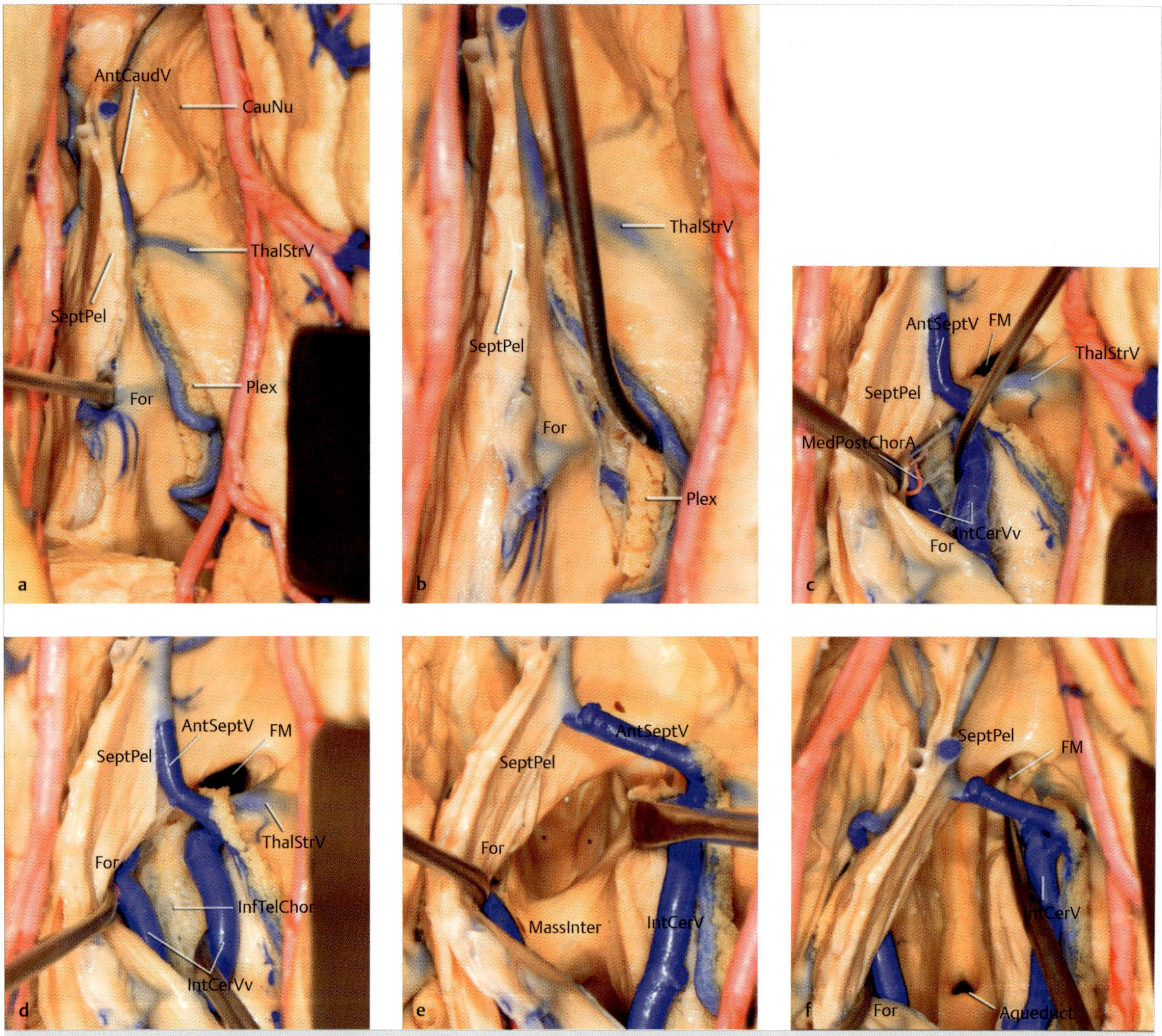


**Fig. 2.4** Stepwise anatomical dissection depicting the transchoroidal surgical approach to the third ventricle. **(a)** The body of lateral ventricle is opened and its inner structures are identified. **(b)** The choroidal fissure is opened at the taenia fornicis, between the fornix medially and the choroid plexus laterally. **(c)** The velum interpositum cistern is reached, and both internal cerebral veins can be identified. **(d)** Inferior and between both internal cerebral veins, the inferior tela choroidea is exposed. **(e)** The inferior tela choroidea is opened, and the third ventricle is approached from its roof. **(f)** The massa intermedia is cut to allow visualization of the posterior part of the third ventricle floor, and the orifice of the aqueduct can be seen. (Anatomical dissections performed by Eduardo Carvalhal Ribas, MD.)

**Table 2.1** Brain structures related with the third ventricle

| | | |
|---|---|---|
| **Anterior wall** | Foramina of Monro | |
| | Pillars or Columns of the fornices | |
| | Anterior commissure | |
| | Lamina terminalis | |
| | Optic recess | |
| | Optic chiasm | |
| **Lateral walls** | Thalami | |
| | Stria medullaris thalami | |
| | Hypothalamic Sulcus | |
| | Hypothalamus | |
| **Floor** | Hypothalamus | Optic chiasm |
| | | Infundibular recess |
| | | Infundibulum |
| | | Tuber cinereum |
| | | Mamillary bodies |
| | | Posterior perforated substance |
| | Mesencephalon | Mesencephalic tegmentum / Roof of interpeduncular fossa |
| | | Posterior perforated substance |
| | | Orifice of aqueduct |
| **Roof** | Foramina of Monro | |
| | Bodies and crura of fornices, hippocampal commissure | |
| | Superior tela choroidea | |
| | Velum interpositum cistern (medial posterior choroidal arteries, internal cerebral veins) | |
| | Inferior tela choroidea | |
| | Choroid plexus | |
| | Suprapineal recess | |
| **Posterior wall** | Suprapineal recess | |
| | Habenula | |
| | Habenular commissure | |
| | Pineal Recess | |
| | Pineal gland | |
| | Posterior commissure | |

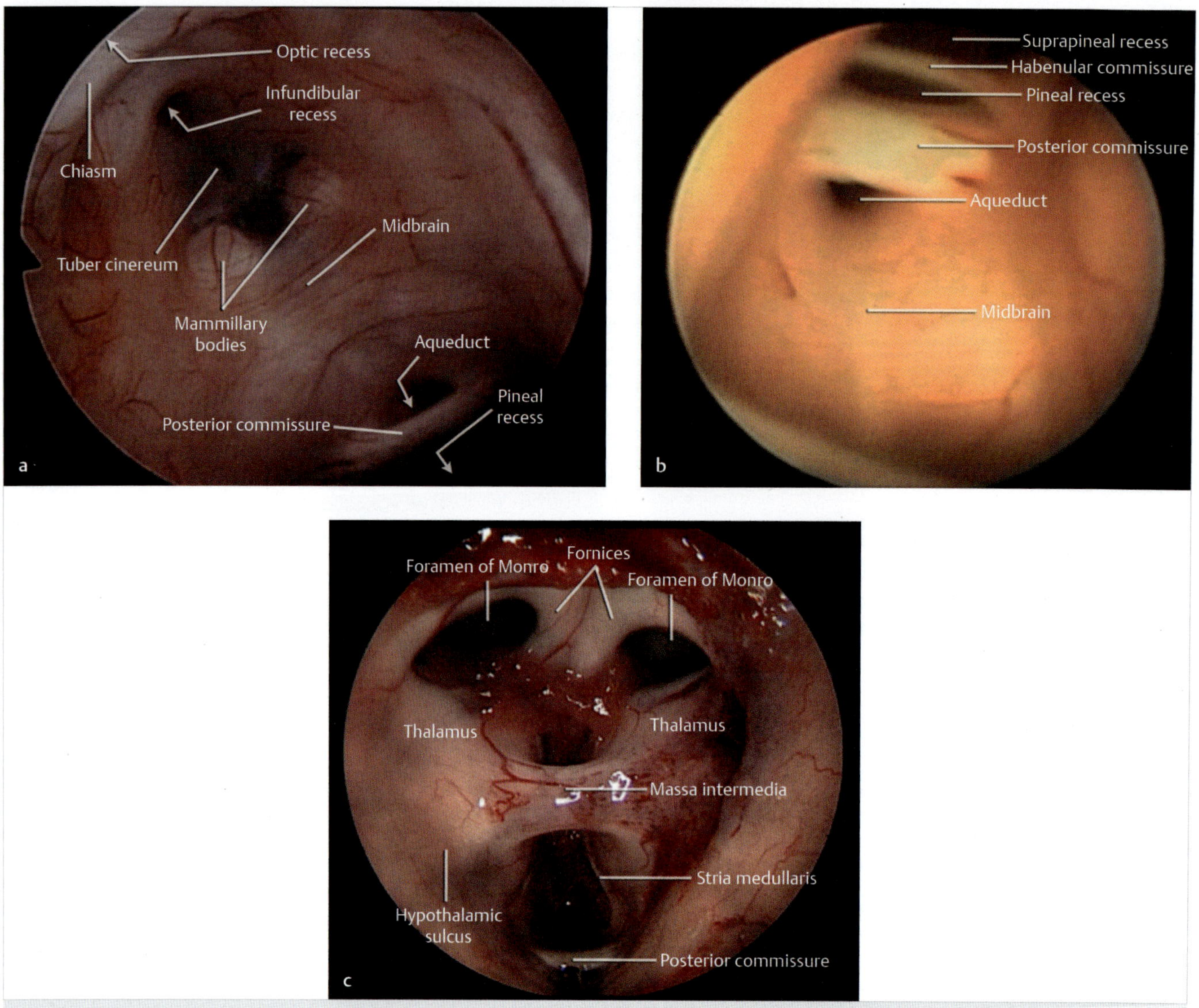


**Fig. 2.5** Endoscopic views of the third ventricle. **(a)** Endoscopic superoanterior view. At this point of view, the endoscope is located at the foramen of Monro and directed toward the floor of the third ventricle. Its anterior part is composed, from anterior to posterior, of the optic chiasm, the infundibulum, the tuber cinereum, and the mammillary bodies, while the posterior part corresponds to the roof of the interpeduncular fossa and is formed by the mesencephalic tegmentum. **(b)** Endoscopic superoposterior view. At this point of view, the endoscope is located at the foramen of Monro and directed toward the posterior wall of the third ventricle. At this region, several structures can be identified from superior to inferior: the suprapineal recess, the habenular commissure, the pineal recess, and the posterior commissure, which is the upper aspect of the opening of the aqueduct. (Parts **a** and **b** used with permisison from Dr. Koshiro Nishikuni.) **(c)** Endoscopic inferior view. The superior and lateral aspects of the third ventricle are seen from an anteroinferior perspective, through an endonasal transsphenoidal approach, after a craniopharyngioma removal. Both the foramina of Monro are identified superiorly, next to each other at the most superior and anterior aspect of the third ventricle, and the massa intermedia is seen at the center of the ventricular cavity connecting both thalami. (Used with permission from Dr. Aldo Stamm.)

# References


[1] Rhoton AL, Jr. Cranial anatomy and surgical approaches. Neurosurgery. 2003; 53:1–746

[2] Yamamoto I, Rhoton AL, Jr, Peace DA. Microneurosurgery of the third ventricle: part I, microsurgical anatomy. Neurosurgery. 1981; 8:334–356

[3] Nieuwenhuys R, Voogt J, Van Huijzen C. The Human Central Nervous. System Berlin: Steinkopff; 2007. ed 4.

[4] Wen HT, Rhoton AL, Jr, Oliveira E. Transchoroidal approach to the third ventricle: an anatomic study of the choroidal fissure and its clinical application. Neurosurgery. 1998; 42:1205–1209


# Suggested Readings


Barber SM, Rangel-Castilla L, Baskin D. Neuroendoscopic resection of intraventricular tumours: a systematic outcomes analysis. Minim Invasive Surg. 2013;2013:898753

Brodal A. Neurological anatomy in relation to clinical medicine. 3rd ed. New York: Oxford University Press; 1981

Duvernoy HM. The human hippocampus. 2nd ed. Berlin: Springer; 1998

Ebeling U, Reulen HJ. Neurosurgical topography of the optic radiation in the temporal lobe. Acta Neurochir (Wien). 1988;92:26–36

Ebeling U, Steinmetz H. Anatomy of the parietal lobe: Mapping the individual pattern. Acta Neurochir (Wien). 1995; 136:8–11

Friedman MA, Meyers CA, Sawaya R. Neuropsychological effects of third ventricle tumour surgery. Neurosurgery. 2008;62(6 Suppl 3):1093–1100

Harkey HL, Al-Mefty O, Haines DE, Smith RR. The surgical anatomy of the cerebral sulci. Neurosurgery. 1989; 24:651–654

Hart MG, Sarkies NJ, Santarius T, Kirollos RW. Ophthalmological outcome after resection of tumours based on the pineal gland. J Neurosurg. 2013;119(2):420–426

Hassaneen W, Suki D, Salaskar AL, Levine NB, DeMonte F, Lang FF, McCutcheon IE, Dorai Z, Feiz-Erfan I, Wildrick DM, Sawaya R. Immediate morbidity and mortality associated with transcallosal resection of tumours of the third ventricle. J Clin Neurosci. 2010;17(7):830–836

Heimer L. The human brain and spinal cord. 2nd ed. New York: Springer Verlag; 1995

Kirollos RW, Javadpour M, May P, Mallucci C. Endoscopic treatment of suprasellar and third ventricle-related arachnoid cysts. Child's Nervous System. 2001;17(12):713–718

Ludwig E, Klinger J. Atlas Cerebri Humani. Basel: S. Karger; 1956

Martino J, Hamer PCD, Vergani F, Bogna C, de Lucas EM, Vazquez-Barquero A, Garcia-Porrero JA, Duffau H. Cortex-sparing fiber dissection: an improved method for the study of white matter anatomy in the human brain. J Anat. 2011; 219(4):1469–7580

Milligan BD, Meyer FB. Morbidity of transcallosal and transcortical approaches to lesions in and around the lateral and third ventricles: a single-institution experience. Neurosurgery. 2010;67(6):1483–1496, discussion 1496

Morris TC, Santoreneos S. Colloid cyst of velum interpositum: a rare finding. J Neurosurg Pediatr. 2012; 9(2):206–208

Nagata S, Rhoton AL Jr, Barry M. Microsurgical anatomy of the choroidal fissure. Surg Neurol. 1988; 20:3–59

Ono M, Kubik S, Abernathey CD. Atlas of cerebral sulci. Stuttgart: Thieme; 1990

Oka K, Rhoton AL Jr, Barry M, Rodriguez R. Microsurgical anatomy of the superficial veins of the cerebrum. Neurosurgery. 1985; 17(5):711–748

Rhoton AL, The lateral and third ventricles. Neurosurgery. 2002; 51(Suppl 1):207–271

Rhoton AL Jr, Yamamoto I, Peace DA. Microsurgery of the third ventricle: Part 2. Operative approaches. Neurosurgery. 1981;8(3):357–373

Ribas GC. Telencéfalo. In: Meneses MS, ed. Neuroanatomia aplicada. Rio de Janeiro: Guanabara Koogan; 1999: 237–272

Ribas GC, Rodrigues AJ. The suprapetrosal craniotomy. J Neurosurg. 2007; 106(3):449–454

Ribas GC, Yasuda A, Ribas EC, Nishikuni K, Rodrigues Junior AJ. Surgical anatomy of microneurosurgical sulcal key-points. Neurosurgery. 2006; 59(ONS Suppl4):ONS-177–ONS-209

Ribas GC. Microanatomia cirúrgica dos pontos-chave dos sulcos e giros cerebrais [tese livre-docência]. São Paulo: Faculdade de Medicina, Universidade de São Paulo; 2005:297

Selvanathan SK, Kumar R, Goodden J, Tyagi A, Chumas P. Evolving instrumentation for endoscopic tumour removal of CNS tumours. Acta Neurochir (Wien). 2013; 155(1):135–138

Symss NP, Ramamurthi R, Kapu R, Rao SM, Vasudevan MC, Pande A, Cugati G. Complication avoidance in transcallosal transforaminal approach to colloid cysts of the anterior third ventricle: an analysis of 80 cases. Asian J Neurosurg. 2014; 9(2):51–57

Szmuda T, Słoniewski P, Szmuda M, Waszak PM, Starzyńska A. Quantification of white matter fibre pathways disruption in frontal transcortical approach to the lateral ventricle or the interventricular foramen in diffusion tensor tractography. Folia Morphol (Warsz). 2014; 73(2):129–138

Timurkaynak E, Rhoton AL Jr, Barry M. Microsurgical anatomy and operative approaches to the lateral ventricles. Neurosurgery. 1986; 19:685–723

Türe U, Yaşargil MG, Al-Mefty O. The transcallosal-transforaminal approach to the third ventricle with regard to the venous variations in this region. J Neurosurg. 1997;87(5):706-715

Türe U, Yasargil MG, Friedman AH, Al-Mefty O. Fibre dissection technique: lateral aspect of the brain. Neurosurgery. 2000;47:417–427

Ulm AJ, Russo A, Albanese E, Tanriover N, Martins C, Mericle RM, Pincus D, Rhoton AL. Limitations of the transcallosal transchoroidal approach to the third ventricle. J Neurosurg. 2009; 111(3):600–609

Villani R, Papagno C, Tomei G, Grimoldi N, Spagnoli D, Bello L. Transcallosal approach to tumours of the third ventricle. Surgical results and neuropsychological evaluation. J Neurosurg Sci. 1997; 41(1):41–50

Wen HT, Rhoton AL Jr, Oliveira E, Cardoso ACC, Tedeschi H, Baccanelli M, Marino Junior R. Microsurgical anatomy of the temporal lobe: part I: mesial temporal lobe anatomy and its vascular relationships and applied to amygdalohippocampectomy. Neurosurgery. 1999; 45:549–592

Williams PL, Warwick R, ed. Gray's anatomy. 36th ed. Philadelphia: Saunders; 1980

Yasargil MG: Microneurosurgery. Stuttgart, Georg Thieme, 1996, vol. IVb

# 3 Neuroimaging of Colloid Cysts

*Franz J. Wippold II*

**Abstract**

Computed tomography (CT) and magnetic resonance (MR) imaging have revolutionized the diagnosis and management of colloid cysts of the third ventricle. An approach to systematically analyzing these lesions is discussed including recognizing notable primary imaging signs, avoiding common pitfalls of interpretation, and evaluating possible alternatives in the differential diagnosis.

*Keywords:* colloid cyst, third ventricle masses, neuroimaging third ventricle, MRI third ventricle, CT third ventricle

## 3.1 Introduction

Cross-sectional imaging using computed tomography (CT) and magnetic resonance (MR) imaging has revolutionized the diagnosis of intraventricular lesions, especially colloid cysts of the third ventricle, and has dramatically increased the discovery of incidental cysts on otherwise routine screening examinations for vague symptoms such as headache.[1,2,3,4] Once discovered, imaging also provides an invaluable tool for noninvasive tracking of the cyst over time, especially when coupled with monitoring of symptoms, and can also assist in therapy planning and post-therapy surveillance.[1,5,6] Finally, imaging can also detect the complications of both treated and untreated colloid cysts, such as hydrocephalus and hemorrhage, especially since these conditions are not easily discovered or evaluated by clinical examination alone.[4,7,8] Although 85% of colloid cysts remain stable over time, over 10% will progress and develop life-threatening symptoms rapidly.[4,9,10] Cysts measuring 7 mm or more in diameter are more commonly associated with deterioration and death.[11] Therefore, immediate access to reliable imaging is crucial for management. Given the complex technical aspects of these imaging techniques and the high stakes for diagnosis and monitoring, accurate analysis of the imaging findings requires the coordinated efforts of both the clinical and imaging specialists of the health care team.

Once confronted with an intraventricular lesion, a systematic approach to image evaluation should be emphasized. First, the location of the lesion should be confirmed by careful analysis of the images in multiple planes. Review of several different planes of orientation establishes an intraventricular site of origin rather than a periventricular or extraventricular site of origin. Confirming the site of origin impacts not only diagnostic considerations but also therapy options. This initial evaluation is especially important for large masses in which the site of origin may be difficult to determine on casual review. For example, potential colloid cyst mimics such as gliomas more commonly arise adjacent to the ventricle and may protrude into the ventricle, whereas another mimic, the choroid plexus papilloma, typically arises within the ventricle and when large may invade the wall of the ventricle. Large cystic lesions such as Rathke's cleft cysts or craniopharyngiomas will often reveal clues of an extraventricular, suprasellar site of origin.

Once intraventricular site of origin is confirmed, the location of the lesion within the ventricle provides the next valuable diagnostic key.[12] Although traditional pathological sorting of diagnostic options, such as congenital, vascular, and neoplastic, remains useful, many of these intraventricular lesions characteristically arise in specific regions within the ventricle, thus providing critical information regarding etiology. For example, the colloid cyst virtually always originates in the anterior third ventricle (although rare exceptions do occur).[13] Other lesions, such as subependymal giant cell astrocytomas, most commonly arise near the foramen of Monro and would be decidedly unusual in the atrium of the lateral ventricle.

Following location, the age of the patient allows for further sorting of diagnostic possibilities. For example, embryonal tumors should be considered for an intraventricular mass in an infant, whereas this diagnosis almost never occurs in a middle-aged adult. Colloid cysts usually present in the third to fourth decades and are rarely seen in young children.

Finally, imaging appearance further narrows the diagnostic considerations. For example, is the lesion cystic or solid? If the lesion is cystic, does the MR imaging appearance suggest hemorrhage or viscous protein content? If the lesion is solid, does it enhance following administration of intravenous contrast agents? Although imaging appearance is rarely pathognomonic for any given entity, the cross-sectional imaging features may point to a limited variety of possibilities. Imaging appearance may also alert the examiner to subtle clues indicating rare mimics of the colloid cyst. With the emphasis on molecular and genetic signatures of tumors introduced in the recent World Health Organization 2016 revision of tumor classification, detailed analysis of the imaging phenotype may intimate the genotype in some colloid cyst impostors.[14] Additionally, the recent advances in machine learning offer exciting opportunities for more specific and highly detailed information derived from CT and MR imaging features.

When analyzing a suspected third ventricle lesion detected on CT or MR imaging, several errors or pitfalls need to be cautiously considered. These pitfalls may lead to misdiagnoses and can be divided into technical, systematic, and cognitive errors. Technical factors include imaging artifacts that may mask important findings or present misleading clues. For example, flow artifacts created by normal cerebrospinal fluid (CSF) pulsations within the ventricles as seen on fluid-attenuated inversion recovery (FLAIR) MR images may mimic lesions. Also, calcium may not be as apparent on MR compared with CT.[7,15,16] For example, calcified portions of a mass on CT suggesting a meningioma may be missed on MR and the lesion incorrectly diagnosed as a noncalcified colloid cyst or other soft tissue tumor. Therefore, consultation with an imaging specialist knowledgeable in scanning techniques may prove invaluable.

Faulty approaches to image analysis give rise to systematic errors. One such hazard is failure to employ a systematic search pattern when evaluating an imaging study. By applying a thorough systematic search pattern, analogous to a pre-flight checklist in the aviation industry, all portions of the study are examined. Subtle findings are more likely to be detected. For example, failure to routinely note the foramen magnum on sagittal T1-weighted MR images may lead to overlooking subtle tonsillar herniation due to mass effect from an intraventricular lesion. Failure to routinely consider the caliber of the temporal horns may lead to overlooking subtle and possibly life-threatening hydrocephalus. Failure to review the scout images may lead to missing an important sign not present on the cross-sectional images. Therefore, clinicians are urged to routinely employ a standard imaging checklist of important findings to minimize this pitfall.

A systematic search pattern should also account for all the images and series of a given imaging study. Today's typical MR imaging study may generate 10 or more imaging series and several thousand individual images. Apparent lack of an important series in a study presented for interpretation should prompt a diligent searching of the electronic file for its whereabouts. Unfortunately, no formatting standardization exists among the thousands of imaging centers nationwide in the US, and the task may appear daunting given the numerous equipment hardware and software options. Nevertheless, the consulting physician must become familiar with various imaging protocols and basic imaging techniques to minimize the chance of an incomplete evaluation.

Failure to systematically evaluate images may also lead to another related pitfall known as "satisfaction of search." In this pitfall, discovery of an obvious imaging finding prompts interruption of the systematic search pattern and may lead to overlooking important additional, but less obvious, findings. For example, a cursory review of the study may identify an obvious anterior third ventricle cystic lesion and prompt a premature diagnosis of a colloid cyst, whereas a closer inspection may reveal additional subtle cystic lesions elsewhere in the brain indicating infection or metastases.[17]

A third category of errors includes cognitive biases or interpretive errors, in which the lesion is appreciated, but its significance is overlooked, and it is subsequently misdiagnosed. A complete discussion of the sources of cognitive bias is beyond the scope of this work; however, a few biases warrant mentioning. Availability bias refers to the tendency to base diagnoses on personal experience.[17] A colloid cyst is the most commonly encountered anterior third ventricular cystic mass for most neurosurgeons; however, few imaging presentations are truly pathognomonic for a single diagnosis. Therefore, consideration of other diagnoses may be important especially if the cyst demonstrates atypical features such as hemorrhage, avid enhancement, or surrounding edema. Anchoring bias reflects the persistence of an initial impression despite subsequent contrary evidence that challenges the initial diagnosis.[17] Therefore, the clinical team should remain open to diagnostic challenges when presented with additional imaging information.

In summary, imaging has provided a rewarding tool in the diagnosis and management of intraventricular masses, especially colloid cysts, when applied in a systematic fashion with attention to potential pitfalls.

## 3.2 CT Imaging

CT continues to provide a rapid, readily available screening tool and is usually the first study for a patient presenting with headache or mental status changes.[18] CT displays calcification and hemorrhage extremely well. Less dense tissues, such as with water, fat, and air, display varying degrees of radiolucency. CT depicts cerebral tissue moderately well, especially when dense material such as protein is present. However, CT poorly differentiates soft tissues with similar densities, such as the gray and white matter.

Administration of intravenous iodinated contrast material improves the conspicuity of many brain lesions, but these agents carry a small but definite risk of anaphylaxis and renal impairment. These adverse effects should be considered carefully when requesting contrast-enhanced CT in the elderly patient. Newly developed nonionic agents are better tolerated than the ionic contrast agents. In the era of widely available MR imaging, most clinicians forego an enhanced CT in favor of MR imaging.

Another major advantage of CT in the screening examination is its rapid scanning speed. Modern scanners can quickly produce multiplanar reformations from the original axially oriented acquisitions. Many of the technical artifacts, which hampered image quality in the early scanners, have been largely remedied with newer scanners.

Although a CT scan is rarely sufficient to thoroughly evaluate the patient with an intraventricular mass, it remains the predominant screening tool and is usually the first imaging examination for a patient presenting to the primary care physician with a nonspecific symptom such as a headache.[18] Moreover, CT is an excellent, readily available tool for monitoring ventricular size. Although CT may be used in the postoperative patient, a normal image does not absolutely preclude recurrence and MR imaging is generally preferred in this population.[1]

Colloid cysts usually display a round or ovoid shape, homogenous density, and sharply defined margins.[16] They tend to be hyperdense or isodense compared with the density of the gray matter of the brain and are usually easily detected within the lucent CSF-filled third ventricle[8,19,20,21] (▶ Fig. 3.1). Only 15% of colloid cysts are hypodense[1,19] (▶ Fig. 3.2, ▶ Fig. 3.3). Radiodensity that is greater than water may be due to hydration status of the cyst, protein concentration, abundancy of cholesterol, or hemorrhage.[2] Atomic spectrometry of cyst mucin has also revealed other factors contributing to the density of the cyst including presence of calcium, magnesium, and traces of silicon, copper, iron, phosphorus, and aluminum.[22,23] The density of colloid cysts may also evolve over time as the protein concentration changes with water resorption.[19] Some authors have proposed that hyperdense cysts may be more solid than radiolucent cysts and not as inclined to grow.[9] Dense colloid cysts tend to be viscous and may be more difficult to aspirate than cysts composed predominantly of water, although CT density as a predictor of ease of aspiration is not always reliable.[1,16,24] Only 10% of lesions display calcification visible on imaging and some authors suggest that calcification should prompt consideration of alternative diagnoses.[7,8,16,20,25] For example, rim calcification, especially if the contents are dense, may imply an aneurysm, whereas solid calcification may imply a tumor such as craniopharyngioma (▶ Fig. 3.4, ▶ Fig. 3.5, ▶ Fig. 3.6). Calcification within the cyst may also develop after hemorrhage.[8,25]

Colloid cysts typically do not enhance following administration of intravenous contrast agents.[16,26] Enhancement, although rarely present, has been attributed to inflammatory components or veins within the cyst wall.[16,19] Thickened rim

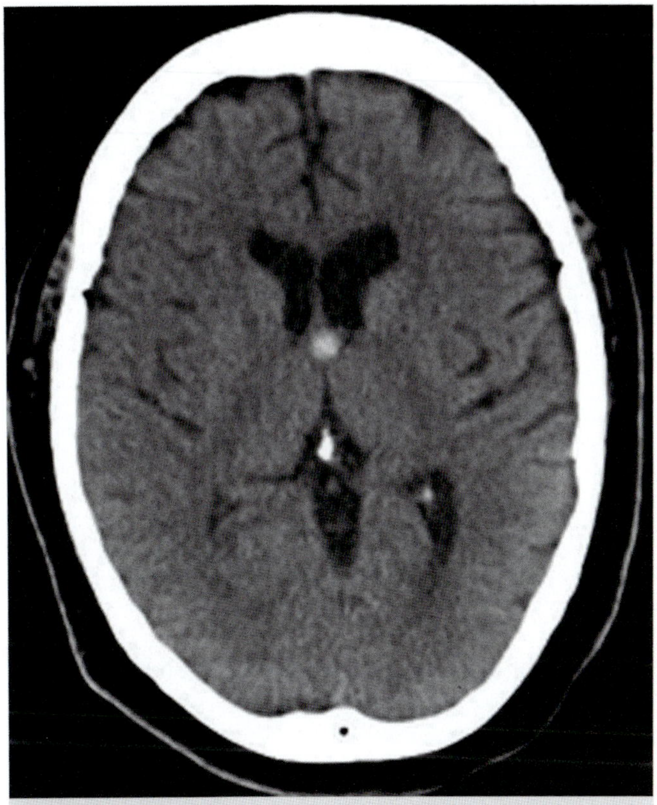

**Fig. 3.1** A 66-year-old female with mental status changes. Computed tomography (CT) demonstrating a hyperdense midline lesion within the anterior third ventricle, immediately posterior to the columns of the fornix, consistent with a colloid cyst. There is mild ventriculomegaly.

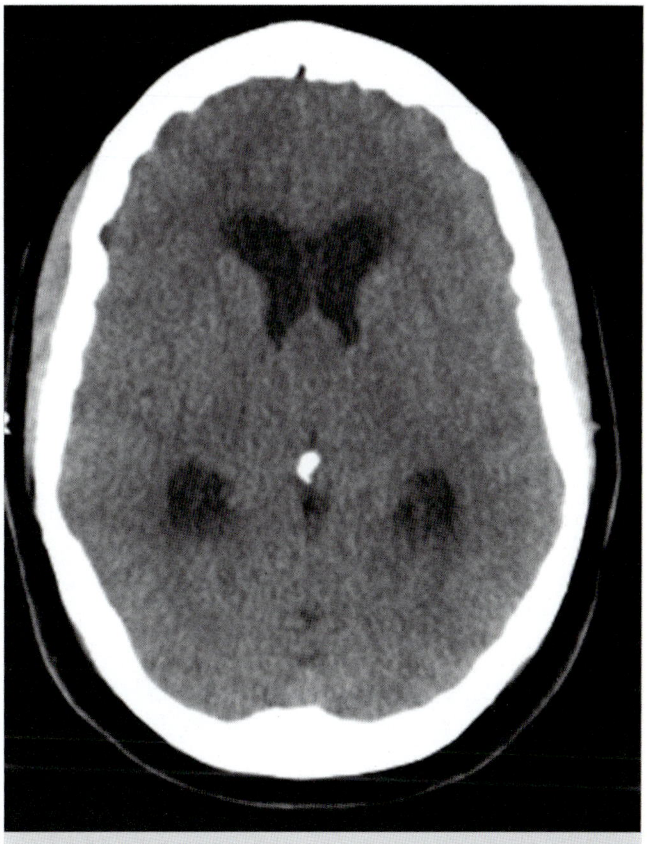

**Fig. 3.2** A 25-year-old female with headaches. Computed tomography (CT) demonstrating an isodense to slightly hypodense midline anterior third ventricular mass consistent with a colloid cyst. The mass is obstructing the foramen of Monro causing hydrocephalus.

or irregular solid enhancement should prompt further evaluation with CT angiography and MR imaging. Rim enhancement may indicate a craniopharyngioma or aneurysm and solid enhancement may suggest a tumor such as an ependymoma, meningioma, or adenoma (▶ Fig. 3.4, ▶ Fig. 3.5). Atypical imaging features include asymmetry and ectopic location (▶ Fig. 3.3). Colloid cysts have been demonstrated in the lateral ventricles and posterior third ventricle and even extraventricular locations, but alternative diagnoses should be excluded prior to intervention.[13]

## 3.3 MR Imaging

MR imaging has emerged as the preferred imaging modality when evaluating intraventricular masses, although CT remains useful for detecting calcifications and hemorrhage and should be considered a complementary tool for validating the causes of MR signal.[15,27] For example, focal hypointensity on MR images can be confirmed as calcium when seen as hyperdensity on corresponding CT slices.[21,28] Most centers now use high-field-strength magnets (1.5–3.0 T) because of improved signal-to-noise ratios, gradient strength, and spatial resolution when compared with low-field units. The axial plane, the primary source of information, is usually supplemented with coronal and sagittal planes. Fundamental sequences include T1-weighted, T2-weighted, and enhanced T1-weighted imaging sequences. Additional sequences may be available on scanners depending on manufacturer options. For example, restriction of water diffusion on diffusion-weighted imaging (DWI) indicates a possible epidermoid cyst (▶ Fig. 3.7) and blooming artifact on susceptibility-weighted imaging (SWI) suggests blood products.

Intravenous contrast enhancement with gadolinium agents has become a standard and invaluable component of the MR examination and is generally safer than iodinated compounds used in CT. However, in recent years the realization that gadolinium can be deposited in tissues over time has warranted caution in its use. In nephrogenic sclerotic systemic fibrosis (NSF), free gadolinium collecting within the soft tissues of the body can cause a potentially fatal sclerosis of these tissues, especially in patients with compromised renal function. Awareness of this complication coupled with evaluation of the renal function and avoidance of some agents have markedly decreased the incidence of NSF.[29] A second more recent finding is the deposition of gadolinium in the dentate nucleus.[30] This appears to be dose dependent; however, to date it has not caused any observable clinical syndromes. Nevertheless, this finding and its potentially latent clinical results are being carefully studied. A rule of thumb is to use gadolinium only when specifically indicated and to limit its use to patients with normal renal function.

As with CT imaging, colloid cysts demonstrate an ovoid shape and smooth walls on MR imaging.[31] MR signal characteristics are variable.[27] On T1-weighted sequences, almost 70% of cysts

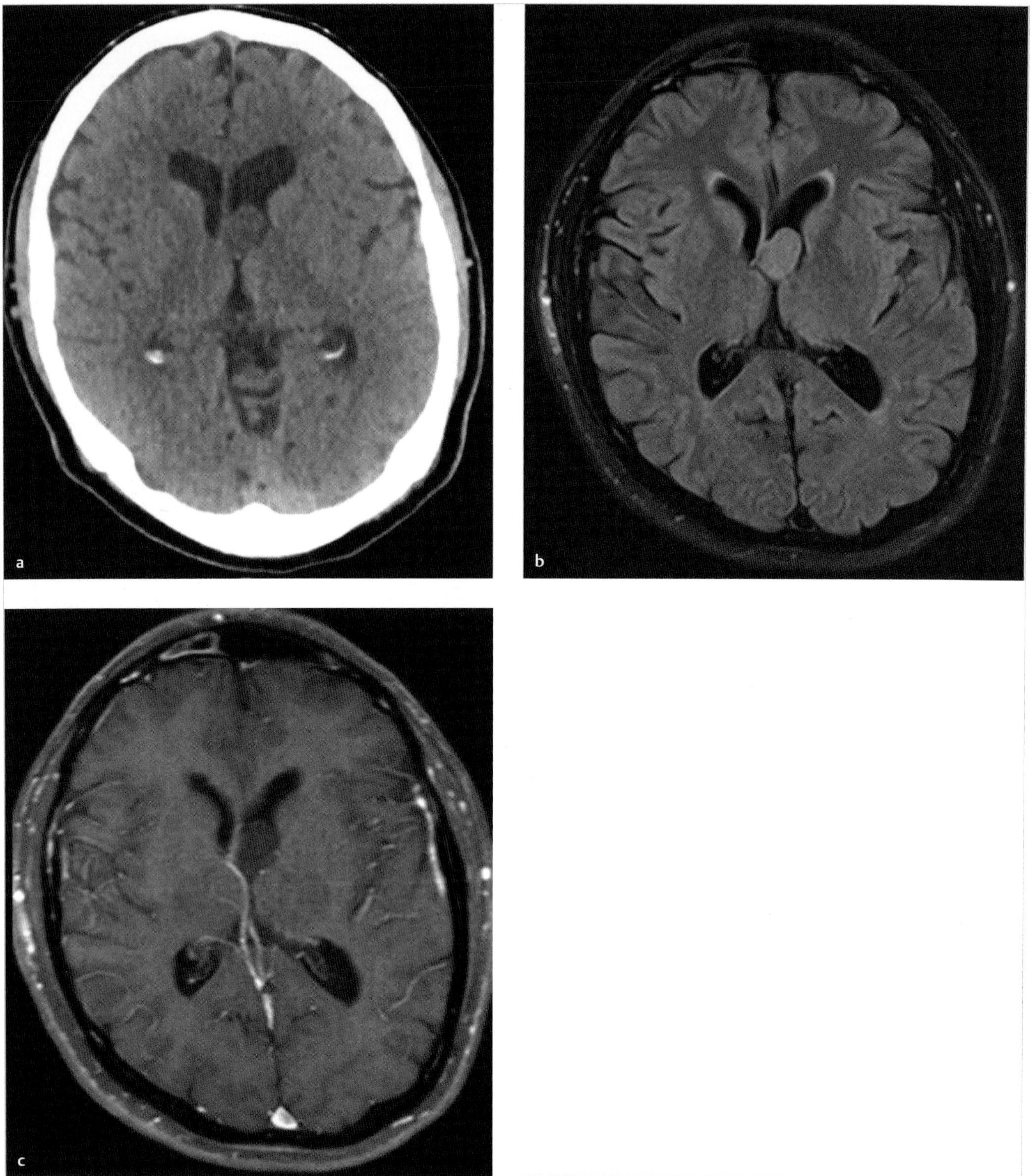

**Fig. 3.3** Colloid cyst. A 62-year-old female with mass incidentally discovered on imaging obtained after unrelated trauma. Computed tomography (CT) demonstrating an eccentric, slightly hypodense, well-defined mass straddling the left foramen of Monro **(a)**. It is projecting into the left frontal horn and the anterior third ventricle. The lesion is slightly hyperintense on fluid-attenuated inversion recovery (FLAIR) **(b)** and hypointense without enhancement on T1-weighted enhanced **(c)** magnetic resonance (MR) images.

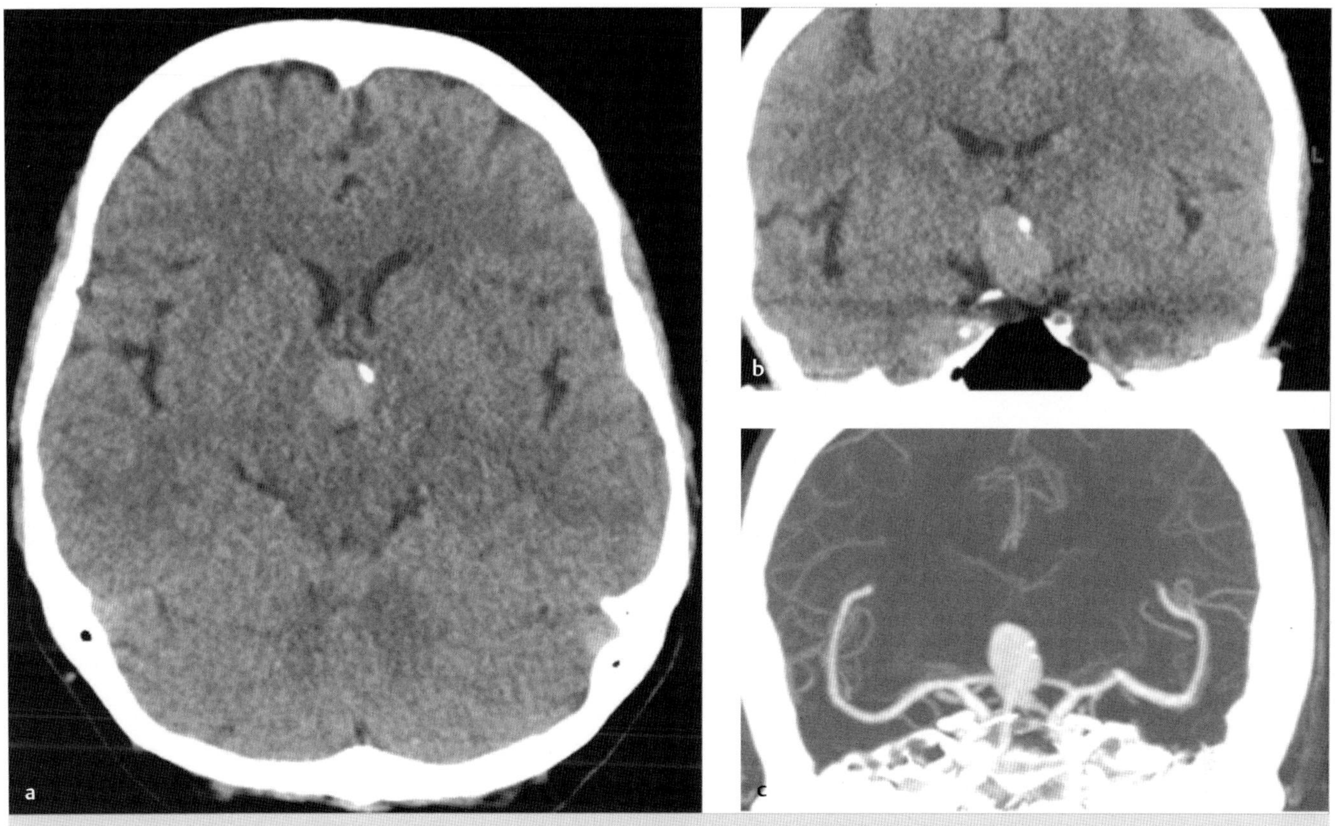

**Fig. 3.4** Aneurysm. A 59-year-old female with headache. Computed tomography (CT) demonstrating a dense mass in the region of the anterior third ventricle superficially resembling a colloid cyst **(a)**. A small peripheral calcification is noted. Coronal reformatted image further reveals that the mass originated within the basilar cistern and is projecting superiorly into the third ventricle deforming its floor **(b)**. Maximum intensity projection (MIP) image from CT angiogram showing dense opacification of the lesion, with intravenous contrast confirming the presence of an aneurysm arising from the terminus of the basilar artery **(c)**.

are hyperintense; however, some cysts may be hypointense or isointense[19,21,26,32] (▶ Fig. 3.8, ▶ Fig. 3.9). The appearance on T2-weighted images is also variable. Almost 80% of cysts are hyperintense with the remainder isointense or hypointense[19,21,32] (▶ Fig. 3.8, ▶ Fig. 3.10, ▶ Fig. 3.11). The MR signal characteristics of some colloid cysts may resemble craniopharyngiomas or hemorrhagic cysts and correlation with CT may be useful in confirming the diagnosis.[21] Although most cysts are homogenous in signal intensity, some may demonstrate a small central area of concentrated hypointensity on FLAIR or T2-weighted images[16,19] (▶ Fig. 3.12, ▶ Fig. 3.13). Interpretation of the FLAIR sequence may pose challenges due to flow artifacts near the foramen of Monro. Small hypointense and isointense cysts may be even missed on MR imaging[3] (▶ Fig. 3.12). Hyperintensity on FLAIR images has been recently associated with an increased risk of obstructive hydrocephalus.[11] FLAIR signal may even evolve over time (▶ Fig. 3.12). Heterogenous signal intensities may pose diagnostic dilemmas by mimicking solid masses, such as gliomas.[32] Cysts usually do not enhance with intravenous administration of gadolinium-based contrast agents, although rim enhancement may be rarely encountered[19,21,27] (▶ Fig. 3.9, ▶ Fig. 3.13).

The causes for the variability in MR signal have been the subject of intense interest. In general, watery fluid tends to display hypointensity on T1-weighted images and hyperintensity on T2-weighted images.[16,32] Some authors have attempted to link the fluid and protein mixture within cysts with viscosity and have suggested that hypointensity on T2-weighted images may imply high protein concentration and potential difficulty with aspiration.[5,24,27,33,34] Others have implied that watery cysts may be inclined to enlarge.[35] Blooming on SWI usually indicates hemorrhage.

Interestingly, fluid collections in other anatomic regions may also demonstrate variable MR signal features prompting Som et al to analyze aspirated, chronically obstructed paranasal sinus secretions using ultraviolet spectrophotometry.[36] Although these data evaluated extracranial mucous collections, the findings may be instructive for colloid cysts. They found that signal intensity on T1-weighted and T2-weighted sequences reflected macromolecular protein concentration, amount of free water, and the specimen viscosity. Iron and methemoglobin did not significantly contribute to signal in their study. Glycoprotein may constitute a major component of the protein. These large, elongated macromolecules

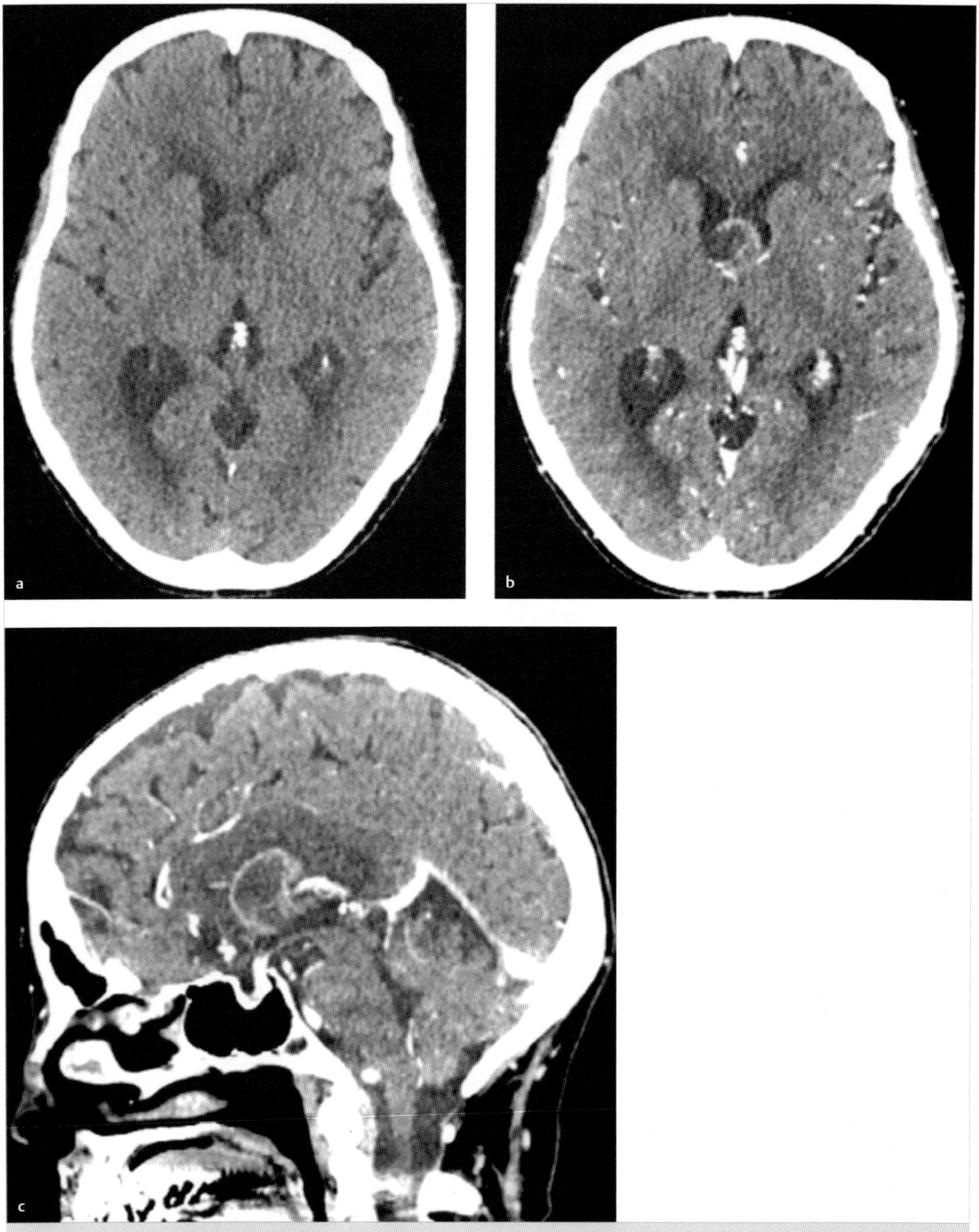


**Fig. 3.5** Glioblastoma. A 72-year-old female with headache. A lesion arising at the foramina of Monro and septum pellucidum displays hypodense cystic and isodense solid components on unenhanced computed tomography (CT) **(a)**. Following administration of intravenous contrast, the solid component enhances mildly; an enhancing rim partially encapsulates the cystic portion of the lesion **(b)**. The rim enhancement is better demonstrated on the sagittal reformatted image **(c)**. Biopsy revealed glioblastoma.

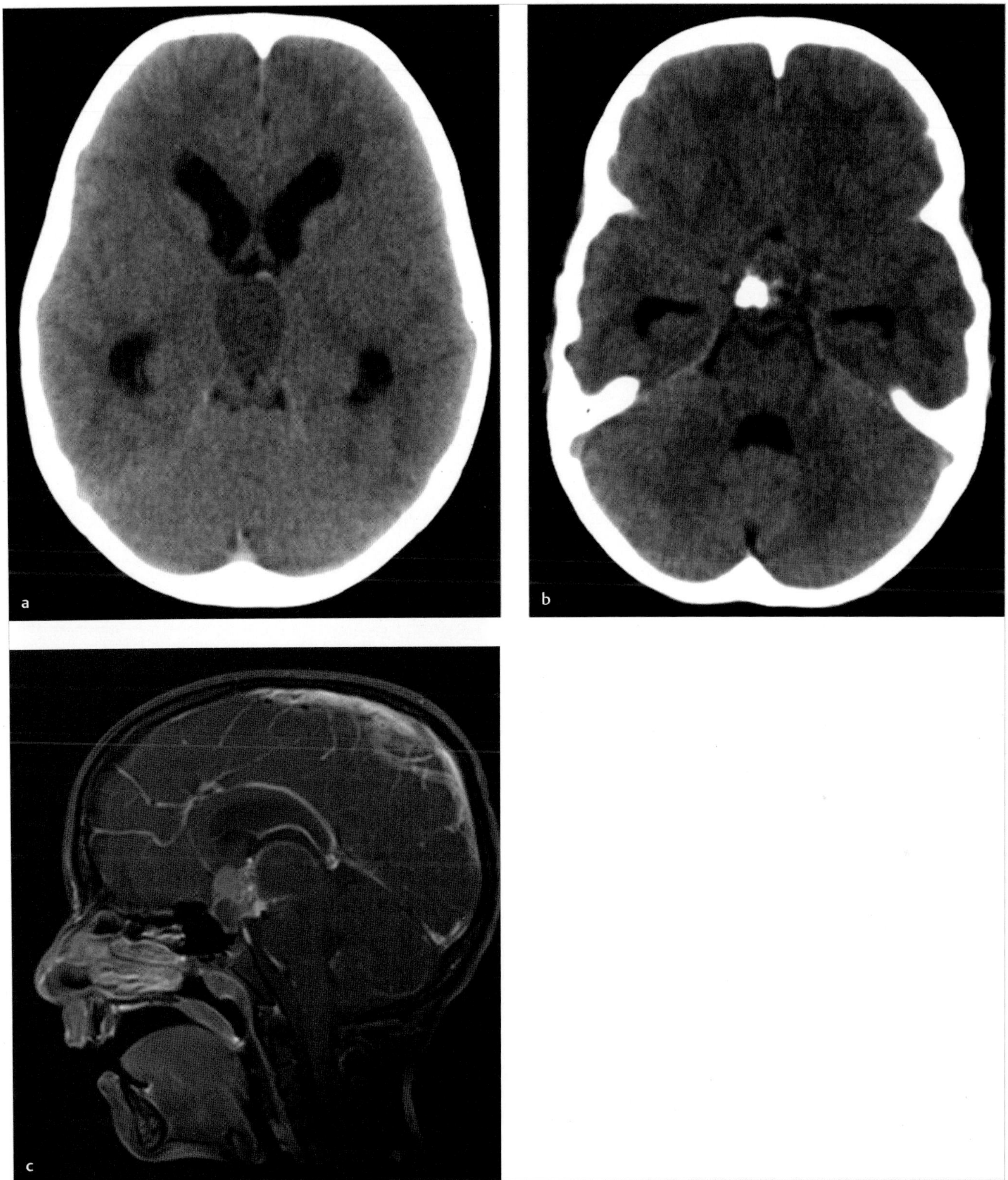

**Fig. 3.6** Craniopharyngioma. A 7-year-old boy with headache. Computed tomography (CT) demonstrating a hypodense cystic mass filling the third ventricle **(a)**. An inferior slice reveals amorphous calcification, which is unusual for a colloid cyst **(b)**. The temporal horns are dilated indicating hydrocephalus. Sagittal, postcontrast, T1-weighted magnetic resonance imaging (MRI) demonstrates a complex cystic and solid mass originating in the suprasellar cistern and extending into the third ventricle **(c)**. The multilocular cysts reveal both hyperintense and hypointense components.

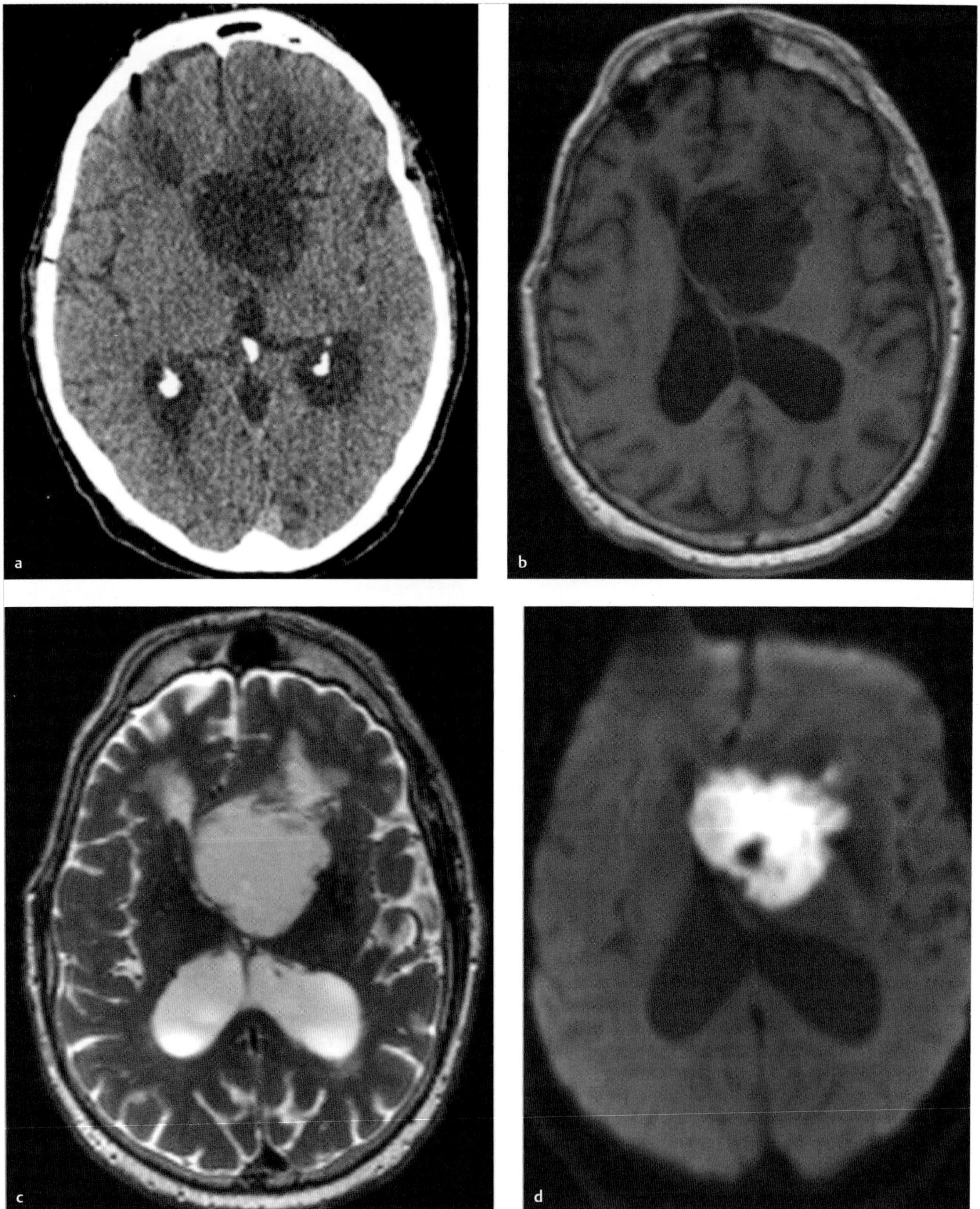

Fig. 3.7 Epidermoid. A 62-year-old man's status post biopsy for a large intracranial mass. Noncontrast computed tomography (CT) reveals a hypodense mass arising in the region of the left foramen of Monro **(a)**. The mass is hypointense on T1-weighted sequences **(b)** and hyperintense on T2 **(c)**. There is transependymal edema adjacent to the frontal horns. The mass displays restricted diffusion on diffusion-weighted imaging (DWI) sequences **(d)**. Compare with colloid cyst in ▶ Fig. 3.9d.

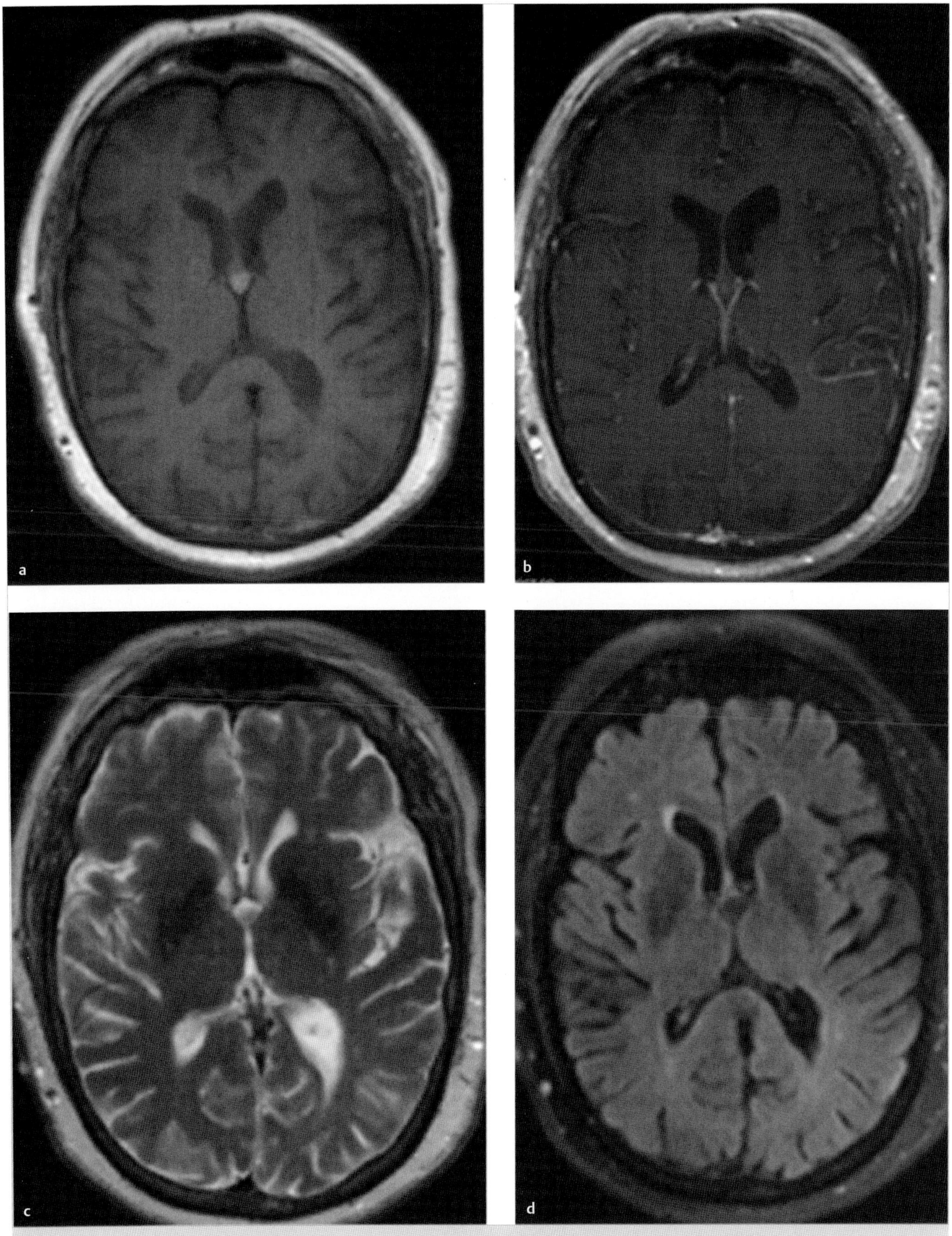


**Fig. 3.8** Magnetic resonance imaging (MRI) of the same patient in ► Fig. 3.1. The cyst is hyperintense on T1-weighted **(a)** and moderately hyperintense on T2-weighted **(b)** sequences. The cyst is hypointense on fluid-attenuated inversion recovery (FLAIR) image **(c)** and there is no enhancement **(d)**.

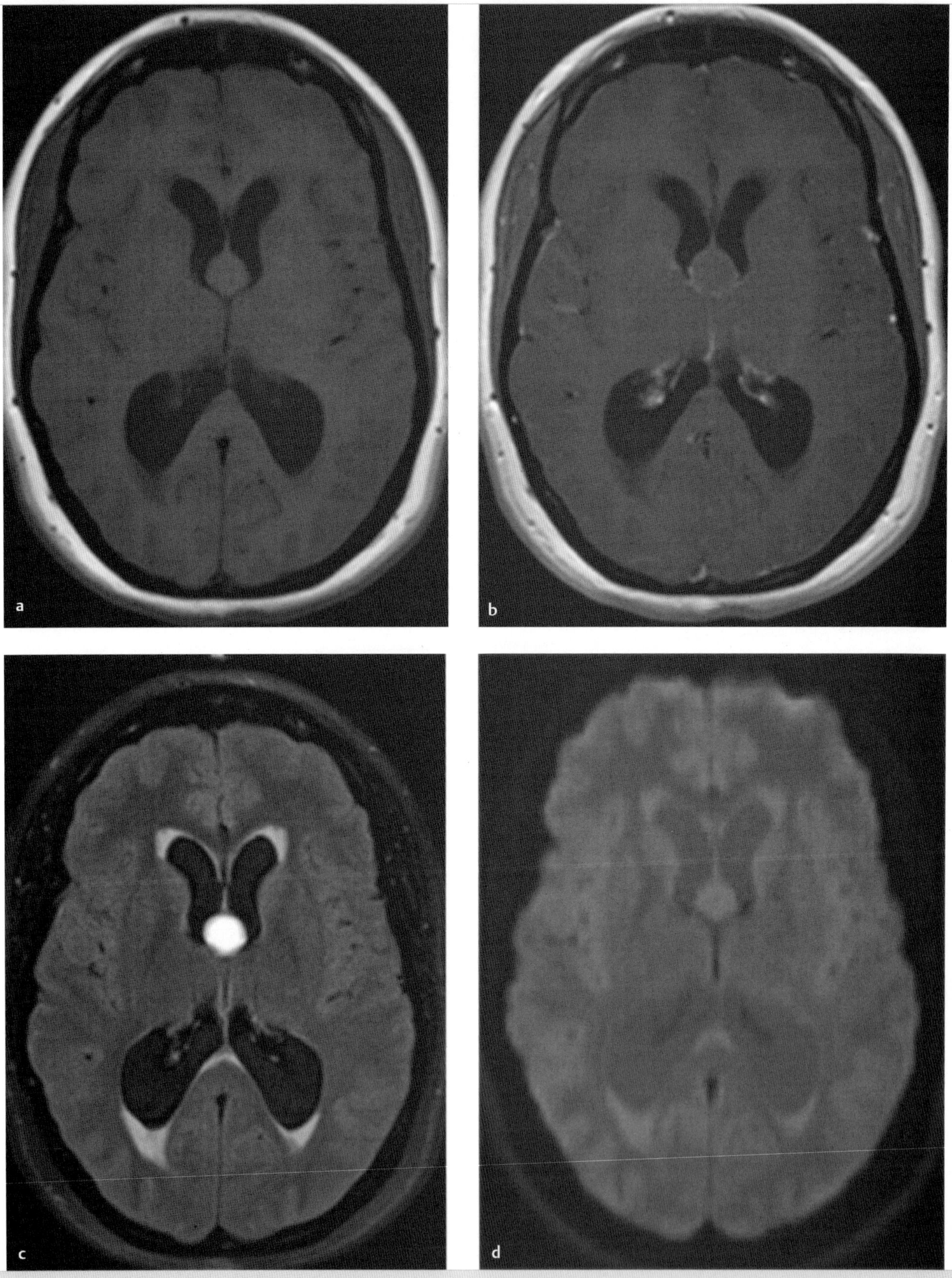


**Fig. 3.9** Magnetic resonance imaging (MRI) of the same patient in ▶ Fig. 3.2. The mass is hypointense to isointense on T1-weighted sequences **(a)** with a faint rim enhancement on postcontrast T1-weighted sequences, in part due to splayed internal cerebral veins **(b)**. There is notable fluid-attenuated inversion recovery (FLAIR) hyperintensity within the lesion along with marked ventriculomegaly and transependymal edema **(c)**. There is no restricted diffusion on diffusion-weighted imaging (DWI) **(d)**.

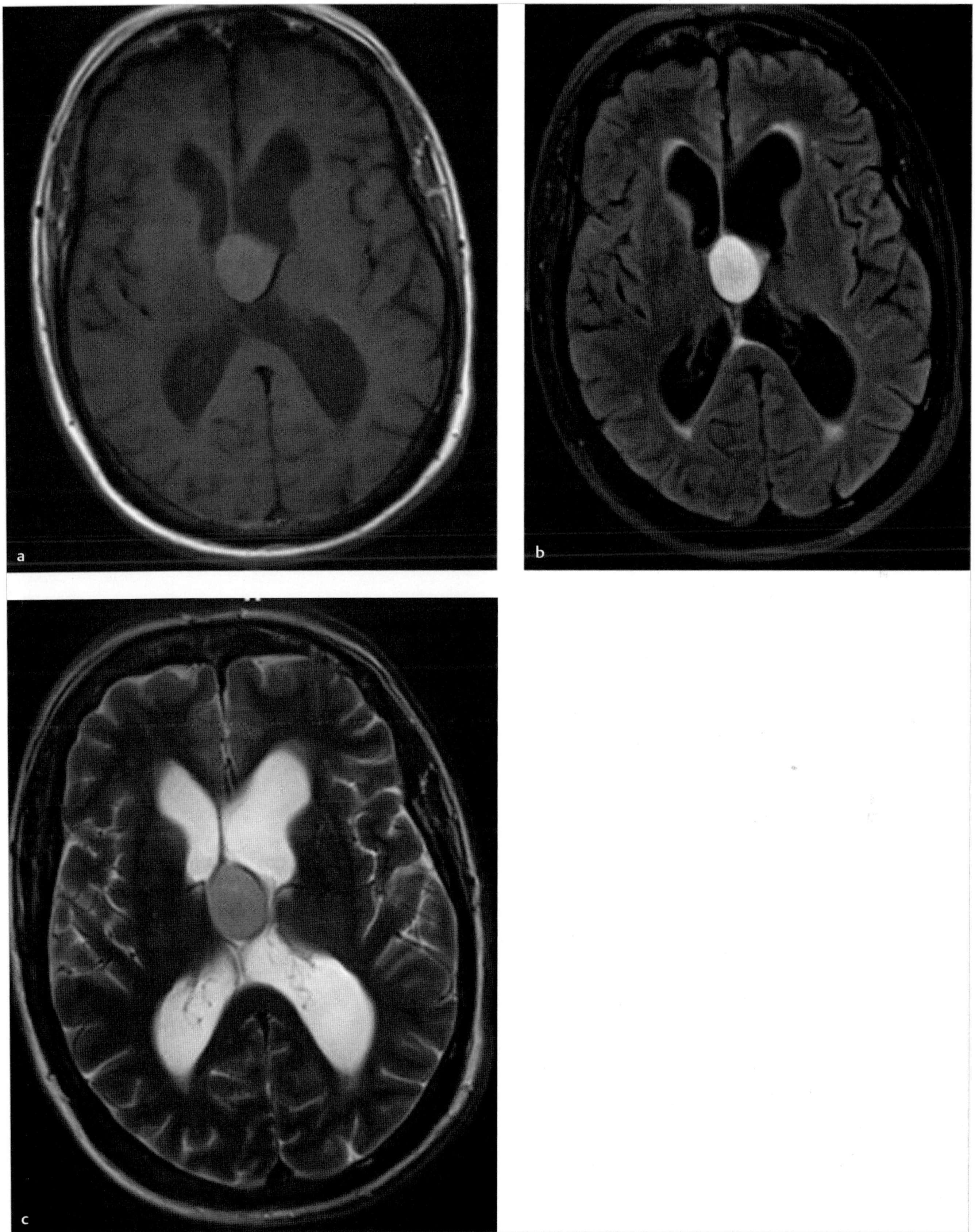

**Fig. 3.10** Colloid cyst. A 52-year-old male with headache and confusion. An anterior third ventricle mass displays hyperintensity on T1-weighted **(a)**, fluid-attenuated inversion recovery (FLAIR) **(b)**, and T2-weighted **(c)** magnetic resonance (MR) images. The lateral ventricles are expanded with hyperintense transependymal edema on FLAIR **(b)** and T2-weighted **(c)** images.

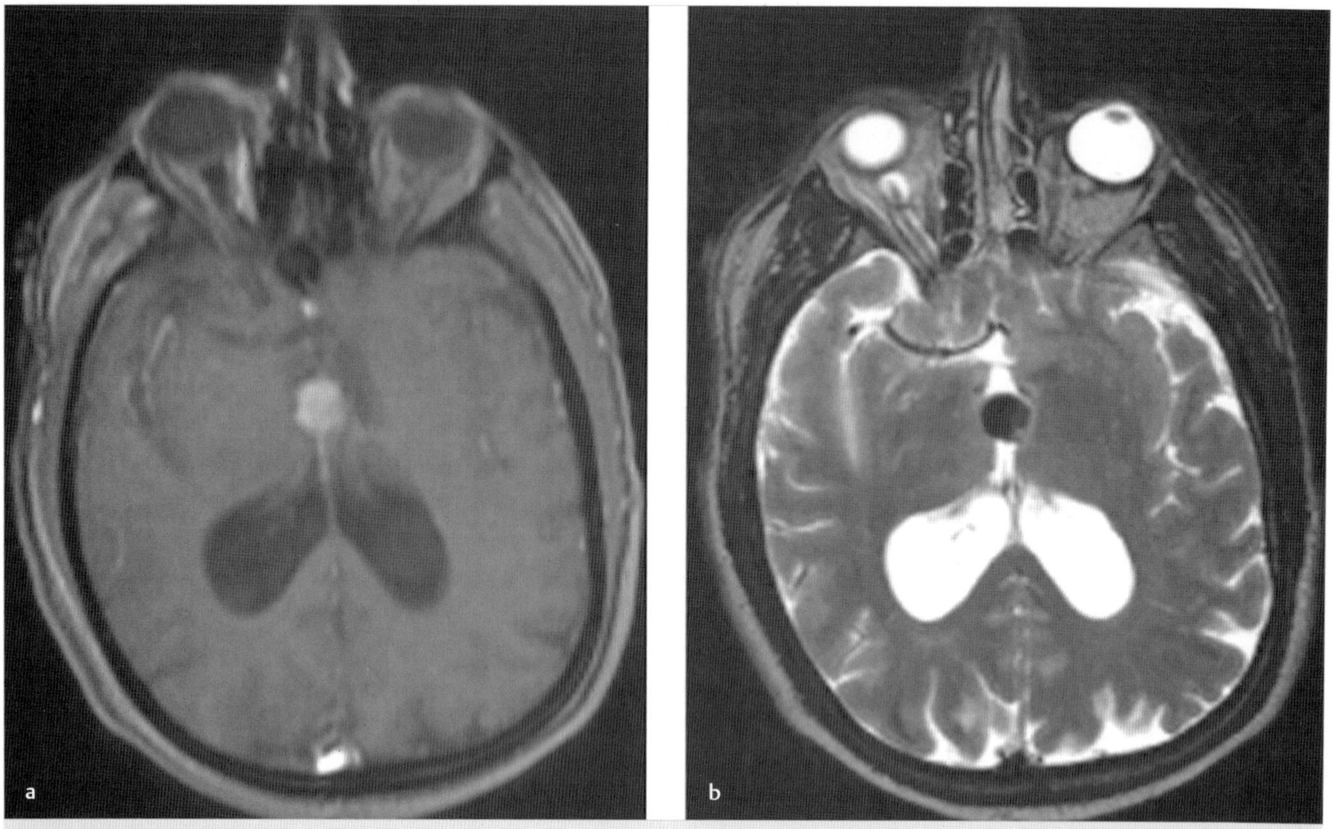


**Fig. 3.11** Colloid cyst. A 60-year-old male with colloid cyst incidentally discovered when he was scanned for recurrent sinusitis. The cyst is hyperintense on T1-weighted **(a)** and hypointense on T2-weighted **(b)** magnetic resonance (MR) images.

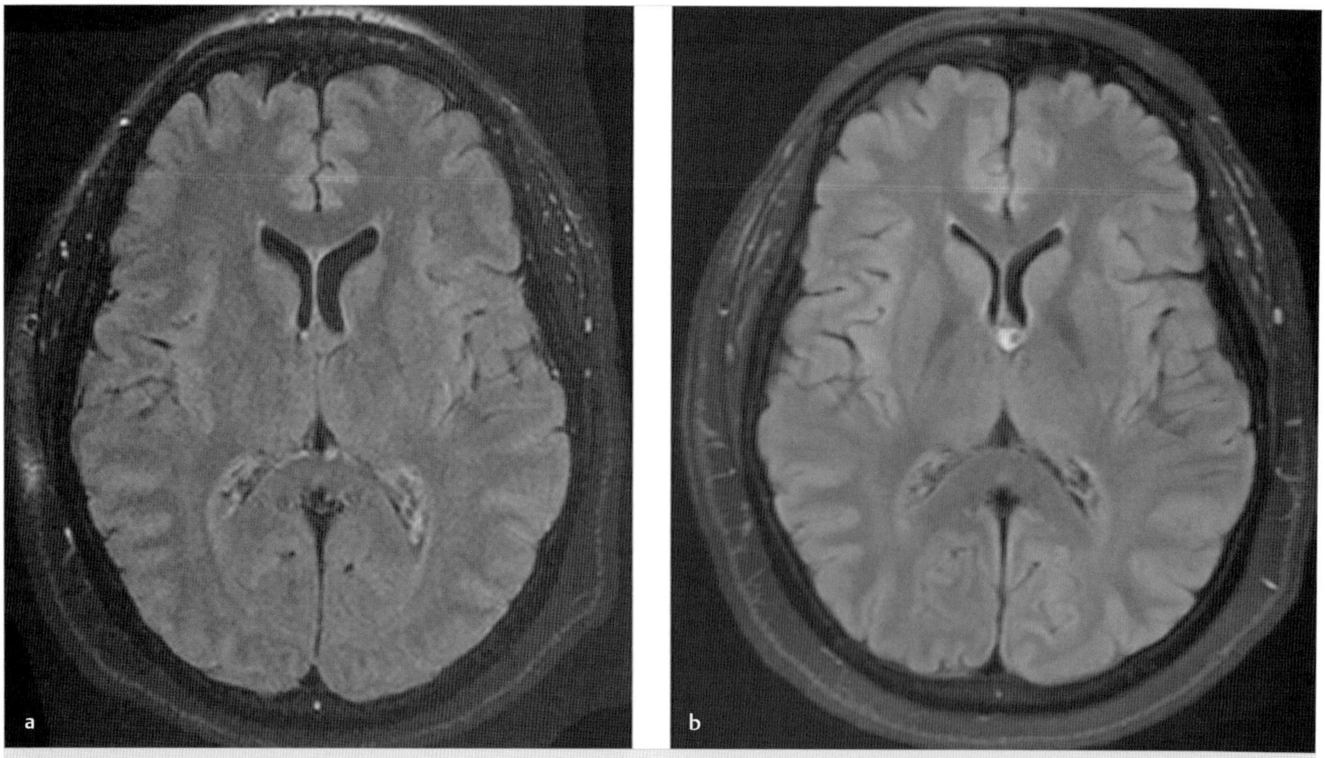


**Fig. 3.12** Colloid cyst. A 51-year-old female with headache. Initial fluid-attenuated inversion recovery (FLAIR) magnetic resonance (MR) image demonstrating a subtle, small, isointensity in the anterior third ventricle **(a)**. The lesion is not easily detected and could be mistaken for the columns of the fornix. After 1 year, the cyst has converted to hyperintensity **(b)**. Note the small hypointensity within the cyst.

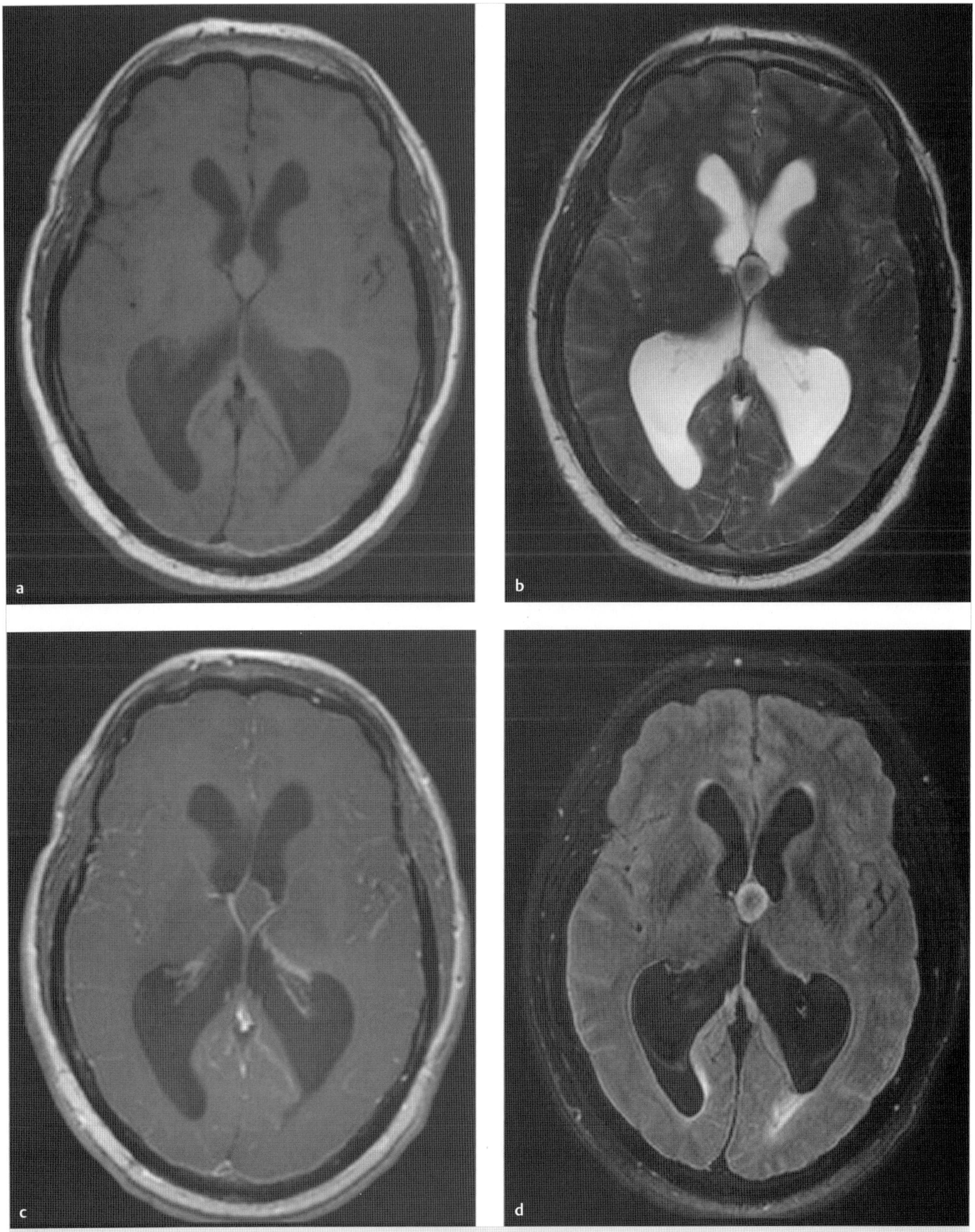


**Fig. 3.13** Colloid cyst. A 49-year-old male with new onset of positional headaches. Magnetic resonance (MR) reveals an anterior third ventricular mass that is isointense on T1-weighted **(a)** and hyperintense on T2-weighted **(b)** and fluid-attenuated inversion recovery (FLAIR) **(c)** images. Note the dilated lateral ventricles, transependymal edema, and the central hypointensity within the cyst on T2-weighted **(b)** and FLAIR **(c)** images. Rim enhancement is due to splayed veins **(d)**.

demonstrated a high affinity to bind free water molecules, and free water slowly resorbed over time as protein concentration and viscosity increased. Secretions with protein concentrations of up to 10% tended to demonstrate hypointensity on T1-weighted images and hyperintensity on T2-weighted sequences with free water as the predominant constituent. As protein concentration increased from approximately 10 to 25%, the signal intensity of the secretions on both T1-weighted and T2-weighted sequences became hyperintense. Signal of the secretions on both T1-weighted and T2-weighted sequences converted to hypointensity when protein secretions exceeded 25%. The signal intensity of the secretions on T1-weighted sequences tended to be more hyperintense than the intensity on T2-weighted sequences until the protein concentration approached 30%, above which the relationship inverted, and the T2-weighted intensity dominated (▶ Fig. 3.14).[36] Other investigators have observed similar relationships between protein concentration, free water, and signal characteristics.[37] Cholesterol esters and old hemorrhage may also contribute to the signal intensity of colloid cysts.[2,16,33,38] A more recent application of MR technique is CSF flow analysis. This is especially useful in evaluating points of obstruction caused by the cyst and in demonstrating patent flow following third ventricular fenestration procedures (▶ Fig. 3.15). Another special application, MR perfusion, has little value in the routine analysis of colloid cysts.

### 3.3.1 Cisternography

Positive contrast cisternography (PCC) entails injecting CT or MR imaging contrast agents intrathecally and subsequently evaluating the patient with cross-sectional imaging. It is largely unnecessary due to the advances in noninvasive MR imaging flow techniques for evaluating CSF dynamics. Moreover, PCC is contraindicated in patients with possible ventricular obstruction because of the danger of acute tonsillar herniation due to CSF pressure gradients. Nevertheless, a small colloid cyst may be rarely discovered by PCC performed for other reasons such as CSF leak studies in CSF hypotensive patients. Because colloid cysts do not communicate with the third ventricle, they do not fill with contrast on PCC and produce a filling defect within the third ventricle.

### 3.3.2 Positron Emission Tomography

Positron emission tomography (PET) uses intravenously injected radioactive positron-emitting metabolite analogs, such as fluorine-18 tagged glucose (FDG), to study the metabolism of tissues, especially neoplasms. PET may be coupled with either CT or MR. Although PET has many uses in cancer staging, it has no role in the routine evaluation of colloid cysts and only rarely in other intraventricular tumors unless metastases are suspected in which case hypermetabolic deposits in other sites of the body suggest the correct diagnosis. Discovery of an FDG-PET avid third ventricular cystic mass should prompt consideration of a neoplasm rather than a benign colloid cyst.

### 3.3.3 Angiography

Catheter angiography (CA) remains the “gold standard” for evaluating cerebral vasculature but has been largely replaced by CT and MR angiography in daily practice. CT angiography uses CT-acquired data to display intracranial and extracranial vessels. The resolution is inferior to catheter angiography and requires intravenous administration of iodinated contrast material but is becoming a preferred modality for vascular screening tool because it is rapid, available, less invasive, and sufficiently detailed for entities such as aneurysms (▶ Fig. 3.4). CA still provides the most detailed and spatially resolved information on vessel anatomy but is invasive and carries higher risk than CT and MR angiography. Therefore, the clinician should carefully balance the desire for information with that of higher risk and determine if noninvasive studies are sufficient in a given clinical setting.

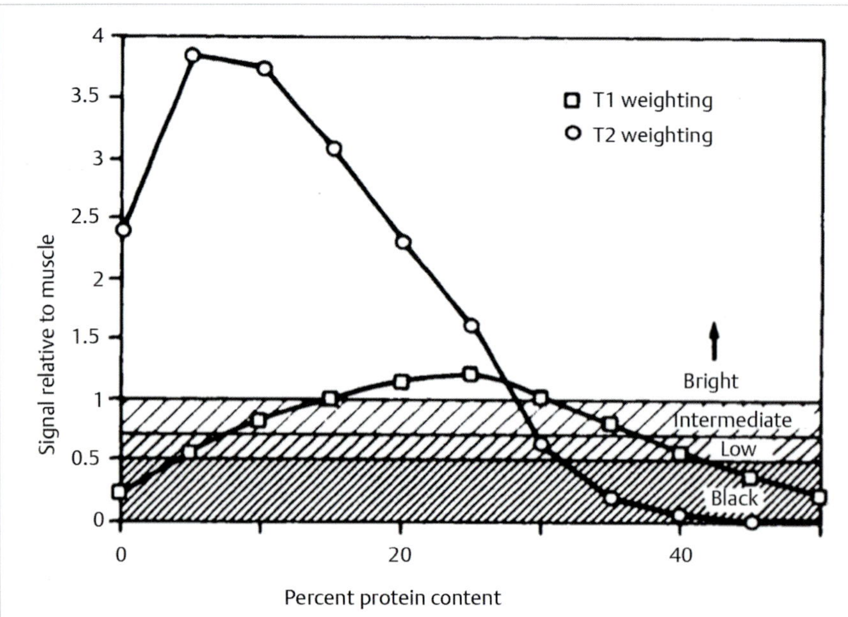


**Fig. 3.14** Graph of signal amplitude (with reference to skeletal muscle) as a function of percentage protein content for T1- and T2-weighted magnetic resonance (MR) sequences in chronically obstructed sinonasal secretions. (Reproduced with permission from Som PM, Dillon WP, Fullerton GD, Zimmerman RA, Rajagopalan B, Marom Z. Chronically obstructed sinonasal secretions: observations on T1 and T2 shortening. Radiology 1989;172:515–520.)

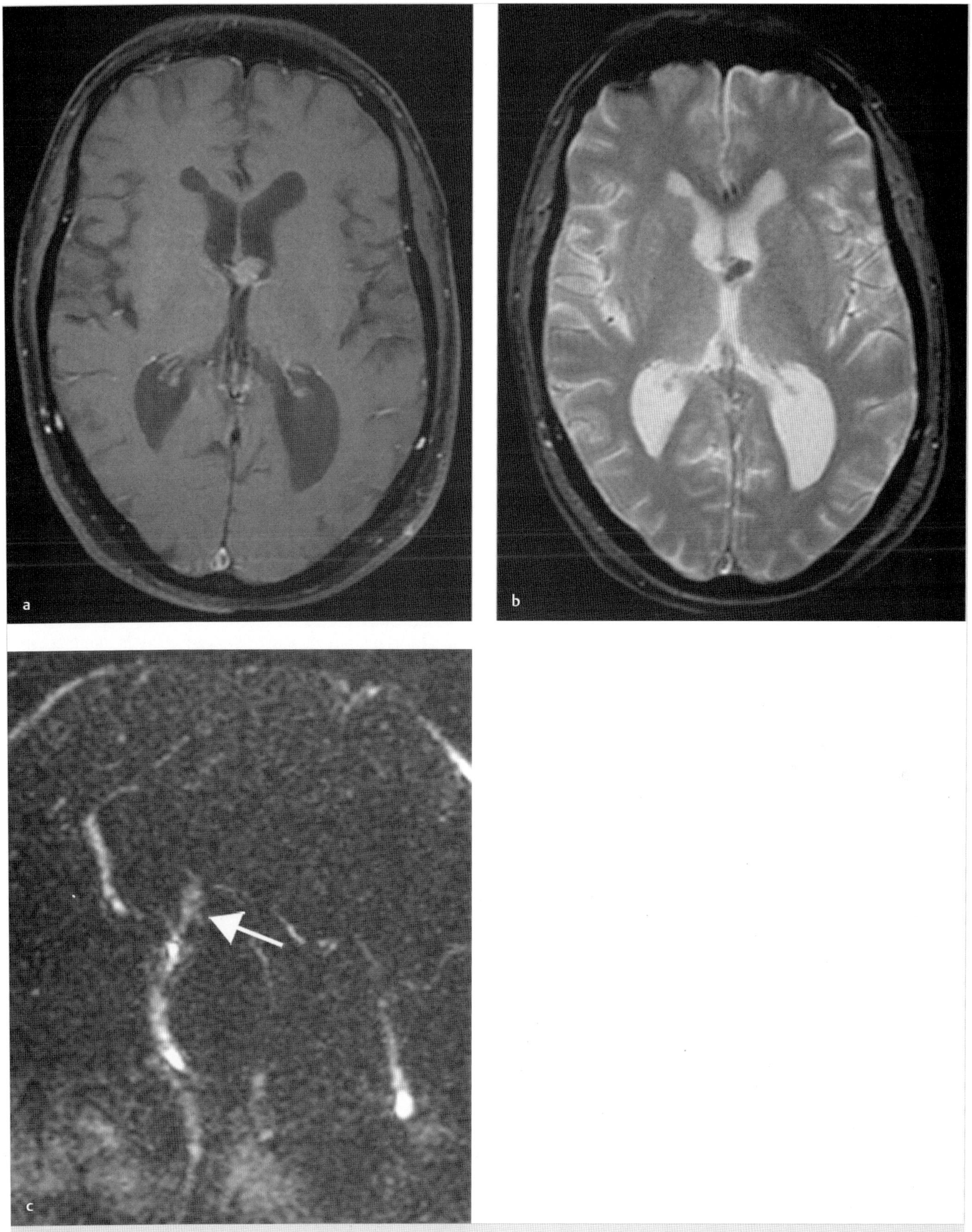


**Fig. 3.15** Colloid cyst. A 77-year-old man with colloid cyst and hydrocephalus treated with third ventricular fenestration. An eccentric anterior third ventricular colloid cyst demonstrating mild hyperintensity on T1-weighted **(a)** and hypointensity on T2-weighted **(b)** magnetic resonance (MR) images. Sagittal cerebrospinal fluid (CSF) flow study reveals flow jet in the floor of the third ventricle (*arrow*) indicating patency with the suprasellar cistern **(c)**; the ventricles have been decompressed.

Although CA provides little primary information for the diagnosis of colloid cysts, it may be useful in excluding alternative diagnoses such as ependymoma or aneurysm, especially when clinical presentation, cross-sectional imaging appearance, or noninvasive vascular studies are atypical or ambiguous. CA may also inform the surgeon about vascular anatomy adjacent to the tumor especially if a percutaneous therapy is an option. The typical anterior third ventricle colloid cyst is located adjacent to the foramen of Monro, which in turn is angiographically located at the junction of the internal cerebral, thalamostriate, and septal veins. This confluence is known as the "venous angle" and can be evaluated on lateral views of the venous phase of internal carotid injections. Colloid cysts are usually avascular and may displace or narrow the venous angle, depending upon the size and location within the third ventricle.[20] Cysts located in the anterior third ventricle focally elevate the anterior portion of the internal cerebral vein in a curvilinear configuration, whereas cysts within the foramen of Monro of the lateral ventricle depress the internal cerebral vein. The angiographic findings are nonspecific and may be produced by any avascular mass within this region.[39]

Of special note, the presence of hydrocephalus and transtentorial and tonsillar herniations should also be carefully evaluated on a cerebral angiogram because ventricular dilation may develop or worsen since the last CT or MR images were performed prior to the catheter study. The lateral ventricles are most commonly involved in hydrocephalus due to the position of the cyst in proximity to the foramina of Monro. Angiographic evidence of hydrocephalus includes elevation of the pericallosal artery, inferior lateral displacement of the lenticulostriate arteries, and lateral bowing of the thalamostriate veins due to lateral ventricle enlargement and steepening of the slope of the middle cerebral arteries due to temporal horn dilatation.[40,41] The tonsillar branches of the posterior inferior cerebellar artery (PICA) are downwardly displaced and the hemispheric branches of PICA are stretched and inferiorly displaced in tonsillar herniation.[42] Angiographic recognition of transtentorial herniation may be more challenging because of the complex and variable relationship of vessels to the tentorium cerebelli. In general, the posterior cerebral artery, posterior communicating artery, anterior choroidal artery, superior cerebellar artery, and the basal vein of Rosenthal may be stretched and inferiorly or medially displaced in downward transtentorial herniation.[43,44,45,46]

## 3.4 Imaging Differential Diagnosis

From a clinical perspective, a colloid cyst should always remain in the differential diagnosis considerations of a patient presenting with a sudden headache, especially if the headache is positional. Although the presence of a colloid cyst is much rarer than a tumor or subarachnoid hemorrhage, imaging is usually able to quickly confirm or eliminate colloid cyst as a diagnostic possibility.

Once imaging is obtained, diagnosis of a colloid cyst within the third ventricle is usually straightforward due to its prevalence and typical appearance. However, challenges may be encountered when the cyst is unusually large, presents in an atypical location, or displays unusual features.[13,47] Differential diagnostic considerations for colloid cysts may be sorted by the age of patient and by imaging appearances (▶ Table 3.1). Because few features of these lesions are pathognomonic when considered in isolation, both patient's age and imaging aspects should be coupled with clinical presentation in formulating the diagnosis (▶ Table 3.2).

Colloid cysts are rarely discovered in children, and a cystic mass in a child should prompt consideration of an alternative diagnosis such as a craniopharyngioma or ependymal cyst. The former is usually complex in appearance and displays enhancement and calcification, whereas the ependymal cyst may pose a more difficult challenge (▶ Fig. 3.6). Examination of the sella and infundibulum may provide clues for entities such as Rathke's cleft cyst.[13,47]

**Table 3.1** Differential diagnoses of anterior third ventricle masses sorted by age

| 0–5 years | 6–30 years | >30 years |
|---|---|---|
| Craniopharyngioma<br>Embryonal tumor<br>Ependymal cyst<br>Langerhans cell histiocytosis | **Colloid cyst**<br>Choroid plexus papilloma<br>Craniopharyngioma<br>Dysembryoplastic neuroepithelial tumor<br>Ganglioglioma<br>Germinoma<br>Ependymal cyst<br>Ependymoma<br>Hamartoma<br>Neurocytoma<br>Oligoastrocytoma<br>Pilocytic astrocytoma<br>Subependymal giant cell astrocytoma<br>*(Rathke's cleft cyst)*<br>*(Neurocysticercosis)* | **Colloid cyst**<br>Aneurysm<br>Chordoid glioma<br>Ependymoma<br>Epidermoid<br>Glioma<br>Granulomatous disease<br>Lymphoma<br>Meningioma<br>Metastasis<br>Subependymal giant cell astrocytoma<br>Subependymoma<br>*(Adenoma)*<br>*(Cavernoma)*<br>*(Rathke's cleft cyst)*<br>*(Neurocysticercosis)* |

Note: Compilation of masses occurring in the anterior third ventricle sorted by age and prevalence and based upon literature review and the Washington University experience. Bold = common; plain text = less common; italics = rare.

Table 3.2 Differential diagnoses of anterior third ventricle masses sorted by MR appearance

| | | T1 | | |
|---|---|---|---|---|
| | | **Hypo** | **Iso** | **Hyper** |
| | **Hypo** | Colloid cyst<br>Aneurysm (flow)*[p]<br>Craniopharyngioma*[c]<br>Dystrophic calcification*<br>Epidermoid[c] | Colloid cyst<br>Craniopharyngioma*[c] | Colloid cyst<br>Adenoma (hemorrhage)<br>Aneurysm (thrombosed)*<br>Craniopharyngioma*[c]<br>Dermoid[c]<br>Epidermoid (rare) [c]<br>Lipoma<br>Rathke's cleft cyst[c] |
| T2 | Iso | Colloid cyst<br>Adenoma<br>Metastasis | Colloid cyst<br>Adenoma<br>Aneurysm (thrombosed)*<br>Granulomatous disease<br>Hamartoma<br>Langerhans cell histiocytosis<br>Meningioma*<br>Metastasis | Colloid cyst<br>Aneurysm (thrombosed)* |
| | **Hyper** | Colloid cyst<br>Adenoma (cystic)[c]<br>Craniopharyngioma*[c]<br>Ependymal cyst[c]<br>Epidermoid[c]<br>Glioma/astrocytoma<br>Rathke's cleft cyst[c] | Colloid cyst<br>Adenoma (cystic)[c]<br>Aneurysm (thrombosed)<br>Craniopharyngioma*[,c]<br>Germinoma<br>Glioma/astrocytoma<br>Hamartoma (rare)<br>Meningioma (rare)* | Colloid cyst<br>Aneurysm (thrombosed)*<br>Craniopharyngioma*[,c]<br>Epidermoid (rare)[c]<br>Rathke's cleft cyst[c] |

Abbreviations: Hyper, hyperintense; Hypo, hypointense; Iso, isointense; MR, magnetic resonance; T1, T1-weighted MR image; T2, T2-weighted image.
Note: Compilation of masses occurring in the anterior third ventricle sorted by MR appearance and based upon literature review and the Washington University experience. *, May calcify; [c], may demonstrate cystic components; [p], phase artifact.

A predominantly solid lesion with cysts found in a child usually poses little difficulty and should prompt consideration for an embryonal tumor. Neoplasms tend to enhance and display irregular borders.

Differential diagnosis considerations for older children and young adults are more extensive and can be divided into predominantly solid lesions with cystic components, such as ganglioglioma, craniopharyngioma, or germinoma, and predominantly cystic lesions with little or no solid components, such as Rathke's cleft cyst and neurocysticercosis. Solid lesions are usually less challenging because of overall appearance and typical enhancement compared with colloid cysts. Most solid tumors, such as gangliogliomas, display avid enhancement and irregular, eccentric cysts (▶ Fig. 3.16). Predominantly cystic lesions may be more challenging; however, cystic mimics of colloid cyst are very rare. Neurocysticercosis is unusual in developed nations; however, it must be considered in immigrant populations arriving from regions with high rates of infection. Intraventricular neurocysticercosis is usually cystic; however, it is often accompanied by calcified extraventricular lesions, which aid in accurate diagnosis[48,49,50] (▶ Fig. 3.17).

Most lesions in the anterior third ventricle in older adults are solid and not easily confused with a colloid cyst. Occasionally, a mixed solid and cystic tumor may mimic a colloid cyst, but usually these lesions enhance (▶ Fig. 3.5). Large aneurysms may project into the ventricle; however, these usually display telltale clues such as blood products, calcifications, and pulsation artifacts. CT angiography or catheter angiography may be necessary to conclusively eliminate or confirm an aneurysm during diagnosis (▶ Fig. 3.4).

Basing the differential diagnoses solely on signal characteristics is difficult because the signal characteristics of colloid cysts are variable. Therefore, some cystic lesions mimicking a colloid cyst may pose challenges. Craniopharyngiomas usually reveal a suprasellar site of origin when the images are carefully inspected (▶ Fig. 3.6). Unlike colloid cysts, epidermoids are usually hyperintense on DWI (▶ Fig. 3.7). Cystic pituitary adenomas extending into the third ventricle often enlarge the sella. Ependymal cysts usually display signal features identical to CSF, which may aid in diagnosis; however, differentiation from a colloid cyst with similar features may be difficult. Fortunately, most of the mimickers are much rarer in prevalence than colloid cysts; nevertheless critical analysis of the imaging should always consider the possibility of such an occurrence.

In summary, the main tools of analysis of colloid cysts of the third ventricle include CT and MR imaging. These modalities complement each other and supplement the clinical examination.

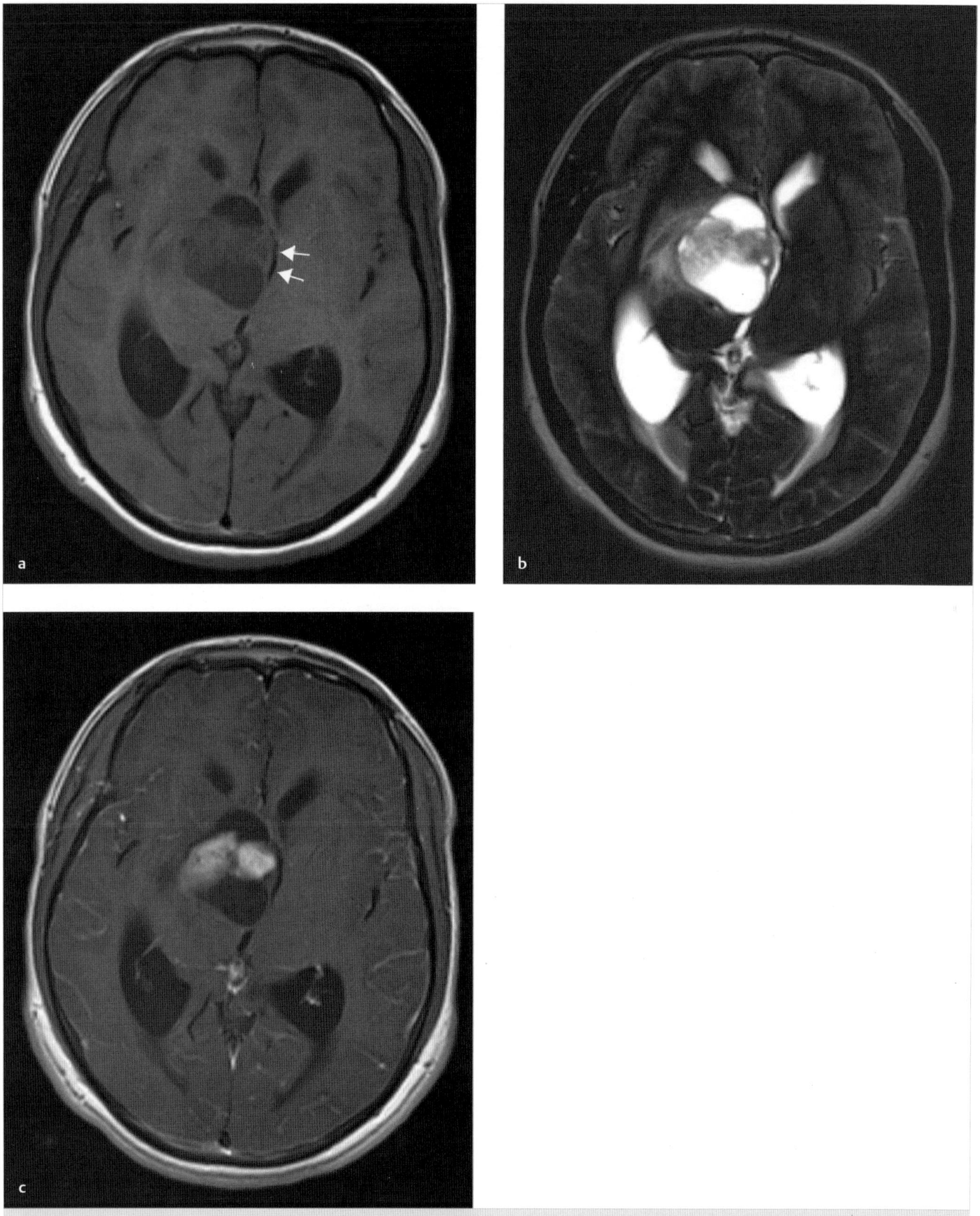


**Fig. 3.16** Ganglioglioma. A 28-year-old male with headache. T1-weighted magnetic resonance (MR) image demonstrating a mixed solid and cystic mass in the region of the third ventricle **(a)**. Closer inspection reveals that the mass is arising from the right basal ganglia and compressing the third ventricle (arrows) causing lateral ventricular enlargement and transependymal edema, best seen adjacent to the occipital horns on the T2-weighted images **(b)**. The solid components of the mass are isointense on the T1-weighted **(a)** and hyperintense on the T2-weighted **(b)** images, and enhance avidly **(c)**. The cystic components are hypointense on the T1-weighted **(a)** and hyperintense on the T2-weighted **(b)** images.

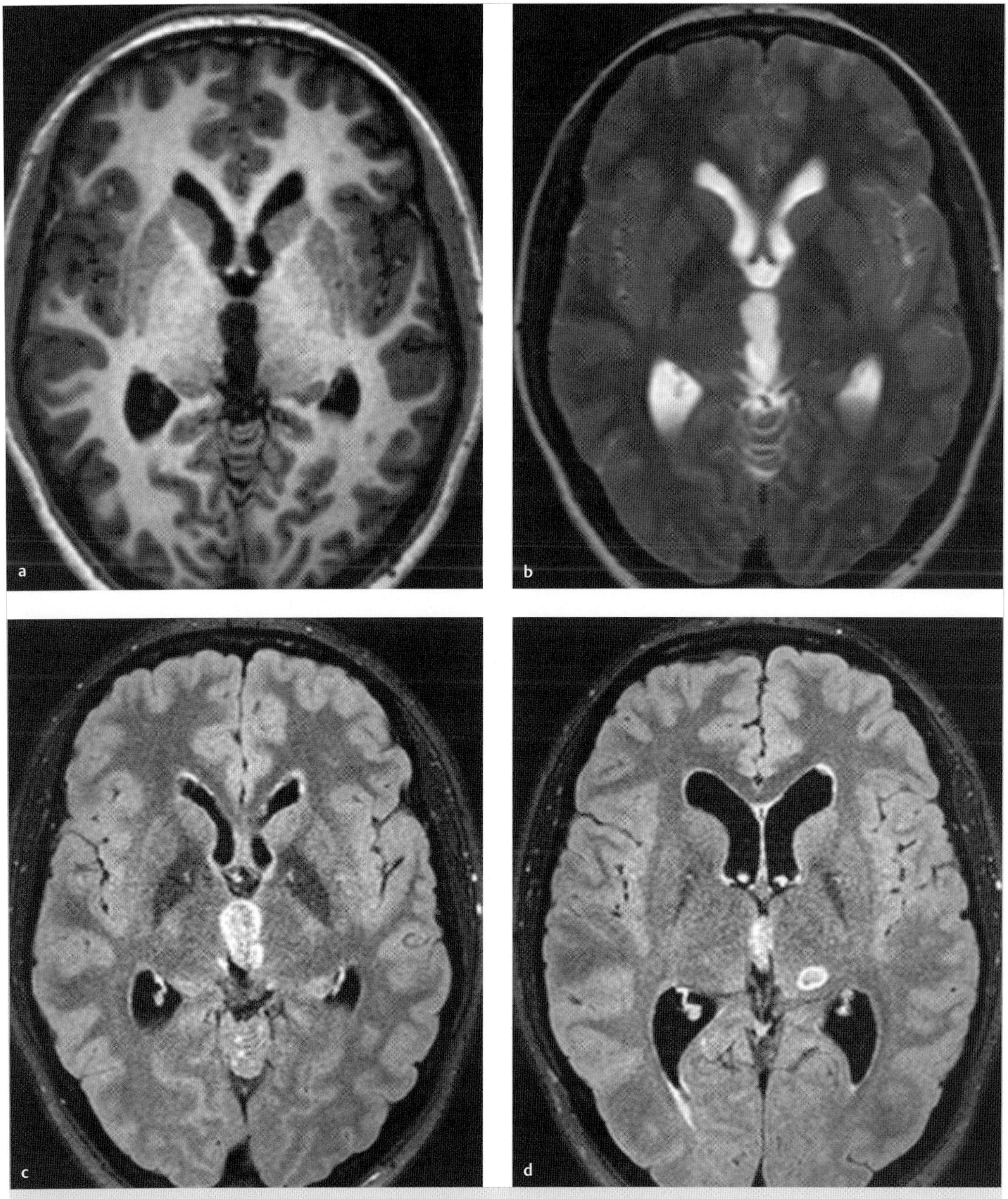


**Fig. 3.17** Neurocysticercosis. A 28-year-old woman with headache, blurry vision, and nausea. Magnetic resonance (MR) scan demonstrating expansion of the third ventricle by a hypointense, cystic lesion on the T1-weighted image **(a)**. The lesion is hyperintense on the T2-weighted image **(b)**. On fluid-attenuated inversion recovery (FLAIR), the lesion is hyperintense **(c)**; an adjacent slice reveals a second hyperintense lesion in the left thalamus **(d)**. FLAIR is extremely useful in detecting intraventricular neurocysticercosis because lesions are often isointense to cerebrospinal fluid (CSF) on T1-weighted and T2-weighted MR images. Careful inspection of the brain parenchyma often reveals extraventricular lesions which suggest the diagnosis.

# References


[1] Mathiesen T, Grane P, Lindgren L, Lindquist C. Third ventricle colloid cysts: a consecutive 12-year series. J Neurosurg. 1997; 86:5–12

[2] Maeder PP, Holtås SL, Basibüyük LN, Salford LG, Tapper UA, Brun A. Colloid cysts of the third ventricle: correlation of MR and CT findings with histology and chemical analysis. AJNR Am J Neuroradiol. 1990; 11(3):575–581

[3] Mortimer AM, Bradley MD, Stoodley NG, Renowden SA. Thunderclap headache: diagnostic considerations and neuroimaging features. Clin Radiol. 2013; 68(3):e101–e113

[4] O'Neill AH, Gragnaniello C, Lai LT. Natural history of incidental colloid cysts of the third ventricle: a systematic review. J Clin Neurosci. 2018; 53:122–126

[5] Horn EM, Feiz-Erfan I, Bristol RE, et al. Treatment options for third ventricular colloid cysts: comparison of open microsurgical versus endoscopic resection. Neurosurgery. 2007; 60(4):613–618, discussion 618–620

[6] Shapiro S, Rodgers R, Shah M, Fulkerson D, Campbell RL. Interhemispheric transcallosal subchoroidal fornix-sparing craniotomy for total resection of colloid cysts of the third ventricle. J Neurosurg. 2009; 110(1):112–115

[7] Batnitzky S, Sarwar M, Leeds NE, Schechter MM, Azar-Kia B. Colloid cysts of the third ventricle. Radiology. 1974; 112(2):327–341

[8] Ganti R. Lesion of the third ventricle. Columbia University College of Physicians and Surgeons Lecture Series 1981; 251–259

[9] Pollock BE, Schreiner SA, Huston J, III. A theory on the natural history of colloid cysts of the third ventricle. Neurosurgery. 2000; 46(5):1077–1081, discussion 1081–1083

[10] Lagman C, Rai K, Chung LK, et al. Fatal colloid cysts: a systematic review. World Neurosurg. 2017; 107:409–415

[11] Beaumont TL, Limbrick DD, Jr, Rich KM, Wippold FJ, II, Dacey RG, Jr. Natural history of colloid cysts of the third ventricle. J Neurosurg. 2016; 125(6): 1420–1430

[12] Jelinek J, Smirniotopoulos JG, Parisi JE, Kanzer M. Lateral ventricular neoplasms of the brain: differential diagnosis based on clinical, CT, and MR findings. AJNR Am J Neuroradiol. 1990; 11(3):567–574

[13] Guduk M, Sun HI, Sav MA, Berkman Z. Pituitary colloid cyst. J Craniofac Surg. 2017; 28(2):e166–e168

[14] Louis DN, Ohgaki H, Wiestler OD, Cavenee WK, eds. WHO Classification of Tumours of the Central Nervous System. 4th ed. Lyon: IARC Press; 2016

[15] Oot RF, New PFJ, Pile-Spellman J, Rosen BR, Shoukimas GM, Davis KR. The detection of intracranial calcifications by MR. AJNR Am J Neuroradiol. 1986; 7 (5):801–809

[16] Waggenspack GA, Guinto FC. MR and CT of masses of the anterosuperior third ventricle. AJNR Am J Neuroradiol. 1989; 10(1):105–110

[17] Itri JN, Patel SH. Heuristics and cognitive error in medical imaging. AJR Am J Roentgenol. 2018; 210(5):1097–1105

[18] Douglas AC, Wippold FJ, II, Broderick DF, et al. ACR Appropriateness Criteria Headache. J Am Coll Radiol. 2014; 11(7):657–667

[19] Kirsch C, Smirniotopoulos J, Olan W, Koeller K. Colloid cysts. International Journal of Neuroradiology. 1997; 6:460–469

[20] Morrison G, Sobel DF, Kelley WM, Norman D. Intraventricular mass lesions. Radiology. 1984; 153(2):435–442

[21] Wilms G, Marchal G, Van Hecke P, et al. Colloid cysts of the third ventricle: MR findings. J Comput Assist Tomogr. 1990; 14(4):527–531

[22] Donaldson JO, Simon RH. Radiodense ions within a third ventricular colloid cyst. Arch Neurol. 1980; 37(4):246

[23] Scotti G, Scialfa G, Colombo N, Landoni L. MR in the diagnosis of colloid cysts of the third ventricle. AJNR Am J Neuroradiol. 1987; 8(2):370–372

[24] El Khoury C, Brugières P, Decq P, et al. Colloid cysts of the third ventricle: are MR imaging patterns predictive of difficulty with percutaneous treatment? AJNR Am J Neuroradiol. 2000; 21(3):489–492

[25] Brooks BS, El Gammal T. Lesions at the foramen of Monro: evaluation by computed tomography, angiography, and pneumoencephalography. South Med J. 1983; 76(12):1515–1523

[26] Glastonbury CM, Osborn AG, Salzman KL. Masses and malformations of the third ventricle: normal anatomic relationships and differential diagnoses. Radiographics. 2011; 31(7):1889–1905

[27] Aygun N, Shah G, Gandhi D. Pearls and Pitfalls in Head and Neck and Neuroimaging. New York: Cambridge University Press; 2013:153–160

[28] Mamourian AC, Cromwell LD, Harbaugh RE. Colloid cyst of the third ventricle: sometimes more conspicuous on CT than MR. AJNR Am J Neuroradiol. 1998; 19(5):875–878

[29] Kaewlai R, Abujudeh H. Nephrogenic systemic fibrosis. AJR Am J Roentgenol. 2012; 199(1):W17–W23

[30] Bond KM, Brinjikji W, Eckel LJ, Kallmes DF, McDonald RJ, Carr CM. Dentate update: imaging features of entities that affect the dentate nucleus. AJNR Am J Neuroradiol. 2017; 38(8):1467–1474

[31] de Castro FD, Reis F, Guerra JG. Intraventricular mass lesions at magnetic resonance imaging: iconographic essay - part 2. Radiol Bras. 2014; 47(4):245–250

[32] Price A, Babigian G. MRI of intraventricular tumours. MRI Decisions. 1991; 5(3): 2–18

[33] Bender B, Honegger JB, Beschorner R, Ernemann U, Horger M. MR imaging findings in colloid cysts of the sellar region: comparison with colloid cysts of the third ventricle and Rathke's cleft cysts. Acad Radiol. 2013; 20(11): 1457–1465

[34] Grondin RT, Hader W, MacRae ME, Hamilton MG. Endoscopic versus microsurgical resection of third ventricle colloid cysts. Can J Neurol Sci. 2007; 34(2): 197–207

[35] Wagner AL. Brain imaging in colloid cyst. Emedicine Medscape. Accessed at: https://emedicine.medscape.com/article/337686-overview. Last updated August 28, 2018

[36] Som PM, Dillon WP, Fullerton GD, Zimmerman RA, Rajagopalan B, Marom Z. Chronically obstructed sinonasal secretions: observations on T1 and T2 shortening. Radiology. 1989; 172(2):515–520

[37] Fullerton GD, Cameron IL, Ord VA. Frequency dependence of magnetic resonance spin-lattice relaxation of protons in biological materials. Radiology. 1984; 151:135–138

[38] Armao D, Castillo M, Chen H, Kwock L. Colloid cyst of the third ventricle: imaging-pathologic correlation. AJNR Am J Neuroradiol. 2000; 21(8): 1470–1477

[39] Rosenbaum AE, Stein RI, Section II. Abnormal supratentorial deep cerebral veins. In: Newton TH, Potts DG, eds. Radiology of the Skull and Brain: Angiography. St. Louis: C.V. Mosby; 1974:1999–2110

[40] Little JR, MacCarty CS. Colloid cysts of the third ventricle. J Neurosurg. 1974; 40(2):230–235

[41] Swischuk LE, Meyer GA, Bryan N. Infantile hydrocephalus and cerebral angiography. Am J Roentgenol Radium Ther Nucl Med. 1972; 115(1):50–61

[42] Margolis MT, Newton TH. An angiographic sign of cerebellar tonsillar herniation. Neuroradiology. 1971; 2(1):3–8

[43] Lindenberg R. Compression of brain arteries as pathogenetic factor for tissue necroses and their areas of prediction. J Neuropath Experimental Neurol. 1955; 14(3):223–243

[44] Azambuja N, Lindgren E, Sjögren SE. Tentorial herniations. III. Angiography. Acta Radiol. 1956; 46(1–2):232–241

[45] Perrett LV, Margolis T. Section II. Angiography. In: Newton TH, Potts DG, eds. Radiology of the Skull and Brain: Angiography. St. Louis: C.V. Mosby; 1974:2671–2699

[46] Rai R, Iwanaga J, Shokouhi G, Oskouian RJ, Tubbs RS. The tentorium cerebelli: a comprehensive review including its anatomy, embryology, and surgical techniques. Cureus. 2018; 10(7):e3079

[47] Niknejad HR, Samii A, Shen SH, Samii M. Huge familial colloid cyst of the third ventricle: an extraordinary presentation. Surg Neurol Int. 2015; 6 Suppl 11: S349–S353

[48] Ginier BL, Poirier VC. MR imaging of intraventricular cysticercosis. AJNR Am J Neuroradiol. 1992; 13(4):1247–1248

[49] Teitelbaum GP, Otto RJ, Lin M, et al. MR imaging of neurocysticercosis. AJR Am J Roentgenol. 1989; 153(4):857–866

[50] Lucato LT, Guedes MS, Sato JR, Bacheschi LA, Machado LR, Leite CC. The role of conventional MR imaging sequences in the evaluation of neurocysticercosis: impact on characterization of the scolex and lesion burden. AJNR Am J Neuroradiol. 2007; 28(8):1501–1504

# Part II

## Natural History, Clinical Decision-Making, and Treatment Overview



II

# 4 Natural History of Colloid Cysts of the Third Ventricle

*Thomas L. Beaumont and Ralph G. Dacey, Jr.*

**Abstract**

Colloid cysts are rare, histologically benign lesions that can cause obstructive hydrocephalus and death. Nearly one-half of patients with symptomatic colloid cysts present with obstructive hydrocephalus which has an associated 3.1% risk of death. Understanding the natural history of colloid cysts has been challenging due to the rarity of the lesion and the relatively small number of cases in most reported series. This has complicated efforts to establish reliable prognostic factors and surgical indications, particularly for asymptomatic patients with incidental lesions. This chapter describes our single-center retrospective review of all cases of colloid cysts of the third ventricle treated over nearly two decades. We identified clinical imaging and anatomic factors associated with symptomatic clinical status and presentation with obstructive hydrocephalus. We then established a simple 5-point risk prediction model referred to as the Colloid Cyst Risk Score (CCRS) that can be used to identify symptomatic lesions and stratify the risk of obstructive hydrocephalus with good predictive capacity.

*Keywords:* colloid cyst, third ventricle, hydrocephalus, natural history

**Table 4.1** Presenting symptoms or indication for neuroimaging of patients with colloid cysts of the third ventricle

| | No. | |
|---|---|---|
| | **Symptomatic** | **Incidental** |
| Headache | 58 (89%) | 24 (25%) |
| Nausea/vomiting | 15 (23%) | 5 (5%) |
| Vision change | 14 (22%) | 2 (2%) |
| Dizziness/ataxia | 13 (20%) | 6 (6%) |
| Cognitive decline | 9 (14%) | 11 (11%) |
| Syncope | 6 (9%) | 5 (5%) |
| Seizure | 4 (6%) | 2 (2%) |
| Bradycardia | 4 (6%) | 0 (0%) |
| Sensory change | 3 (5%) | 1 (1%) |
| Memory decline | 3 (5%) | 0 (0%) |
| Trauma | 1 (2%) | 27 (28%) |
| General medical | 1 (2%) | 12 (12%) |
| General neurological | 0 (0%) | 8 (8%) |
| Stroke | 0 (0%) | 8 (8%) |
| Cancer staging | 0 (0%) | 6 (6%) |

Source: Adapted from Beaumont TL, Limbrick DD Jr, Rich KM, Wippold FJ II, Dacey RG Jr. Natural history of colloid cysts of the third ventricle. J Neurosurg 2016;125(6):1420–1430. An Open Access or Creative Commons publishing model conveys no rights to use this material in any format without written permission from the JNS Publishing Group.

## 4.1 Introduction and Historical Perspective

Colloid cysts of the third ventricle are rare, histologically benign lesions that can cause obstructive hydrocephalus, rapid clinical deterioration, and death. The incidence has been estimated at 3.2 per million per year, accounting for approximately 2% of all intracranial tumors.[1] Defining the natural history of colloid cysts has been challenging due to both the low incidence and the small number of cases in most reported series. Most patients present with symptoms of hydrocephalus including headache, nausea, vomiting, blurred vision, gait ataxia, and cognitive decline (▶ Table 4.1).[2] Approximately 50% of patients with colloid cysts of the third ventricle are symptomatic at the time of diagnosis and ultimately undergo neurosurgical intervention.[2,3,4,5,6] Notably, a small proportion of symptomatic patients present with acute obstructive hydrocephalus and progress to brain death, despite rapid cerebrospinal fluid (CSF) diversion and appropriate supportive care. Historically, this observation has strongly influenced clinical decision-making and resulted in a relatively low threshold for surgery, often in asymptomatic patients. Nonetheless, estimates of the risk of rapid clinical deterioration due to acute hydrocephalus in patients with colloid cysts varied widely, ranging from 3 to 35%, with the associated risk of death ranging from 5 to 38%.[5,7,8,9] Two more recent well-powered studies suggested the rate of acute hydrocephalus to be 0.25% per year or 5% overall with a 3% associated risk of death.[2,10] In addition, although these patients were often described to experience "sudden deterioration and death," studies using modern neuroimaging techniques have demonstrated that nearly all patients with acute obstructive hydrocephalus have progressive symptoms that precede precipitous clinical deterioration. Potential exceptions are the rare instances of acute intralesional hemorrhage and after trauma.[2,4,11]

Incomplete understanding of the natural history of colloid cysts of the third ventricle has impeded efforts to establish evidence-based prognostic factors and objective surgical indications, particularly for asymptomatic patients with incidental lesions. Early studies have focused on patient demographics, presenting symptoms, and cyst diameter in an attempt to identify patients most at risk for rapid deterioration and death. Although no pathognomonic findings were identified, patients with colloid cysts of the third ventricle who experience rapid deterioration and death tended to be younger, to have longstanding symptoms, and to have cysts at least 8 mm in diameter.[3,7,9] As a result, asymptomatic patients with lesions less than 7 mm have historically undergone observation with serial imaging, while those with larger lesions have undergone surgical resection or shunting.[12]

With widespread use of modern neuroimaging, an increasing number of incidental colloid cysts are being identified. Thus, new emphasis was placed on understanding the natural history of asymptomatic lesions and identifying risk factors associated with symptomatic colloid cysts. Two consecutive studies from the Mayo Clinic provided several key insights. Importantly, the 10-year incidence of cyst-related symptoms in asymptomatic patients undergoing follow-up with serial imaging was 8%, with only two patients demonstrating cyst enlargement, one of whom also developed progressive ventriculomegaly and underwent surgical resection of the lesion.[13] Symptomatic patients were significantly younger (44 vs. 57 years) and had more frequent headaches (78 vs. 28%), larger cysts (13 vs. 8 mm), and frequent ventriculomegaly (83 vs. 31%) and hyperintensity on T2-weighted magnetic resonance imaging (MRI) (44 vs. 8%).[6,13] Although several case series have corroborated these findings, risk prediction algorithms for patients with colloid cysts remained undefined until 2016, leaving surgical decision-making primarily to clinician gestalt.[14,15,16]

More recently, the Colloid Cyst Risk Score (CCRS) was developed based on a large retrospective cohort of patients with colloid cysts managed at a large tertiary care hospital over 2 decades.[2] Consistent with the abovementioned case series, the most common presenting complaints included sequelae of hydrocephalus such as headache, nausea/vomiting, blurred vison or diplopia, dizziness, ataxic gait, cognitive decline, and syncope (▶ Table 4.1).[5,6,8,13,17] Interestingly, all symptomatic patients with hydrocephalus had colloid cysts with axial diameter ≥ 7 mm (▶ Fig. 4.1). Also consistent with prior published data, hydrocephalus was common, occurring in 46.2% of symptomatic patients, eight of whom (12.3%) presented with acute symptoms. Specific emphasis was placed on natural history, presenting symptoms, neuroimaging findings, and morphological characteristics that could be used as potential prognostic factors to identify symptomatic colloid cysts and better understand the risk of obstructive hydrocephalus.

## 4.2 The Colloid Cyst Risk Score

The CCRS was developed based on a retrospective cohort of 163 patients with colloid cyst of the third ventricle diagnosed in the setting of symptomatic presentation ($n = 65$, 40%) or identified incidentally ($n = 98$, 60%).[2] Patients with colloid cysts remained in the incidental group if their symptoms were attributable to an alternative cause and no ventriculomegaly was identified on neuroimaging. Univariate analysis of symptomatic versus incidental cases evaluated variables including age at presentation, presence of headache, cyst diameter and volume, as well as signal intensity on several MRI sequences. The symptomatic group was further subdivided based on the presence of hydrocephalus ($n = 30$, 46.2%) and acute hydrocephalus ($n = 8$, 12.3%), with the latter defined as hydrocephalus with symptom onset or acute progression from baseline within 24 hours of presentation.[8] Additionally third ventricle risk zones were defined, as not all cyst locations within the third ventricle were similarly associated with the risk of hydrocephalus (▶ Fig. 4.2).

### 4.2.1 Incidental Patients

A total of 57 patients (58%) with incidental colloid cysts underwent serial neuroimaging with mean follow-up of 5.1 years (range 0.5–23 years); 10 patients were followed for at least 10 years. Over the study period, five patients (8.8%) followed with serial neuroimaging experienced progression and underwent surgical resection. Importantly, no patient with an incidentally discovered, asymptomatic colloid cyst experienced acute obstructive hydrocephalus or sudden neurological deterioration in the absence of antecedent trauma. Two patients (3.5%) demonstrated cyst regression, both with greater than 30% decrease in diameter of their lesions. A third patient was assaulted and underwent imaging that demonstrated an 8-mm colloid cyst with ventriculomegaly. Although the patient had no complaints

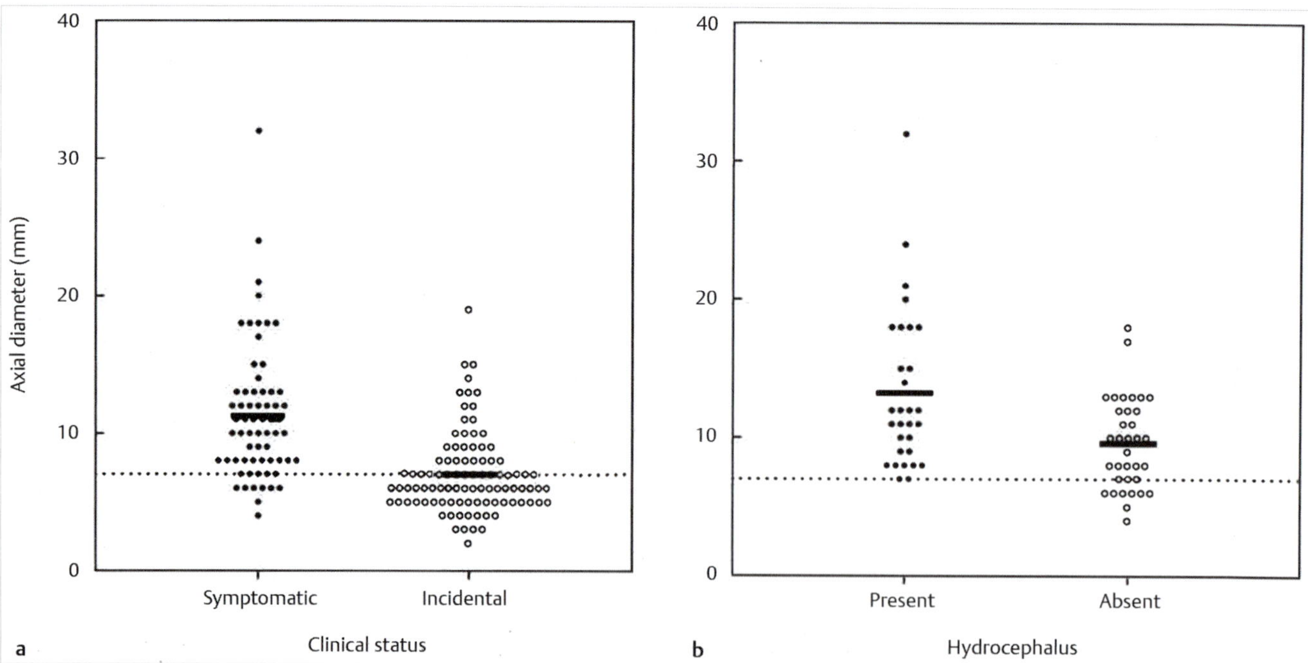


**Fig. 4.1** Scatter plots of colloid cyst axial diameters. **(a)** Patients with symptomatic colloid cysts demonstrated a wide range of axial diameter, while the majority of those with incidental cysts (86.7%) had diameter ≤ 7 mm (*dashed line*). The mean axial diameter was significantly different between the two groups (11.3 ± 5.0 mm and 7.0 ± 3.0 mm, respectively, $p < 0.0001$, *solid bars*). **(b)** Symptomatic patients with hydrocephalus had colloid cysts with axial diameter ≥ 7 mm (*dashed line*). These lesions had significantly larger mean axial diameter compared to the group of symptomatic patients without hydrocephalus (13.2 ± 5.8 mm and 9.6 ± 3.4 mm, respectively, $p < 0.004$, *solid bars*). (Reproduced with permission from Beaumont TL, Limbrick DD Jr, Rich KM, Wippold FJ II, Dacey RG Jr. Natural history of colloid cysts of the third ventricle. J Neurosurg 2016;125(6):1420–1430. An Open Access or Creative Commons publishing model conveys no rights to use this material in any format without written permission from the JNS Publishing Group.)

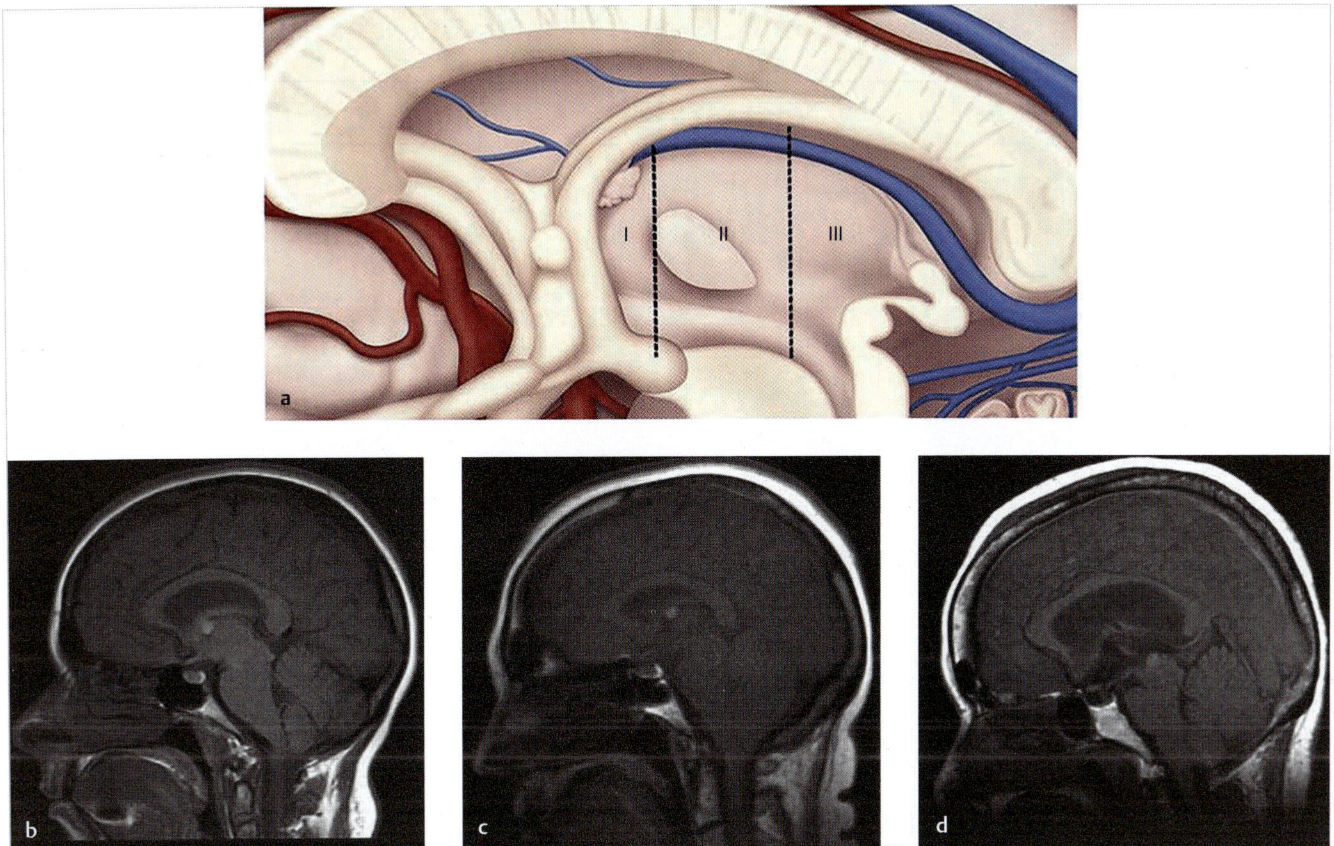


**Fig. 4.2** Anatomic risk zones for colloid cysts of the third ventricle. **(a)** The third ventricle was divided into three zones along the sagittal axis. Zone I—from lamina terminalis to a vertical line drawn from the mammillary body and tangential to the massa intermedia; Zone II—from the posterior boundary of Zone I to the rostral apex of the midbrain tegmentum at the inlet of the cerebral aqueduct; Zone III—from the posterior boundary of Zone II to the posterior limit of the third ventricle. The term "*Risk Zone*" refers to Zones I and III collectively. **(b–d)** Sagittal noncontrast T1-weighted magnetic resonance imaging (MRI) demonstrating Zone I, II, and III lesions, respectively. (Reproduced with permission from Beaumont TL, Limbrick DD Jr, Rich KM, Wippold FJ II, Dacey RG Jr. Natural history of colloid cysts of the third ventricle. J Neurosurg 2016;125(6):1420–1430. An Open Access or Creative Commons publishing model conveys no rights to use this material in any format without written permission from the JNS Publishing Group.)

and was previously asymptomatic, he demonstrated marked sinus bradycardia while supine. Cardiac evaluation revealed no underlying cause, and the patient therefore underwent surgical resection. Notably, the patient's bradycardia fully resolved following surgery.

## 4.2.2 Symptomatic Patients

Nearly all patients with symptomatic colloid cysts underwent surgical resection ($n = 59$, 91%). Several observed demographic, morphologic, and neuroimaging features were significantly different when patients with symptomatic colloid cysts were compared with patients with incidental cysts. These included: age at presentation (37.9 vs. 54.2 years), the proportion of patients with age < 65 years (96.9 vs. 70.4%, relative risk [RR] 7.4), headache on presentation (92.3 vs. 21.9%, RR 11.9), cyst diameter (11.3 vs. 7.0 mm), proportion of patients with cyst diameter ≥ 7 mm (87.7 vs. 45.8%, RR 4.2), cyst volume (1718.7 vs. 365.5 mm$^3$), proportion of patients with cyst volume ≥ 180 mm$^3$ (90.9 vs. 50.9%, RR 4.0), and cyst hyperintensity on fluid-attenuated inversion recovery (FLAIR) MRI sequences (76.9 vs. 38.3%, RR 2.6) (▶ Table 4.2). These results are consistent with the abovementioned Mayo Clinic studies by Pollock et al, with the exception that cyst hyperintensity on T2-weighed MRI did not achieve statistical significance in the CCRS study (50.0 vs. 34.5%, $p = 0.080$).[13] Interestingly, the proportion of symptomatic patients with cyst hyperintensity on FLAIR MRI sequences was highly significant when compared to incidental patients (▶ Fig. 4.3).

**Table 4.2** Factors associated with symptomatic colloid cysts

| | Relative risk |
|---|---|
| Headache | 11.9 |
| Age < 65 years | 7.4 |
| Cyst diameter ≥ 7 mm | 4.2 |
| Cyst volume > 180 mm$^3$ | 4.0 |
| Hyperintensity on FLAIR | 2.6 |
| Hyperintensity on T2 | 2.3 |
| Location in the third ventricle | - |

Abbreviation: FLAIR, fluid-attenuated inversion recovery.
Source: Adapted from Beaumont TL, Limbrick DD Jr, Rich KM, Wippold FJ II, Dacey RG Jr. Natural history of colloid cysts of the third ventricle. J Neurosurg 2016;125(6):1420–1430. An Open Access or Creative Commons publishing model conveys no rights to use this material in any format without written permission from the JNS Publishing Group.

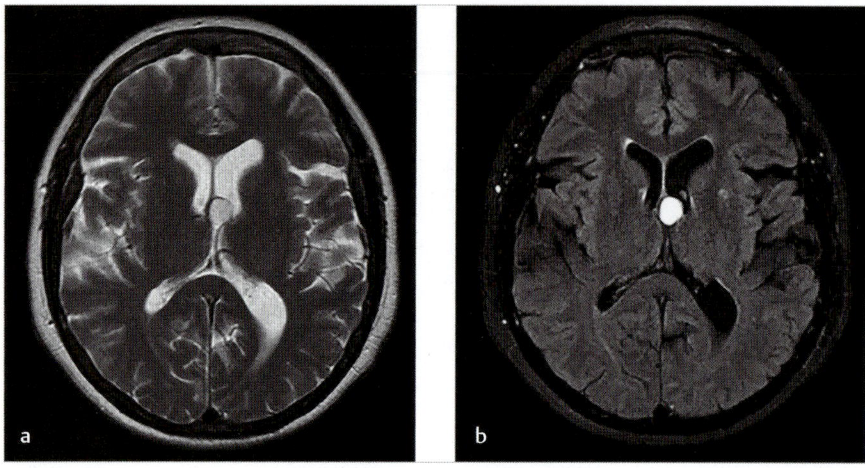


**Fig. 4.3** Neuroimaging of a symptomatic colloid cyst. **(a)** Axial T2-weighted magnetic resonance imaging (MRI) demonstrating cyst hyperintensity and mild asymmetric ventriculomegaly involving the left lateral ventricle. **(b)** Axial fluid-attenuated inversion recovery (FLAIR) MRI demonstrating marked cyst hyperintensity. (Reproduced with permission from Beaumont TL, Limbrick DD Jr, Rich KM, Wippold FJ II, Dacey RG Jr. Natural history of colloid cysts of the third ventricle. J Neurosurg 2016;125(6):1420–1430. An Open Access or Creative Commons publishing model conveys no rights to use this material in any format without written permission from the JNS Publishing Group.)

## 4.2.3 Risk Factors for Hydrocephalus

Several statistically significant factors were identified when the subset of symptomatic patients with and without hydrocephalus were compared. These included mean cyst diameter (13.2 vs. 9.6 mm), proportion of patients with cyst diameter ≥ 7 mm (100 vs. 77.1%, RR 4.7), the proportion of patients with cyst volume ≥ 180 mm$^3$ (100 vs. 82.8%, RR 3.1), Evans ratio (0.36 vs. 0.27), cyst hyperintensity on T2-weighted (70.0 vs. 36.7%, RR 2.3), and FLAIR MRI (94.4 vs. 61.9%, RR 5.1). In all but one patient with hydrocephalus, the colloid cyst was located in Zone I, the classic location within the foramen of Monro at the anterior aspect of the third ventricle. Importantly, in the Washington University CCRS study, no patient with a Zone II lesion presented with hydrocephalus or progressive symptoms.

## 4.2.4 Acute Hydrocephalus and Death

Eight patients in the Washington University CCRS study presented with acute hydrocephalus defined as acute progression of baseline symptoms or onset of new, rapidly progressive symptoms of hydrocephalus within 24 hours of presentation. These patients represented 12.3% of symptomatic patients and 4.9% of all patients in the study. There was no significant difference in age, cyst diameter, or cyst volume between symptomatic patients with and without acute hydrocephalus. Importantly, 50% of the patients presenting with acute hydrocephalus experienced the onset of new, progressive symptoms over 3 to 4 days prior to acute neurological deterioration. Two additional cases of acute hydrocephalus described in the study are noteworthy. The first was a teenage male who experienced a concussion with 2 to 3 minutes loss of consciousness while playing organized football. Neuroimaging demonstrated an 18-mm colloid cyst without ventriculomegaly. Over the subsequent 12 hours, the patient experienced severe, rapidly progressive headache and developed new ventriculomegaly on repeat neuroimaging. In the second case, a patient with a known asymptomatic colloid cyst of the third ventricle complained of slowly progressive gait instability after a fall from standing 1 week prior, with progressive cognitive decline over 24 hours prior to presentation. Neuroimaging demonstrated a hyperdense lesion obstructing the cerebral aqueduct and an absence of the previously identified colloid cyst at the foramen of Monro. These findings were best explained by translocation of the cyst from the foramen magnum to the dependent portion of the posterior third ventricle.[18,19] Taken together, these two cases suggest traumatic translocation as a rare, but possible, mechanism of acute obstructive hydrocephalus in patients with colloid cysts of the third ventricle. Considering all cases together, the CCRS study suggests the risk of death in symptomatic patients with a colloid cyst of the third ventricle is 3.1%.

## 4.2.5 Clinical Decision-Making and the CCRS

The most significant risk factors for symptomatic colloid cysts identified on univariate testing were age at presentation, presence of headache, cyst diameter ≥ 7 mm, cyst hyperintensity on FLAIR MRI, and cyst location in an anatomic Risk Zone. These variables were subsequently combined and assessed for their predictive capacity using logistic regression. The authors elected to use axial cyst diameter instead of cyst volume, as both had similar strong statistical association with symptomatic lesions and the former does not require orthogonal imaging and volume computation. The model demonstrated significant predictive capacity, achieving sensitivity and specificity of 92 and 93%, respectively, for symptomatic clinical status, and 88 and 82% for the subset of symptomatic patients presenting with obstructive hydrocephalus. These risk factors were therefore combined into the simple five-point risk score referred to as the CCRS (▸ Table 4.3). Further analysis of the CCRS with receiver-operator characteristics (ROC) confirmed significant predictive capacity with area under the curve of 0.917 for symptomatic patients and 0.845 for patients presenting with hydrocephalus. The CCRS provided statistically significant stratification of symptomatic patients across the five CCRS levels (▸ Table 4.4). Importantly, all patients presenting with hydrocephalus had CCRS ≥ 4 which demonstrated strong statistical association with hydrocephalus ($p < 0.0001$, RR 19.4). In addition, only incidental patients with CCRS ≥ 3, based on initial imaging, experienced progression over the study period. Taken together, these data suggest that patients with CCRS ≥ 4 represent the "high-risk" subgroup, while CCRS of ≤ 2 represents the "low-risk" subgroup.

Table 4.3 Colloid Cyst Risk Score

| Criterion | Points |
|---|---|
| **Age < 65 years** | |
| Yes | 1 |
| No | 0 |
| **Headache** | |
| Yes | 1 |
| No | 0 |
| **Axial diameter ≥ 7 mm** | |
| Yes | 1 |
| No | 0 |
| **FLAIR hyperintensity** | |
| Yes | 1 |
| No | 0 |
| **Risk Zone** | |
| Yes | 1 |
| No | 0 |

Abbreviation: FLAIR, fluid-attenuated inversion recovery.

Table 4.4 Patient stratification based on CCRS

| | No. | |
|---|---|---|
| CCRS | Symptomatic | Hydrocephalus |
| 0 | 0 | 0 |
| 1 | 0 | 0 |
| 2 | 1 (6%) | 0 |
| 3 | 4 (22%) | 0 |
| 4 | 10 (67%) | 3 (20%) |
| 5 | 24 (96%) | 15 (60%) |

Abbreviation: CCRS, Colloid Cyst Risk Score.

CCRS 3 is considered "intermediate risk," as three of five incidental patients that demonstrated progression on surveillance neuroimaging were CCRS 3 on initial presentation, but progressed to CCRS 5 within 5 years.

In 2020, the CCRS subsequently underwent external validation and demonstrated good intra- and inter-rater reliability as well as comparable predictive capacity.[20,21] Using an independent cohort of 156 patients with colloid cysts of the third ventricle, the CCRS demonstrated area under the curve of 0.914 and 0.892 for symptomatic status and obstructive hydrocephalus, respectively.

## 4.3 Conclusion

Colloid cysts of the third ventricle may undergo expansion with symptom progression or, less commonly, may undergo regression. Patients with incidentally discovered asymptomatic colloid cyst do not experience acute obstructive hydrocephalus or sudden neurological deterioration in the absence of antecedent trauma. Hydrocephalus occurs in nearly one-half of patients with symptomatic colloid cysts, where there is an overall 3.1% risk of death. Several risk factors for symptomatic lesions were identified, including age < 65 years, presence of headache on presentation, cyst diameter ≥ 7 mm on axial imaging, hyperintensity on FLAIR MRI, and location of the colloid cyst within third ventricle Risk Zone. The CCRS can be used to identify symptomatic lesions and stratify the risk of obstructive hydrocephalus during clinical decision-making. Surgical intervention should be considered for all patients with CCRS ≥ 4, as they represent the "high-risk" subgroup.

## References

[1] Hernesniemi J, Leivo S. Management outcome in third ventricular colloid cysts in a defined population: a series of 40 patients treated mainly by transcallosal microsurgery. Surg Neurol. 1996; 45(1):2–14

[2] Beaumont TL, Limbrick DD, Jr, Rich KM, Wippold FJ, II, Dacey RG, Jr. Natural history of colloid cysts of the third ventricle. J Neurosurg. 2016; 125(6):1420–1430

[3] Camacho A, Abernathey CD, Kelly PJ, Laws ER, Jr. Colloid cysts: experience with the management of 84 cases since the introduction of computed tomography. Neurosurgery. 1989; 24(5):693–700

[4] Jeffree RL, Besser M. Colloid cyst of the third ventricle: a clinical review of 39 cases. J Clin Neurosci. 2001; 8(4):328–331

[5] Mathiesen T, Grane P, Lindgren L, Lindquist C. Third ventricle colloid cysts: a consecutive 12-year series. J Neurosurg. 1997; 86(1):5–12

[6] Pollock BE, Huston J, III. Natural history of asymptomatic colloid cysts of the third ventricle. J Neurosurg. 1999; 91(3):364–369

[7] Büttner A, Winkler PA, Eisenmenger W, Weis S. Colloid cysts of the third ventricle with fatal outcome: a report of two cases and review of the literature. Int J Legal Med. 1997; 110(5):260–266

[8] de Witt Hamer PC, Verstegen MJ, De Haan RJ, et al. High risk of acute deterioration in patients harboring symptomatic colloid cysts of the third ventricle. J Neurosurg. 2002; 96(6):1041–1045

[9] Ryder JW, Kleinschmidt-DeMasters BK, Keller TS. Sudden deterioration and death in patients with benign tumors of the third ventricle area. J Neurosurg. 1986; 64(2):216–223

[10] Margetis K, Christos PJ, Souweidane M. Endoscopic resection of incidental colloid cysts. J Neurosurg. 2014; 120(6):1259–1267

[11] Godano U, Ferrai R, Meleddu V, Bellinzona M. Hemorrhagic colloid cyst with sudden coma. Minim Invasive Neurosurg. 2010; 53(5–6):273–274

[12] Kondziolka D, Lunsford LD. Stereotactic management of colloid cysts: factors predicting success. J Neurosurg. 1991; 75(1):45–51

[13] Pollock BE, Schreiner SA, Huston J, III. A theory on the natural history of colloid cysts of the third ventricle. Neurosurgery. 2000; 46(5):1077–1081, discussion 1081–1083

[14] Boogaarts HD, Decq P, Grotenhuis JA, et al. Long-term results of the neuroendoscopic management of colloid cysts of the third ventricle: a series of 90 cases. Neurosurgery. 2011; 68(1):179–187

[15] Horn EM, Feiz-Erfan I, Bristol RE, et al. Treatment options for third ventricular colloid cysts: comparison of open microsurgical versus endoscopic resection. Neurosurgery. 2007; 60(4):613–618, discussion 618–620

[16] Sampath R, Vannemreddy P, Nanda A. Microsurgical excision of colloid cyst with favorable cognitive outcomes and short operative time and hospital stay: operative techniques and analyses of outcomes with review of previous studies. Neurosurgery. 2010; 66(2):368–374, discussion 374–375

[17] Desai KI, Nadkarni TD, Muzumdar DP, Goel AH. Surgical management of colloid cyst of the third ventricle—a study of 105 cases. Surg Neurol. 2002; 57(5): 295–302, discussion 302–304

[18] Rosenstengel C, Baldauf J, Müller JU, Schroeder HW. Sudden intraaqueductal dislocation of a third ventricle ependymoma causing acute decompensation of hydrocephalus. J Neurosurg Pediatr. 2011; 8(2):154–157

[19] Zabihyan S, Etemadrezaie H, Baharvahdat H, et al. Remote transplantation of a third ventricle colloid cyst: case report. J Neurosurg. 2015; 122(6): 1406–1410

[20] Alford EN, Rotman LE, Lepard JR, Agee BS, Markert JM. Interrater and intrarater reliability of the colloid cyst risk score. Neurosurgery. 2020; 86(1): E47–E53

[21] Alford EN, Rotman LE, Shank CD, Agee BS, Markert JM. Independent validation of the colloid cyst risk score to predict symptoms and hydrocephalus in patients with colloid cysts of the third ventricle. World Neurosurg. 2020; 134: e747–e753

# 5 Overview of Surgical Management for Colloid Cysts of the Third Ventricle

Peter Nakaji

**Abstract**

There are multiple surgical options for management of colloid cysts of the third ventricle, including transcallosal craniotomy, transcortical craniotomy, endoscopic transventricular resection, ventricular shunting, and stereotactic drainage. The goals of treatment are focused on complete removal of the cyst wall and contents, management of hydrocephalus, and prevention of complications such as damage to the fornices. An overview of the pros and cons of each of the approaches is separately detailed by way of introducing the more detailed treatment to follow in subsequent chapters.

*Keywords:* transcallosal craniotomy, transcortical craniotomy, endoscopic resection, ventricular shunting, stereotactic drainage, hydrocephalus

## 5.1 Introduction

The colloid cyst of the third ventricle presents a particular surgical challenge due in large part to the complicated adjacent anatomy and its relationship to acceptable entry points. The classic location for a colloid cyst is deep in the brain at the apex of the third ventricle, surrounded by the fornices and the thalamus, which are both highly eloquent. The colloid cyst is a benign mass with a thin membrane distended with mucinous or solid material and with the wall itself attached to the roof of the third ventricle; they are intimately involved with the choroid plexus and the thalamostriate and septal veins and the velum interpositum. Through their growth they often obstruct the foramen of Monro, causing acute or chronic hydrocephalus. When very large, they can stretch the fornices, causing memory problems. The goals of surgical treatment are focused on management of hydrocephalus, reduction in mass effect, and elimination of the cyst itself to effect cure from future risk. They are generally too high to reach from below or subfrontally, making some kind of approach from above preferable.

Although initially addressed microsurgically, over time a great diversity of approaches has been offered to accomplish each of the surgical goals in whole or in part.[1] These include cerebrospinal fluid (CSF) diversion, stereotactic drainage, microsurgical removal, and endoscopic removal, each of which we will briefly review here, and review in greater detail in other parts of this volume (▶ Fig. 5.1).

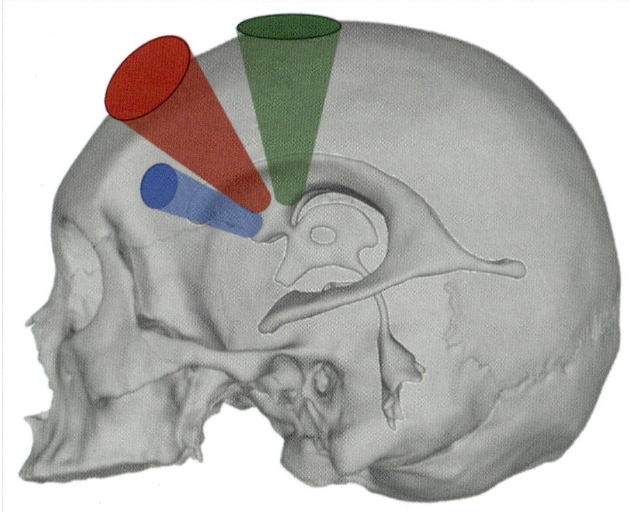

**Fig. 5.1** Various approach trajectories of the major modalities of colloid cyst removal. Typical transcallosal (*green cone*), transcortical (*red cone*), and endoscopic (*blue cone*) corridors are shown.

Natural history and the decision-making process with respect to whether to offer treatment are also discussed in other chapters. Therefore, we will not focus on this question, except as it may pertain to the influence of choice of one specific treatment over others. This is because our focus here is on the treatment options: we acknowledge that while for the colloid cyst patient who presents acutely, there is little debate about *if* treatment should be offered, for many other patients whose cysts are found incidentally or in the setting of mild headaches of unclear etiology, a healthy amount of consideration about whether to treat may be due before acting. That consideration represents a substantial part of the focus of the rest of this volume. Accordingly, we will focus only on an overview of the surgical treatments individually and relative to one another.

## 5.2 Management of Obstructive Hydrocephalus and Cerebrospinal Fluid Dynamics

Since the principal and most feared cause of morbidity and mortality from colloid cysts derives from obstructive hydrocephalus at the level of the foramen of Monro, management of CSF dynamics remains the most important part of treatment. Management may be in the form of CSF diversion, creation of alternative pathways, or restoration of normal flow. In the presence of acute hydrocephalus, the placement of an external ventricular drain into the lateral ventricles may be lifesaving. In some cases, even bilateral drainage may be required.[2] Once the fluid has been drained to maintain pressures and volumes in the ventricle at physiological levels, the rest of treatment can be managed at a more leisurely pace. On rare occasion, particularly where the patient is not a good surgical candidate for a definitive surgery, CSF shunting may serve as a sole treatment.

In the acute setting, placement of an external ventricular drain should not be delayed. The presence of crushing headache and any degree of compromise of level of consciousness makes emergent drainage essential. The drain can be placed in the frontal area at the traditional Kocher's point location in most patients with good efficacy. However, consideration should be given for the planned route for more definitive treatment. A standard right frontal location may conflict with an ipsilateral transcallosal or transcortical craniotomy. A rigid catheter passing through the brain may pose a risk to the brain if the frontal lobe is moved to accommodate an open approach trajectory. In a contralateral approach, there should be no such conflict as the catheter will not move with respect to the brain. In an endoscopic approach, the brain also moves little, and as long as one of the recommended anterolateral trajectories is used, there should be no conflict with an external ventricular drain.

In the setting of whatever surgery is performed, restoration of equilibrium in CSF dynamics is essential. In a craniotomy, the cyst is removed, and the foramen of Monro is unobstructed. In an endoscopic approach, the same is true. Blood clots from surgery as well as cyst contents should be evacuated. Great care should be taken not only to preserve the fornices to preserve the memory but also not to disrupt the pia in the way that can lead to scarring. Consider performing septum pellucidotomy in a way that does not endanger the fornices, as this will give two corridors for CSF egress from both the lateral ventricles. In many patients who present with enlarged ventricles, auto-fenestration has already occurred, obviating the need for further intervention. Although obstruction of the aqueduct with debris is rare, it behooves the surgeon to briefly inspect the posterior third ventricle and gently irrigate it at the end of whichever approach is chosen to ensure patency of the pathways.

CSF shunting as a definitive treatment is not often practiced at present. CSF diversion alone puts the patient at risk of acute deterioration in the setting of shunt failure, does not prevent growth of the cyst with potential deformation of the fornices, and leaves the patient subject to intermittent dilation and contraction of the ventricles depending upon the degree of drainage of the lateral ventricles by the shunt. If it is performed, bilateral drainage must be ensured, whether through a catheter with holes on both sides or surgical or spontaneous fenestration of the septum pellucidum. To which patients might this strategy be applicable? An elderly patient who is not a good candidate for a more prolonged surgery or with a larger cyst with thinned fornices that might not tolerate a more definitive surgery. In this setting, pure CSF drainage with or without drainage of the cyst without an attempt to remove it from the foramen of Monro may be appropriate. Again, this is a rare circumstance.

## 5.3 Stereotactic Drainage

Those familiar with colloid cyst treatment today rarely give the idea of stereotactic drainage much thought. However, it is a strategy with an established history.[3,4,5,6] Because advances in stereotactic drainage kept pace with (or even exceeded those of) microsurgery in their early years, the ability to accurately place a needle stereotactically into a colloid cyst and drain it became an option before sufficiently delicate microsurgical removal was a widespread option. Faced with the devastating neuropsychological consequences of severe memory loss in some open surgical patients, stereotactic drainage gained some adherents. There are naturally many challenges with this strategy, including the possibility of missing the target, difficulty with accessing the interior of the cyst, causing intraventricular hemorrhage, failure to un-obstruct the foramen of Monro, failure to provide longstanding relief, and causing damage upon the fornix, among others. The advent of neuroendoscopic techniques to directly visualize the cyst and achieve the goals of surgery has relegated this approach mostly to the annals of history. However, one should be aware that stereotactic drainage was carried out with some success and efficacy for many years.

## 5.4 Transcranial Open Microsurgical Approaches

The advantages of direct removal of a colloid cyst through an open cranial route are obvious: the techniques are familiar, the dexterity of microdissection is the highest, and the access affords many options in case the cyst proves adherent to critical structures. The principal concern with the open approaches is with the morbidity they entail; mitigation of this morbidity is one of the chief aims of the technical evolution and mastery of open surgery. There are two basic routes that are practiced routinely for colloid cyst removal, namely, the *interhemispheric transcallosal* and the *transcortical* approaches. Each is discussed in greater detail by their adherents later in this book.

Briefly, the *interhemispheric transcallosal* approach involves a standard craniotomy that allows access down one surface of the falx cerebri to the corpus callosum, which is opened to afford access to the lateral ventricle.[7,8] The cyst is identified at the foramen of Monro and removed through the foramen, with or without some degree of opening of the choroidal fissure (▶ Fig. 5.2). Its main advantage is violation of very little brain tissue. From the perspective of trajectory, it comes down directly on the fornices and therefore does not offer an ideal angle to see the underside of the fornices. Traditionally this approach is performed in the straight supine position with the head neutral. However, a significant number of authors have pointed out the advantages of the lateral position with the approach side being the low side (e.g., left side down), which causes the frontal lobe to fall away under gravity retraction without fixed retractors and the contralateral (in this example, right) fornix to slump contralaterally, exposing the foramen of Monro better, facilitating cyst exposure and removal.

Adherents of the *transcortical* approach favor a more frontal and lateral approach directly through the cortex, with or without a tubular retraction system.[9] From a purely anatomical standpoint, much more brain is traversed and disrupted by this approach. In its favor, the angle onto the cyst at the foramen of Monro is superior and especially with the use of image guidance, there is very little risk of getting lost. For those who place the goal of protection of the fornices well above that of the "noneloquent" right frontal cortex, the advantages are worth it. However, the lateral position discussed above for the contralateral interhemispheric transcallosal approach overcomes this concern by offering a similar forniceal-cyst configuration at exposure.

## 5.5 Endoscopic Surgery

The conceptual appeal of endoscopic removal of colloid cysts lies in the notion that the approach is minimally invasive in the sense of "low impact."[10] Neuroendoscopic removal is a form of transcortical surgery, albeit with a much smaller footprint in

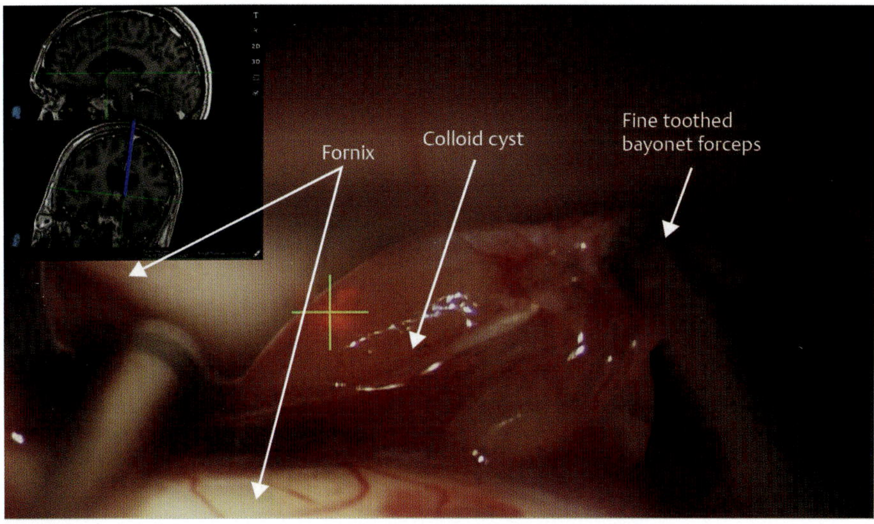


Fig. 5.2 A microscopic view of the right foramen of Monro from a left transcallosal approach, with anterior on the left and posterior on the right, showing the colloid cyst being drawn up into the right lateral ventricle.

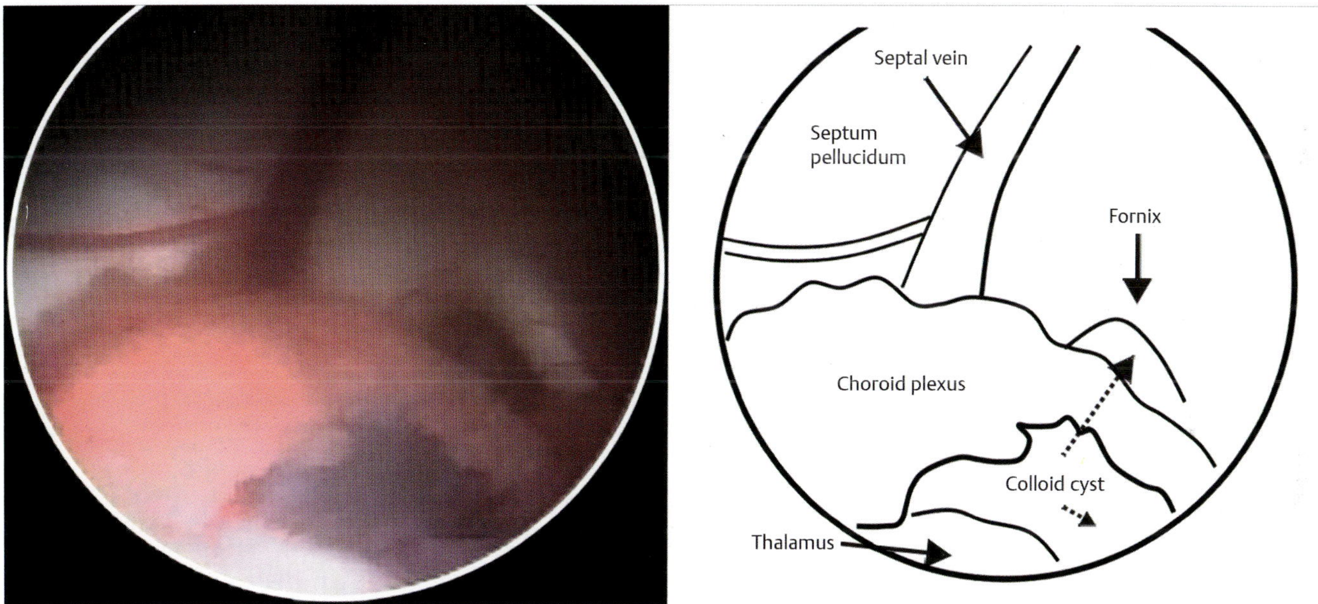


Fig. 5.3 An endoscopic view of the right foramen of Monro showing how much more lateral view is gained through the endoscopic trajectory. Posterior to left, anterior to right.

terms of cortical transgression. Coupled with image guidance and a strict adherence to maintaining a limited degree of excursion of the endoscope shaft, the effective anatomical impact on the brain can be kept low. From the standpoint of patient tolerance and recovery, it offers superior results in the best case.[11] However, concerns persist among its detractors about the high degree of technical facility required, the relative difficulty of microdissection in the way that one is used to do in two-handed microsurgery, the need for two people to handle the endoscope and instruments, and concerns about the higher probability of incomplete removal due to the preceding limitations. The first modern reports used a flexible neuroendoscope, but most modern removal is done with rigid endoscopes. There is a substantial diversity of opinion about the nuances of endoscopic colloid cyst removal technique. Most current reports describe an anterolateral approach through the nondominant frontal lobe that approaches the cyst in the foramen of Monro (▶ Fig. 5.3), devascularizes the exterior, drains its contents, frees it from the choroid plexus, and ultimately dissects and removes the cyst wall from the roof of the third ventricle. For many colloid cysts, this strategy can be carried out very satisfactorily and with reasonable ease. Image guidance is helpful to obtain the optimal entry and trajectory.[12] The endoscope has limitations that create more difficulty with cysts which are densely adherent to the fornices, are very large, or contain a great deal of inspissated materials. It is more difficult to open the choroidal fissure with the endoscope than the microscope, but it is possible to do.[13] Some people have managed the challenges for bimanual dissection posed by the endoscope by a dual-port approach.[14,15] Larger ventricles facilitate the application of the endoscope for colloid cyst removal, although endoscopic removal of colloid cysts can be successfully performed in patients with small ventricles.[16] In some cases, authors have used endoscopic removal when prevention of obstruction is the goal with the intention to forgo complete removal in favor of more limited goals.[17]

## 5.6 Comparative Analysis

Published reports which attempt to compare the strategies discussed above mostly attempt to compare endoscopic and microsurgical removal.[18,19] These studies are comparative in an observational sense but suffer from being largely retrospective and not randomized. Generally speaking, we can say that most series show that open removal has a higher success rate in terms of "complete" cyst removal and lower recurrence, while endoscopic removal has lower complications and a faster recovery.[20,21,22,23] There is not sufficient evidence to establish whether one technique is uniformly "better" than another. In fact, it would be difficult to distinguish whether the technique or the technician is the key to any good results that are reported. A strong facility with all the surgical options and a nuanced decision-making process whose pivot points can be refined with the content of this book will afford the patient the best chance of a good outcome.

## 5.7 Conclusion

A diversity of surgical strategies exists for the surgical management of colloid cysts of the third ventricle, each of which prioritizes a certain aspect of the surgical goals which they all share in common. Exponents of each base their preferences on the how they prioritize each goal and their personal facility with the technique they prefer, customized to the needs of the individual patient. Familiarity with all the techniques and the ability to offer one or more with high efficacy and low morbidity is the key. The following chapters demonstrate the experience of talented experts explaining how they achieve their results.

## References


[1] Kondziolka D, Lunsford LD. Stereotactic techniques for colloid cysts: roles of aspiration, endoscopy, and microsurgery. Acta Neurochir Suppl (Wien). 1994; 61:76–78

[2] Zhou JJ, Mooney MA, Farber SH, Bohl MA, Little AS, Nakaji P. Bedside iohexol ventriculography for patients with obstructive colloid cysts: a protocol to identify auto-fenestration of the septum pellucidum. World Neurosurg. 2019; 122:e279–e284

[3] Bosch DA, Rähn T, Backlund EO. Treatment of colloid cysts of the third ventricle by stereotactic aspiration. Surg Neurol. 1978; 9(1):15–18

[4] Kondziolka D, Lunsford LD. Stereotactic management of colloid cysts: factors predicting success. J Neurosurg. 1991; 75(1):45–51

[5] Musolino A, Fosse S, Munari C, Daumas-Duport C, Chodkiewicz JP. Diagnosis and treatment of colloid cysts of the third ventricle by stereotactic drainage. Report on eleven cases. Surg Neurol. 1989; 32(4):294–299

[6] Kumar K, Kelly M, Toth C. Stereotactic cyst wall disruption and aspiration of colloid cysts of the third ventricle. Stereotact Funct Neurosurg. 1998; 71(3): 145–152

[7] Symss NP, Ramamurthi R, Rao SM, Vasudevan MC, Jain PK, Pande A. Management outcome of the transcallosal, transforaminal approach to colloid cysts of the anterior third ventricle: an analysis of 78 cases. Neurol India. 2011; 59(4): 542–547

[8] Shapiro S, Rodgers R, Shah M, Fulkerson D, Campbell RL. Interhemispheric transcallosal subchoroidal fornix-sparing craniotomy for total resection of colloid cysts of the third ventricle. J Neurosurg. 2009; 110(1):112–115

[9] Desai KI, Nadkarni TD, Muzumdar DP, Goel AH. Surgical management of colloid cyst of the third ventricle—a study of 105 cases. Surg Neurol. 2002; 57 (5):295–302, discussion 302–304

[10] Greenlee JD, Teo C, Ghahreman A, Kwok B. Purely endoscopic resection of colloid cysts. Neurosurgery. 2008; 62(3) Suppl 1:51–55, discussion 55–56

[11] Levine NB, Miller MN, Crone KR. Endoscopic resection of colloid cysts: indications, technique, and results during a 13-year period. Minim Invasive Neurosurg. 2007; 50(6):313–317

[12] Rangel-Castilla L, Chen F, Choi L, Clark JC, Nakaji P. Endoscopic approach to colloid cyst: what is the optimal entry point and trajectory? J Neurosurg. 2014; 121(4):790–796

[13] Iacoangeli M, di Somma LG, Di Rienzo A, Alvaro L, Nasi D, Scerrati M. Combined endoscopic transforaminal-transchoroidal approach for the treatment of third ventricle colloid cysts. J Neurosurg. 2014; 120(6):1471–1476

[14] Mishra S, Chandra PS, Suri A, Rajender K, Sharma BS, Mahapatra AK. Endoscopic management of third ventricular colloid cysts: eight years' institutional experience and description of a new technique. Neurol India. 2010; 58(3): 412–417

[15] Bergsneider M. Complete microsurgical resection of colloid cysts with a dual-port endoscopic technique. Neurosurgery. 2007; 60(2) Suppl 1:ONS33–ONS42, discussion ONS42–ONS43

[16] Wait SD, Gazzeri R, Wilson DA, Abla AA, Nakaji P, Teo C. Endoscopic colloid cyst resection in the absence of ventriculomegaly. Neurosurgery. 2013; 73 1 Suppl Operative:ons39–ons46

[17] Zymberg ST, Riechelmann GS, da Costa MDS, Ramalho CO, Cavalheiro S. Third ventricle colloid cysts: an endoscopic case series emphasizing technical variations. Surg Neurol Int. 2021; 12:376

[18] Horn EM, Feiz-Erfan I, Bristol RE, et al. Treatment options for third ventricular colloid cysts: comparison of open microsurgical versus endoscopic resection. Neurosurgery. 2007; 60(4):613–618, discussion 618–620

[19] Sheikh AB, Mendelson ZS, Liu JK. Endoscopic versus microsurgical resection of colloid cysts: a systematic review and meta-analysis of 1,278 patients. World Neurosurg. 2014; 82(6):1187–1197

[20] Lewis AI, Crone KR, Taha J, van Loveren HR, Yeh HS, Tew JM, Jr. Surgical resection of third ventricle colloid cysts. Preliminary results comparing transcallosal microsurgery with endoscopy. J Neurosurg. 1994; 81(2):174–178

[21] Grondin RT, Hader W, MacRae ME, Hamilton MG. Endoscopic versus microsurgical resection of third ventricle colloid cysts. Can J Neurol Sci. 2007; 34 (2):197–207

[22] Elshamy W, Burkard J, Gerges M, et al. Surgical approaches for resection of third ventricle colloid cysts: meta-analysis. Neurosurg Rev. 2021; 44(6): 3029–3038

[23] Sethi A, Cavalcante D, Ormond DR. Endoscopic versus microscopic transcallosal excision of colloid cysts: a systematic review in the era of complete endoscopic excision. World Neurosurg. 2019; 132:e53–e58

# 6 Consensus Panel Regarding the Diagnosis and Surgical Management of Colloid Cysts

*Thomas L. Beaumont, Ralph G. Dacey, Jr., Arthur Day, Costas Hadjipanayis, Peter Nakaji, Henry W.S. Schroeder, and Robert Spetzler*

**Abstract**

Neurosurgeons typically have strongly held beliefs regarding the surgical management of colloid cysts of the third ventricle. This includes determining which patients are appropriate for surveillance imaging, the specific indications for surgery, and the use of a particular surgical approach with one or more surgical adjuncts. In this chapter, we sought to explore these positions with a group of international experts who have considerable experience managing colloid cyst of the third ventricle. Our specific goal was to understand the factors contributing to firmly held opinions and assess the inherent biases toward either an open or endoscopic approach preference. Further we sought to establish whether there should be equipoise for approach selection or if there are particular anatomic and lesion-specific nuances that dictate the optimal surgical strategy. Finally, it was our specific aim to establish consensus indications for surgery and approach selection for colloid cysts of the third ventricle, even though our expectation was that such a consensus likely would not exist.

*Keywords:* colloid cyst, consensus recommendations, craniotomy, endoscopic, neuroendoscopy, third ventricle

## 6.1 Historical Perspective

Colloid cysts of the third ventricle have been classically managed via two standard transcranial approaches, most commonly the interhemispheric transcallosal (IHTC) approach and less frequently by the transcortical transventricular (TCTV) approach. More recently, single burr hole endoscopic (SBHE) approaches have offered a minimally invasive alternative that offers a reduced rate of complications and improvement in nearly all procedure-related outcomes (see Chapters 5, 10, 11, and 12). However, in early case series there was an increased frequency of coagulated cyst wall remnants, and this seemed to be associated with increased rate of cyst recurrence, although the data were comprised primarily of small retrospective case series and were somewhat anecdotal.[1,2,3] More recent series using a flexible endoscopic technique suggest coagulated cyst wall remnants are not associated with an increased rate of cyst recurrence with more than 10-year median follow-up.[4] Nonetheless, neurosurgeons often remain firmly adherent to a "one approach for all" or "open versus endoscopic" position when considering approach selection for colloid cysts, despite compelling evidence that neither notion is warranted.

There are strongly held beliefs regarding indications for surgery, use of various surgical adjuncts, and which patients with colloid cysts are appropriate for surveillance imaging. In this chapter, we sought to explore these positions with a group of international experts who have considerable experience managing colloid cyst of the third ventricle. Our specific goal was to understand the factors contributing to firmly held opinions and assess the inherent biases toward either an open or endoscopic approach preference. Further we sought to establish whether there should be equipoise for approach selection or if there are particular anatomic and lesion-specific nuances that dictate the optimal surgical strategy. Finally, it was our specific aim to establish consensus indications for surgery and approach selection for colloid cysts of the third ventricle, even though our expectation was that such a consensus likely would not exist.

### 6.1.1 General Points

Intraventricular tumors are one of the greatest technical challenges in neurosurgery. Despite their benign histology, colloid cysts are anatomically complex and technically challenging lesions that carry extreme risk during surgery. Mastery of the salient anatomy and meticulous surgical technique is critical, as even small mistakes are poorly tolerated and can have devastating consequences. Approach selection must be guided not only by surgeon's preference but also by imaging characteristics such as T2 signal within the lesion, anatomical consideration such as the size of the cyst relative to the foramen of Monro, and importantly, the location of the fornicies relative to the lesion. Indeed, knowing the location of the forncies is critical to all steps of clinical and surgical decision-making for colloid cysts. One must be able to clearly visualize these critical structures during surgical manipulation, regardless of the favored surgical approach.

Dr. Day: *"Neurosurgeons interested in doing colloid cysts must commit themselves to being really good, as there is a steep learning curve. Colloid cysts are curable lesions, but slight mistakes can be devastating."*

Most on-call community neurosurgeons will not have the neuroendoscopy expertise or team cohesiveness necessary to safely manage colloid cysts endoscopically. Thus, endoscopy cannot be (and should not be perceived to be) a universal standard. If an institution desires to perform endoscopic resection of colloid cysts, one or two endoscopic experts should be identified and should manage all such cases at the institution. If a patient with a colloid cyst requires acute surgery and endoscopy is felt to be the optimal approach but a neuroendoscopist is not available, single or bilateral external ventricular drains (EVDs) can be placed to stabilize the patient until surgery. Alternatively, patients can be managed by transcranial microsurgery if an appropriately experienced neurosurgeon with experience in the approach is available.

Dr. Dacey: *"Most neurosurgeons with a long experience of managing colloid cysts of the third ventricle will remember adverse outcomes related to sudden deterioration in patients who were undergoing 'observation,' or a failure to manage acute hydrocephalus in the most timely and effective way. In this regard, basic principles of providing appropriately timed neurosurgical care are probably as important as nuanced discussions of various surgical approaches and techniques."*

## 6.2 Surveillance Imaging for Asymptomatic Patients

Surveillance imaging for asymptomatic lesions should address not only the natural history of the colloid cyst but also the patient's anxiety related to the presence of the lesion. Given historical data regarding the risk of acute neurological decline and "sudden death" that continues to influence discussions with healthcare providers, it is important for neurosurgeons to reassure patients and explain that the overall risk is small, perhaps 3% for symptomatic patients.[5] Nonetheless, the lesion must be followed over time to ensure that the patient's risk is not changing. Neurosurgeons must ensure that patients are mindful of the potential symptoms and warning signs, while at same time, be careful not to let the patient become overly focused on the fact that something catastrophic could happen at any moment. A stable long-term clinical relationship with the patient is helpful in understanding each individual patient and whether the patient may be developing new symptoms.

*Dr. Day: "How long does it take for a colloid cyst to grow to 12 millimeters?"*

Factors to consider in establishing an appropriate imaging interval include the size of the cyst, the patient's age, T2/FLAIR signal characteristics, and the reliability of the patient to complete imaging and follow-up. Clinicians should consider using the Colloid Cyst Risk Score (CCRS)[5] to assist with risk stratification but recognize that risk prediction scales are not absolute. The combination of risk prediction tools such as the CCRS and clinician's impression is an optimal strategy and remains firmly rooted in the "art" of medicine. In this way, both the patient and the neurosurgeon must be comfortable with the plan. Despite these many considerations, a near-consensus was identified among the panelists regarding the surveillance imaging interval for asymptomatic patients. The following recommendations were therefore made:

**Surveillance imaging for asymptomatic patients**

- Young patient, T2 hyperintense cyst, no ventriculomegaly—6-month initial interval scan and then every 12 months.
- Young patient, T2 hypointense cyst, no ventriculomegaly—12-month initial interval scan and then every 24 months.
- Patient > 65 years old, T2 hyperintense cyst, no ventriculomegaly—12-month initial interval scan and then every 24 months.
- Patient > 65 years old, T2 hypointense cyst, no ventriculomegaly—12- to 24-month initial interval scan and then every 24 months.

**Expert insight**

Panelists have followed patients with T2 hypointense cysts for > 15 years with no clinical or radiographic change.

Although there is no absolute threshold for cyst diameter that increases risk, there was strong consensus that both published data and panelist experience suggest cysts > 7 mm axial diameter warrant increased scrutiny. However, it is important to note that the size of the cyst must be considered relative to the diameter of the foramen of Monro and the position within the third ventricle. See Chapter 4 on Natural History for a detailed discussion of these relationships.

## 6.3 Indications for Surgery

Given the myriad causes of headaches, together with the fact that colloid cysts are often identified on workup for headaches, it becomes critical to identify characteristics of headaches thought to be specifically referable to colloid cysts. These factors include headaches that are paroxysmal, undulating, pressure-like, and occasionally positional. While classically headaches were said to be worse when upright and improved by lying supine, panelists have also noted the converse. Colloid cyst–related headaches often have a reproducible series of precipitating factors, symptoms, and time to resolution, with a consistent cadence. If such headaches occur in the setting of mild unilateral ventricular enlargement, panelists agreed that there is high likelihood the symptoms are referable to the colloid cyst and surgery should be considered.[6]

*Dr. Dacey: "Patients who present with headaches due to colloid cysts will often relate unusual symptoms, including unusual precipitants or a peculiar crescendos of pain and/or pain relief. It is important that the neurosurgeon carefully interpret the symptoms as decisions are made regarding surgical indications."*

There was no clear consensus on the etiology of syncope in the setting of colloid cysts. However, there was agreement that it often leads to the consideration of surgery, particularly if the patient is young and otherwise healthy, the cyst is large, and there is no other explanation for the syncopal event. If the colloid cyst is small and there are no other referable symptoms, observation is reasonable. Despite the inherent management bias based on larger cyst diameter, most panelists did not believe hypothalamic dysfunction plays a role in syncope in the setting of colloid cysts.[7]

**Consensus indications for surgery**

There are several consensus indications for surgery. These include:

- Referable headaches not clearly attributable to another cause.
- Syncope in an otherwise healthy patient with an unrevealing workup.
- Cysts > 7 mm axial diameter with referable symptoms or ventriculomegaly (unilateral or bilateral).
- Patients with asymptomatic cysts but who have unrelenting anxiety despite stable imaging studies and appropriate counseling.

## 6.4 Timing of Surgery

Patients with concerning colloid cysts that have mild symptoms without progressive ventriculomegaly or transependymal flow and stable surveillance imaging require semi-elective surgery. Factors to consider regarding the timing of semi-elective surgery include the severity of patient's symptoms, the presence of symptom progression, colloid cyst diameter, patient's sophistication, patient's reliability, and proximity to a major medical center. The CCRS (see Chapter 4) was discussed in detail for each of the cases reviewed by the panelists. Although there was no clear consensus on whether or how to use the tool, it was thought to be helpful, although still somewhat preliminary. It was stressed that the CCRS, like all risk prediction tools, ultimately requires clinician's judgment. Risk prediction tools cannot be used in an absolute fashion. The "art" of the diagnosis relates to the ability to talk to the patients and discern whether they may be having transient elevations in intracranial pressure (ICP) that explain their symptoms, or whether they are likely asymptomatic but their quality of life seems severely affected by the presence of the lesion due to the concern for rapid neurological decline and death. It is therefore recommended that the CCRS be used together with clinician's impression to make an individualized decision for each patient. As with any clinical risk prediction tool, the CCRS should not be used in isolation, but rather in an integrated rational process taking into account each individual patient's symptoms, ability to clearly convey changes in symptoms, changes in the imaging data, and the patient's overall surgical risk.

*Dr. Spetzler: "There is always value in measuring something; it just may not be entirely clear what that value is."*

## 6.5 Approach Selection

At the outset, it was our expectation that there would be no consensus on a single approach for all colloid cysts (see Chapter 5). Through the specific case discussions and more general dialogue, three groups of neurosurgeons with regard to approach preference seemed to emerge: neurosurgeons who recommend microsurgical approach only; strongly endoscopic biased neurosurgeons; and those with mastery in both open transcranial microsurgery and neuroendoscopy. In the latter category, however, there was a clear bias toward endoscopy whenever possible due to excellent patient outcomes, reduced length of stay (LOS), reduced complications, and improved patient satisfaction. Conversely, some expert microsurgeons stated categorically that they would not recommend endoscopy, as they had no endoscopic training or experience, and have had decades of excellent outcomes with open transcranial microsurgery.

*Dr. Nakaji: "For experienced surgeons, it is really the surgeon's experience with the preferred approach that leads to favorable outcomes."*

It was frequently emphasized that colloid cysts are technically challenging lesions regardless of the approach. Experienced microsurgeons tend to favor the approach that has offered the best outcome in their hands and are less likely to have developed an interest or expertise in endoscopic approaches. The spectrum of panelist experience and their preferred approach offered a rich discussion pertaining to the following surgical approaches: interhemispheric transcallosal (IHTC), transcortical transventricular (TCTV), and single burr hole endoscopic (SBHE). The decision-making pertaining to these three approaches is presented below. We also briefly discuss the use of port-based approaches for salvage during SBHE, but this is not discussed as a primary surgical strategy. The use of various surgical adjuncts such as EVD placement, septostomy, third ventriculostomy, transchoroidal exposure, and interforniceal exposure is also discussed in context of the approaches below. This will be presented independently for ease of quick access and review. Finally, the importance of bimanual surgical technique is also discussed.

### 6.5.1 Interhemispheric Transcallosal Approach

*Dr. Spetzler: "The veins can be quite tricky, but for an experienced midline neurosurgeon it is a much safer way to go."*

The IHTC was the favored open microsurgical approach for all but one panelist. It was felt that the absence of brain transgression and access to both ventricles make the approach more favorable than the TCTV. However, it was clearly stated that large draining veins can increase the complexity of the approach and must be respected. Care must be taken to identify the superior anastomotic veins during preoperative planning to place the craniotomy optimally. In addition, one must avoid retraction injury, particularly if fixed retractors are used. Most panelists use dynamic retraction and avoid the use of fixed retractors whenever possible. A semi-lateral position with the side of approach down facilitates gravity retraction of the frontal lobe and obviates the need for fixed retractors. There is no left versus right consideration for the interhemispheric approach, as both ventricles are accessible from the side of approach, typically the right.

### 6.5.2 Transcortical Transventricular Approach

A single panelist strongly preferred TCTV approach and has used this strategy successfully for more than three decades with excellent results (see Chapters 8 and 14). Using a 15-mm cortical incision, performed meticulously without any subarachnoid hemorrhage, it was suggested that the approach is not much different from passage of a 19-French introducer (6.3 mm) used during the SBHE approach. The TCTV approach offers a favorable anterolateral trajectory that, together with opening of the choroidal fissure, allows safe and complete resection of even the most challenging colloid cysts. It was suggested that there should be a low threshold for opening the choroidal fissure to optimize this approach. With meticulous surgical technique, it was also argued that there is no increase in the frequency of postoperative seizures with the transcortical corridor. The approach is typically performed from the right, although a left side approach can be safely performed but is rarely required. When a left side approach is performed, the smallest possible corticotomy that allows safe and complete resection of the lesion should be performed.

### 6.5.3 Single Burr Hole Endoscopic Approach

For the majority of panelists, SBHE was the primary approach of choice for appropriately selected patients. However, it should be emphasized that this is not absolute, and there are several circumstances that make the endoscopic approach less favorable. In these situations, an IHTC was universally the preferred second option. Approach from the side of the largest ventricle and/or where the fornix was most favorable was recommended. An anterolateral burr hole with a 30-degree endoscope is universally used (see Chapters 10, 11, and 12). Large cysts that are T2 hypointense on imaging and/or have posterior attachments to the tela choroidia and velum interpositum can be challenging with an endoscopic approach. The cyst wall can be markedly adherent requiring fine bimanual sharp dissection that can be challenging to perform using the endoscope. In addition, firm cyst contents can be tedious and time consuming to remove endoscopically, even with the use of a suction-morcellation device. Although not a direct contraindication for endoscopy, in such cases, an open microsurgical approach is more expeditious and should be considered.

Conversely, cysts that have T2/FLAIR hyperintense contents on imaging typically have viscous fluid that can be easily evacuated with a suction cannula or using a suction-morcellation device, resulting in immediate internal decompression (see Chapter 16). Following this, the cyst wall can be more easily manipulated, transposed through the foramen, and sharply dissected. Although sharp bimanual dissection can be performed during the SBHE approach using modern ventriculoscopes such as the Lotta (Karl Stroz, Germany) by taking advantage of both the working channel and one of the side ports (see Chapter 17), the learning curve is quite steep. Also, there must be a fluid working relationship between the primary neurosurgeon and the neurosurgeon driving the endoscope. Even under optimal conditions, the instruments are constrained and there is instrument conflict that must be managed. Another commonly employed technique is to use a suction-morcellation device such as the Myriad (Nico Corp, Indianapolis, IN, USA) to gently cytoreduce the lesion (see Chapter 16). Extreme care must be taken to avoid excessive traction on the fornicies and internal cerebral veins, as injury to either structure can have catastrophic consequences. If gross total resection of the cyst wall cannot be achieved, complete coagulation of the cyst wall remnant must be performed to reduce the likelihood of recurrence.

*Dr. Dacey: "Endoscopists must recognize that there is a risk of inadvertently introducing the endoscope or other instruments into the fornix, thalamus, or brainstem. Care must be taken to mitigate this risk, particularly for neurosurgeons with relatively limited endoscopic experience."*

*Dr. Spetzler: "As Dr. Drake would say, 'Everyone must have a first case'."*

There is a steep and unforgiving learning curve associated with any intraventricular approach, particularly the SBHE approach. As stated earlier, colloid cysts are curable lesions, but neurosurgeons must recognize that even slight mistakes can be devastating for the patient. As such, SBHE resection should only be attempted by experienced endoscopists. Ideally, there is a progression of skills development from CSF leaks and encephaloceles, to routine pituitary surgery, larger pituitary tumors with lateral and suprasellar extension, to chordoma, chondrosarcomas, and ultimately to intradural lesions such as meningiomas and colloid cysts. Given this steep and protracted learning curve, most neurosurgeons will not have the necessary training and expertise to safely perform SBHE resection of colloid cysts. It should be emphasized that just because the endoscopic technique seems relatively benign when patients do well in the hands of expert neuroendoscopists, one must not be seduced into operating on a patient without clear indications and appropriate expertise.

## 6.6 Surgical Adjuncts

Several surgical adjuncts are discussed including septostomy, transchoroidal exposure, endoscopic third venriculostomy (ETV), and the use of EVDs. Each will be reviewed below in the context with the salient surgical approach. Perhaps not surprisingly, there were strong preferences based on whether the neurosurgeon performed primarily endoscopic resection, microsurgery, or a balanced combination of both approaches.

### 6.6.1 Septostomy

Septostomy was routinely used by neurosurgeons who perform endoscopic resection of colloid cysts. Panelists describe rare cases of foraminal webs causing symptomatic unilateral obstruction at the foramen of Monro that required delayed return to the operating room. Although the frequency of such events is rare, they are preventable. Septostomy is a relatively low risk procedure that can be performed quickly and safely at the end of the surgical procedure. Several endoscopic neurosurgeons always perform septostomy following endoscopic resection of colloid cysts, and there was near-consensus among them that the procedure should be considered a standard part of the endoscopic approach. One neurosurgeon skilled in both open and endoscopic resection of colloid cysts suggested septostomy be performed selectively, only when foramen is small and choroid plexus is hypertrophic.

*Editor's note: Thorough choroid plexus coagulation should be performed to uncover the colloid cyst prior to resection, and following cyst removal to ensure there are no choroidal appendages within the foramen of Monro that can give rise to obstructive webs.*

Neurosurgeons who perform open transcranial microsurgery exclusively either by IHTC or TCTV do not routinely perform septostomy, and there was no clear consensus among this group on when it should be employed. Expert opinion ranged from never performing septostomy to having a low threshold but not performing the procedure routinely. In the latter case, it was suggested that if the neurosurgeon has high confidence that gross total resection (GTR) has been achieved and the foramen is open, septostomy is not necessary. This particular panelist went on to state that as long as the clinician's impression "is good" at the completion of the procedure, septostomy is not performed. There was dissent to this metacognitive strategy, based on cases of foraminal webs causing symptomatic obstruction at the foramen of Monro following transcranial microsurgery, even when complete removal had been achieved. Although these events are rare, delayed return to the operating room was required and could have been avoided with simple adjunctive procedure.

### 6.6.2 Transchoroidal Approach

Transchoroidal exposure is commonly employed during open transcranial microsurgery. It was suggested that neurosurgeons should have very low threshold to open the choroidal fissure, as it offers clear visualization of the internal cerebral veins and medial posterior choroidal artery (MPCA) that are commonly adherent to or intimately associated with the cyst. It was emphasized that the neurosurgeon must recognize that following opening of the taenia fornicis, the plane of dissection must remain medial to the junction of the internal cerebral, thalamostriate, and anterior caudate veins to avoid catastrophic venous infarction. Once the choroidal fissure is opened, these critical neurovascular structures are "right there in front of you" (see Chapter 12, ▶ Fig. 12.1). Further, transchoroidal exposure provides superior access to the cyst attachments on the tela choroidea and velum interpositum, particularly in the setting of more posteriorly positioned lesion. One proponent suggested that opening of the choroidal fissure is analogous to opening the Sylvian fissure wherein it is advantageous to have wide exposure, but there is increasing risk as one moves posteriorly.

### 6.6.3 External Ventricular Drain Placement after Surgery

There was wide agreement, particularly among the endoscopic surgeons, that EVDs are not required after the uncomplicated resection of colloid cysts. Among these surgeons, there was consensus agreement that the occurrence of significant bleeding during surgery was an indication for EVD placement, even if the bleeding was controlled and the ventricles cleared. In this setting, the decision of whether the EVD remains clamped and is used only for ICP monitoring, or it is allowed to drain and further clear the ventricular system is based on the extent of intraventricular hemorrhage encountered. Interestingly, one panelist who strongly advocated for placement of an EVD at the end of the procedure historically has not routinely performed postoperative imaging in the absence of intraoperative complications. In this situation, the EVD was used to demonstrate normal ICP and thus, to infer the resolution of obstructive hydrocephalus. With further discussion, there was consensus agreement that following the uncomplicated resection of a colloid cyst, an EVD is not required as long as postoperative imaging is performed. It is recommended that all patients who undergo resection of a colloid cyst have a CT scan of the head within 2 hours of surgery. Postoperative MRI prior to discharge from hospital is recommended but there was no clear consensus on this recommendation.

#### Endoscopic Third Ventriculostomy

There was clear consensus that ETV is rarely, if ever, indicated during the resection of colloid cysts of the third ventricle and almost never performed. This primarily relates to the fact that obstruction to CSF flow is at the foramen of Monro, not the cerebral aqueduct. The only situation in which this may be necessary is when there is aqueductal obstruction from a Zone 3 colloid cyst (see Chapter 4, ▶ Fig. 4.2). However, it is recommended that the cyst be removed endoscopically, as such lesions are thought to have dislodged from their attachments at the foramen of Monro and translocated to the cerebral aqueduct. In such cases, the cyst can be retrieved with relative ease. If the cyst cannot be removed from the aqueduct and there is concern for ongoing obstruction, ETV would be indicated.

## 6.7 Extent of Resection and Cyst Wall Remnants

*Dr. Day: "Can you ensure gross total resection by microsurgical standards?"*

Among neurosurgeons who exclusively perform transcranial microsurgery, there is an inherent bias that the probability of gross total resection is reduced using the SBHE approach. This is in part related to several early reports in the literature and some more recently that describe coagulated cyst wall remnants in more than half of the patients at the conclusion of endoscopic surgery. Several institutional cohorts and meta-analysis confirm this notion and this fact is not contested. However, the endoscopic procedure has continued to evolve, particularly in the hands of experts, resulting in significantly increased rates of complete resection that approach that of open microsurgery (see Chapter 17). Further contributing to this bias, published data do not clearly demonstrate how the presence of coagulated cyst wall remnants relate to cyst recurrence. In fact, the most recent data suggest there may be no relationship between coagulated cyst wall remnants and cyst recurrence, with median follow-up of more than 10 years.[4] It was emphasized, however, that while complete cyst removal should be the goal of surgery with either approach, whenever it can be done safely, with the endoscopic approach, if the cyst is firmly adherent to critical neurovascular structures, one must be prepared to leave a small coagulated cyst wall remnant to avoid potential catastrophic injury. The importance of balancing the relatively low risk of recurrence of a benign lesion with the dynamic risk of high consequence neurovascular complications throughout a particular case must be thoroughly appreciated by neurosurgeons, particularly when using the SBHE approach.

## 6.8 Follow-Up and Outcome Measures

Based on panelist experience and recently published data, there was consensus that most recurrences occur within 10 years of surgery. Thus, it is recommended that postoperative surveillance imaging should be performed for at least one decade.

However, citing reports of late recurrences as much as 15 years postoperatively, it is suggested that extended interval imaging (every 2–3 years) be performed for an additional 5 to 10 years. Thus, a total 20 years of postoperative surveillance imaging is recommended. In addition, it is recommended that all patients with colloid cysts who will undergo elective surgery have neuropsychological testing preoperatively and 6 to 12 months postoperatively, with additional testing performed if persistent deficits are identified.

## 6.9 Cases Reviewed

### 6.9.1 Case 1 (▶ Fig. 6.1)

Panelist recommendations: There was clear majority recommendation of endoscopic resection (71%) followed by microsurgical resection (29%). Observation was not recommended. All except one neurosurgeon recommended endoscopic resection should approach from the left (see ▶ Table 6.1).

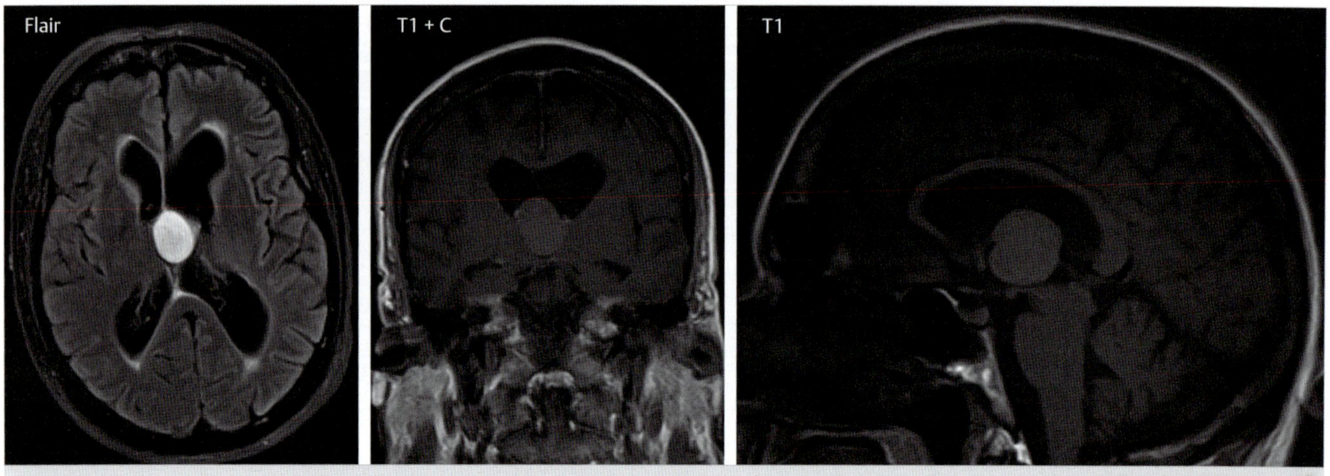


**Fig. 6.1** A 52-year-old male presented with chronic headaches and slowly progressive cognitive decline. Neuroimaging demonstrated a 2.7-cm T2-hyperintense colloid cyst of the third ventricle, Colloid Cyst Risk Score (CCRS) 5. The patient had stable vital signs and a nonfocal neurological examination.

**Table 6.1** Consensus panel participant recommendations for reviewed cases of colloid cysts of the third ventricle

| | 1 | 2 | 3 | 4 | 5 | 6 | 7 | 8 | 9 | 10 | 11 |
|---|---|---|---|---|---|---|---|---|---|---|---|
| Beaumont | Endo L | Endo | Obs | Endo R | Endo | Endo | Endo R | Endo L | Endo | Obs | Obs (IHTC-IF) |
| Dacey | Endo R | Endo | Obs | Endo | Obs | Endo R, poss IHTC | Obs vs. Endo R, survival? | Endo L | Endo | Obs | Obs |
| Day | TCTV-TC R | TCTV-TC R | Obs | TCTV-TC R | TCTV-TC | TCTV-TC R | Obs vs. TCTV or Endo L | TCTV-TC R | TCTV-TC | Obs | Obs (TCTV not IF) |
| Hadjipanayis | Endo R/L | Obs | Obs | Endo R | Obs | Endo TS R | Obs | Endo L | obs vs. IHTC | Obs | Obs |
| Nakaji | Endo L | Obs vs. IHTC R | Obs | Obs vs. Endo R | Obs | IHTC possible IF | Obs vs. Endo R | Endo L | IHTC vs. Endo | Endo vs. Obs | Endo R, start w/ septostomy |
| Schroeder | Endo L, urgent | Obs | Obs | Endo R | Obs | IHTC-IF vs. port | Obs vs. Endo R | Endo L | obs vs. IHTC | Obs | Obs (IHTC-IF) |
| Spetzler | IHTC | IHTC | IHTC | IHTC | Obs vs. IHTC | IHTC | Obs vs. IHTC, survival? | IHTC R | IHTC | Obs | Obs |

Abbreviations: Endo, endoscopic; IF, interforniceal; IHTC, interhemispheric transcallosal; Obs, observation with serial imaging; R and L indicate side of approach; TCTV, transcortical transventricular.
Note: "( )" indicates approach if surgery is necessary.

### 6.9.2 Case 2 (▶ Fig. 6.2)

Panelist recommendations: There was no clear majority recommendation. Panelist recommendations included observation (43%), microsurgical resection (29%), and endoscopic resections (29%). One panelist recommended observation stating that if surgery was pursued an IHTC approach would be recommended. Another who recommended surgery stated it would be done electively but commented that the ventricular asymmetry increased concern (see ▶ Table 6.1).

### 6.9.3 Case 3 (▶ Fig. 6.3)

Panelist recommendations: There was clear majority recommendation for observation. One panelist recommended microsurgical resection (14%) (see ▶ Table 6.1).

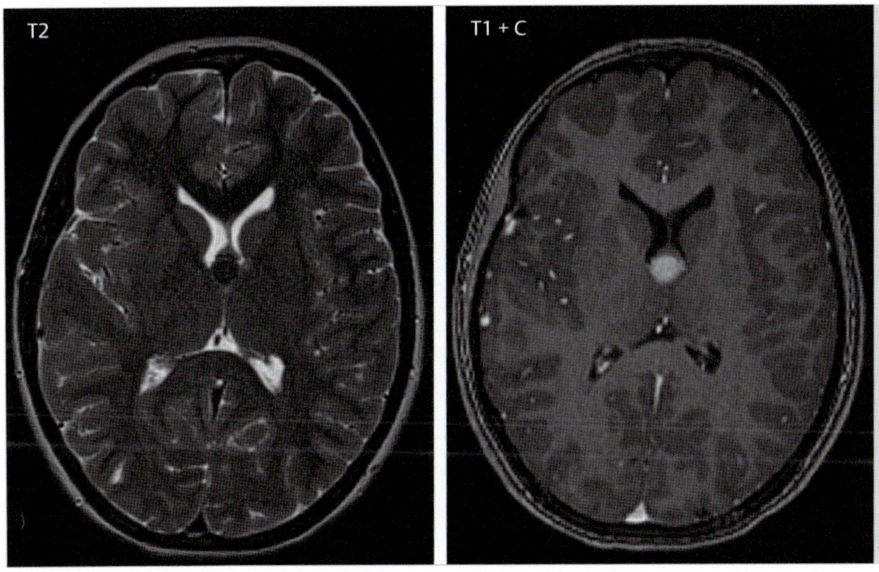


**Fig. 6.2** A 16-year-old female with a history of chronic migraine headaches presented with new frontal holocephalic headache, dizziness, and presyncope. Neuroimaging demonstrated a 12-mm T2-hypointense colloid cyst without ventriculomegaly, but with mild asymmetric ventricular enlargement on right, Colloid Cyst Risk Score (CCRS) 4.

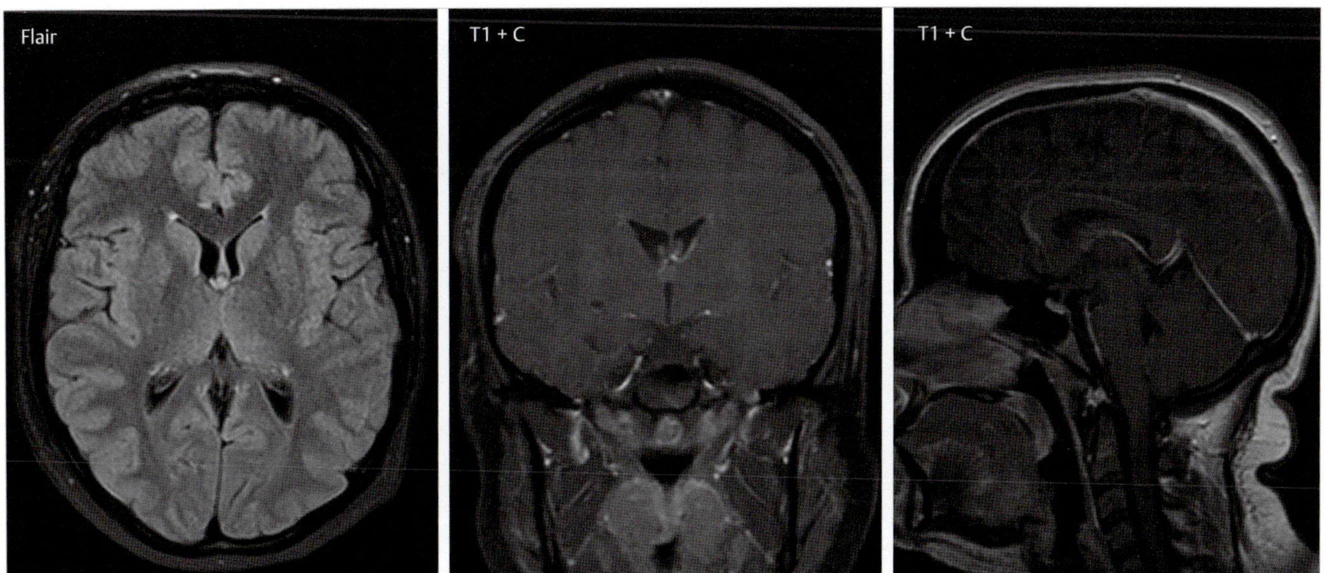


**Fig. 6.3** A 22-year-old female presented with recurrent frontal headaches without migranous features. She was neurologically intact. Neuroimaging demonstrated a 6-mm colloid cyst with mild unilateral ventriculomegaly, Colloid Cyst Risk Score (CCRS) 3. It was not clear to the treating neurosurgeon whether her headaches were related to the cyst.

## 6.9.4 Case 4 (► Fig. 6.4)

Panelist recommendations: There was slight majority in favor of endoscopic resections (57%) followed by microsurgical resection (29%). One panelist recommended observation but suggested a low threshold for endoscopic resection (see ► Table 6.1).

## 6.9.5 Case 5 (► Fig. 6.5)

Panelist recommendations: There was clear majority recommendation for observation (71%) with one panelist each recommending microsurgical resection (14%) and endoscopic resection (14%). Observation was not recommended (see ► Table 6.1).

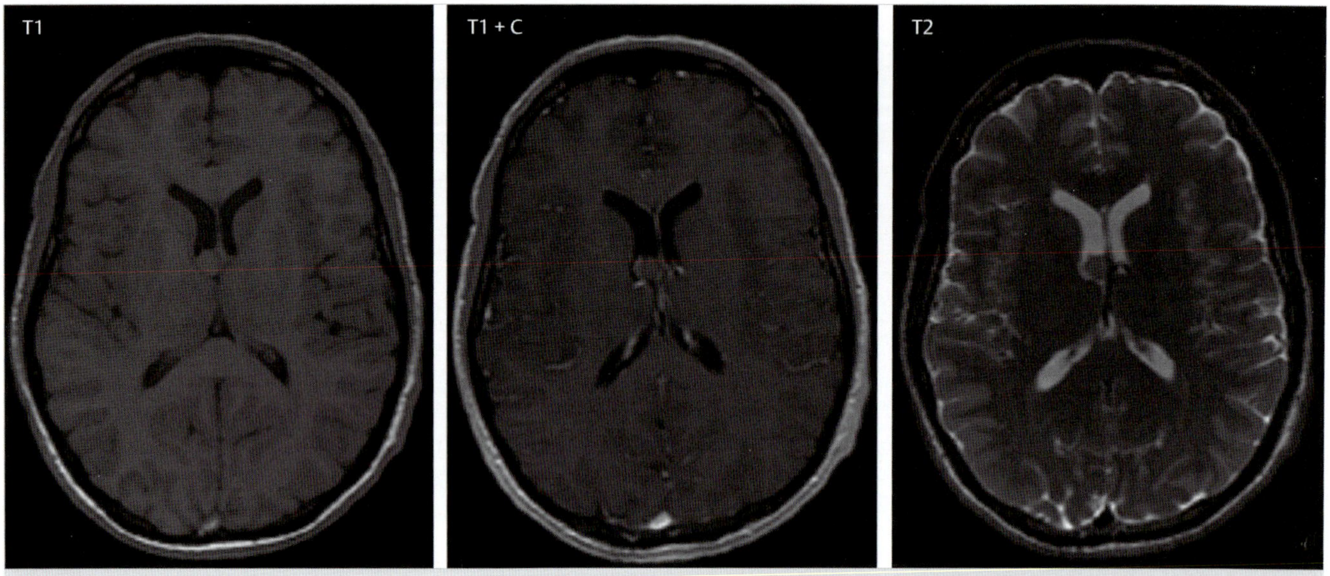


Fig. 6.4 A 42-year-old male presented with progressive headaches and dizziness, prompting neuroimaging that demonstrated a 9-mm colloid cyst with mild ventriculomegaly, Colloid Cyst Risk Score (CCRS) 3. The headaches were worse when lying down on his side and better when upright. He was neurologically intact on examination.

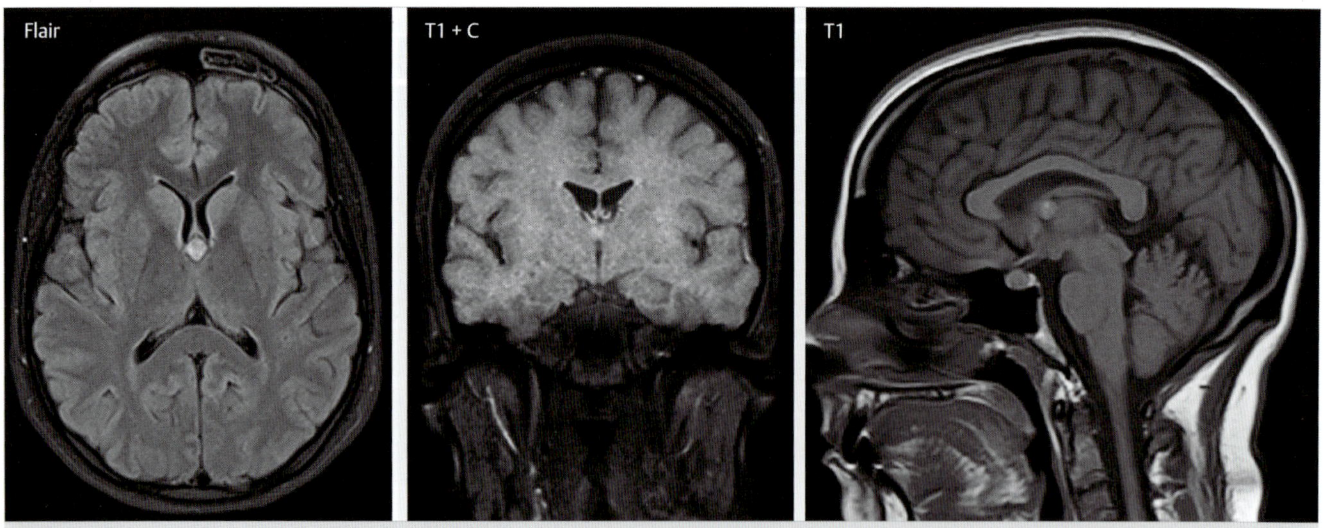


Fig. 6.5 A 25-year-old female presented with headache and blurred vision prompting neuroimaging that demonstrated an 8-mm colloid cyst of the third ventricle, Colloid Cyst Risk Score (CCRS) 4/5. Her symptoms spontaneously resolved suggesting the lesions may have been any incidental finding.

### 6.9.6 Case 6 (▶ Fig. 6.6)

Panelist recommendations: There was a consensus recommendation for surgery with near equipoise for approach. There was a slight majority recommendation for microsurgical resection (57%) over endoscopic resection (43%). There was agreement that surgery be expedited but need not be performed emergently. Observation was not recommended (see ▶ Table 6.1).

### 6.9.7 Case 7 (▶ Fig. 6.7)

Panelist recommendations: There was consensus recommendation for observation, given unknown survival related to oropharyngeal squamous cell carcinoma (100%). If patient had stable local control of cancer with favorable prognosis, surgery would be recommended. If surgery was pursued, there was majority recommendation for endoscopic resection (57%) over microsurgical resection (29%) (see ▶ Table 6.1).

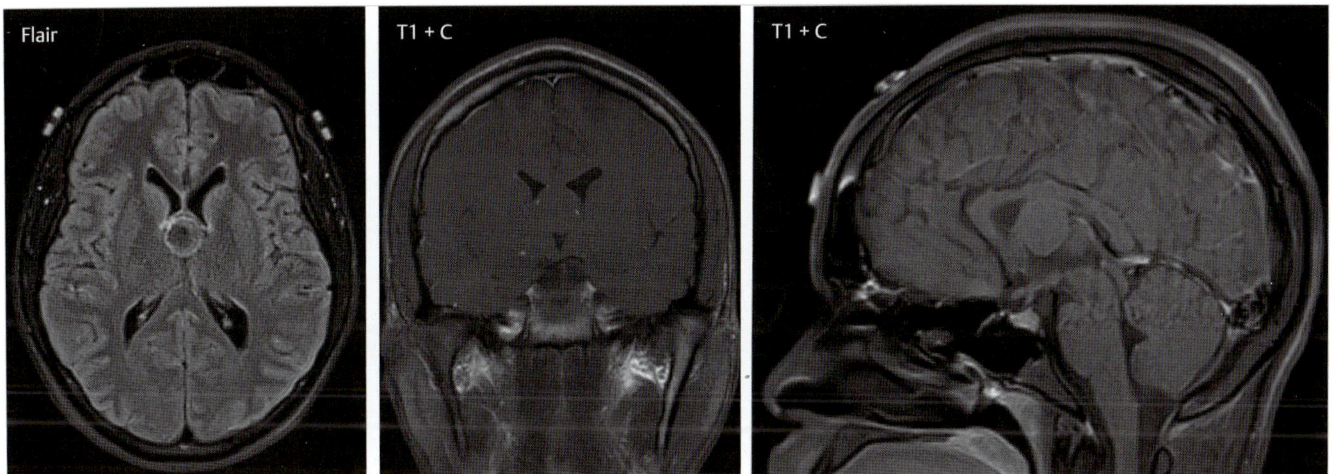


**Fig. 6.6** An 18-year-old male presented with frontal headaches. He was found to have an 18-mm colloid cyst of the third ventricle without hydrocephalus, Colloid Cyst Risk Score (CCRS) 4.

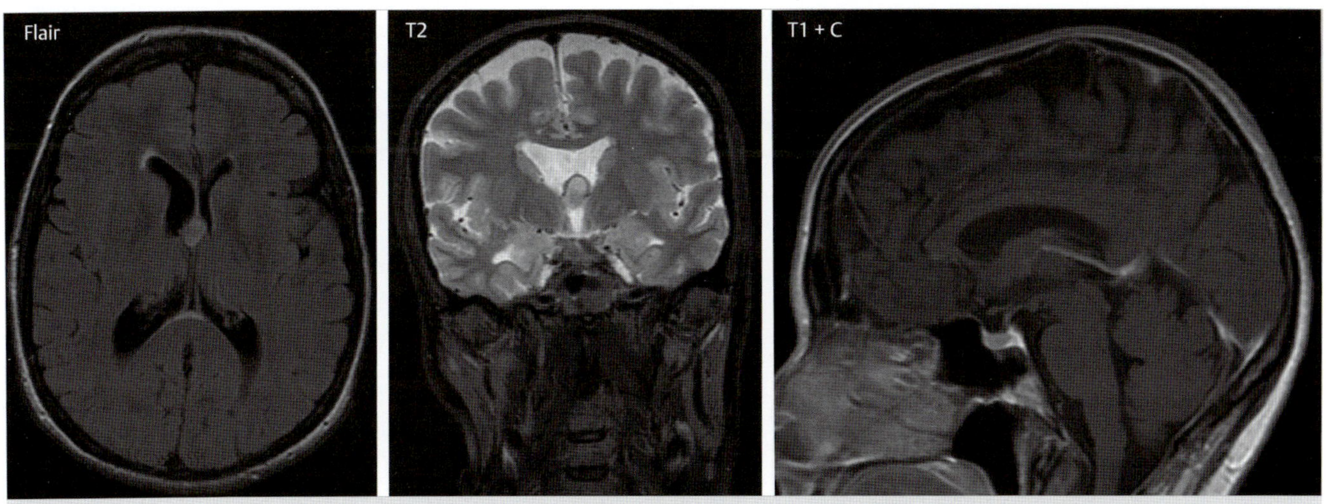


**Fig. 6.7** A 52-year-old female with a history of oropharyngeal squamous cell carcinoma underwent neuroimaging for staging and a 12-mm colloid cyst was incidentally discovered. The cyst was T2 hyperintense and there was unilateral ventricular enlargement, Colloid Cyst Risk Score (CCRS) 4.

### 6.9.8 Case 8 (▶ Fig. 6.8)

Panelist recommendations: There was a consensus recommendation for surgery with a majority recommendation for endoscopic resection (71%) with two panelist recommending microsurgical resection (29%). Observation was not recommended (see ▶ Table 6.1).

### 6.9.9 Case 9 (▶ Fig. 6.9)

Panelist recommendations: There was near equipoise on this case with endoscopic resection slightly favored (43%). Two panelists each recommend microsurgery (29%) and observation (29%). There was strong agreement that syncope in an otherwise healthy young adult with a colloid cyst increases concern, and can be a relative indication for surgery (see ▶ Table 6.1).

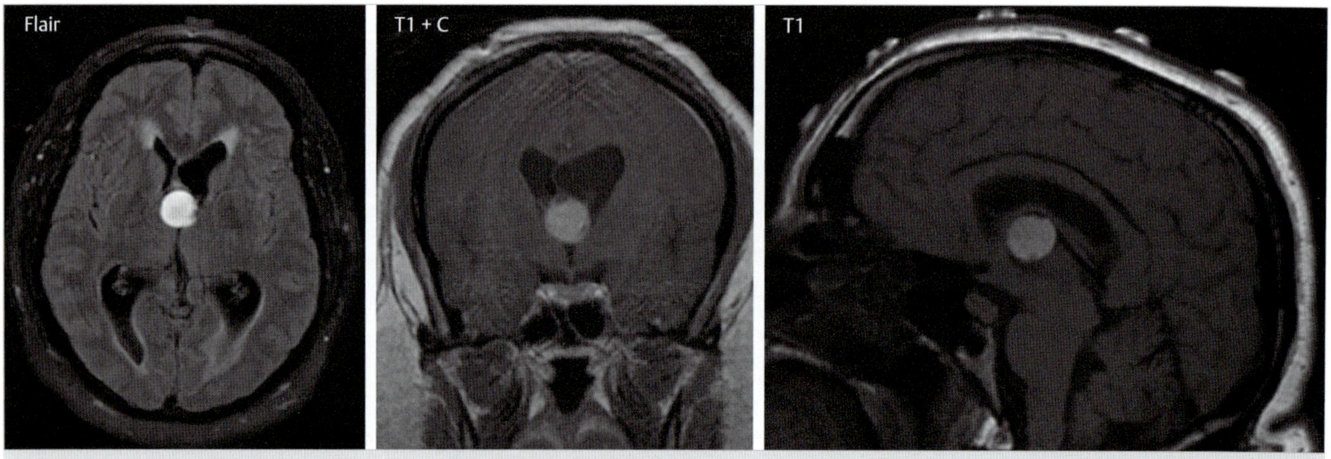


**Fig. 6.8** A 45-year-old male with poorly controlled diabetes presented with acute onset of headache, nausea, vomiting, and ataxia. He also described chronic decline in memory. Imaging revealed an 18-mm T2-hyperintense colloid cyst with marked ventriculomegaly and transependymal flow, Colloid Cyst Risk Score (CCRS) 5.

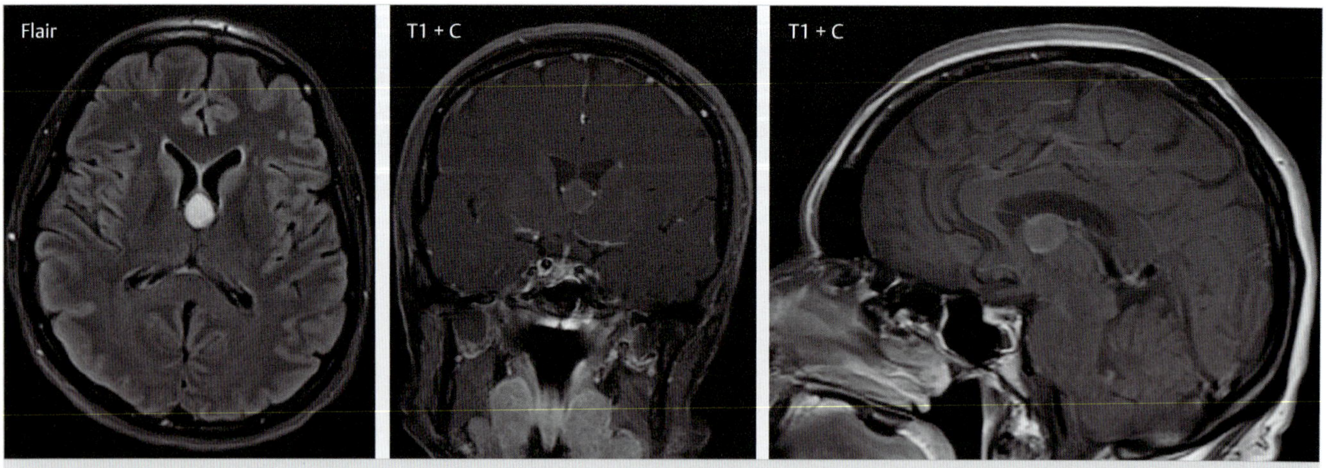


**Fig. 6.9** A 47-year-old female with chronic headaches presented with a presyncopal event. Neuroimaging demonstrated an 11-mm colloid cyst, T2/FLAIR hyperintense, with mild ventriculomegaly without transependymal flow, Colloid Cyst Risk Score (CCRS) 5.

## 6.9.10 Case 10 (▶ Fig. 6.10)

Panelist recommendations: There was near-consensus recommendation for observation (86%) with a single surgeon recommending endoscopic resection (14%). Several panelists felt strongly that there was no indication for surgery (see ▶ Table 6.1).

## 6.9.11 Case 11 (▶ Fig. 6.11)

Panelist recommendations: There was near-consensus recommendation for observation (86%), with a single surgeon recommending endoscopic resection with upfront septostomy for transseptal approach (14%). If the lesion became symptomatic or the patient developed ventriculomegaly, two surgeons stated they would recommend IHTC with interforniceal approach. One additional panelist would recommend TCTV without interforniceal approach. There was spirited discussion about the interforniceal approach, and one senior neurosurgeon stated categorically that this should never be done given the risk of catastrophic complications. On the contrary, one panelist in favor of the interforniceal approach countered that in cases such as this, where the fornicies are widely splayed by the cyst, the interforniceal approach can be (and is) done safely (see ▶ Table 6.1).

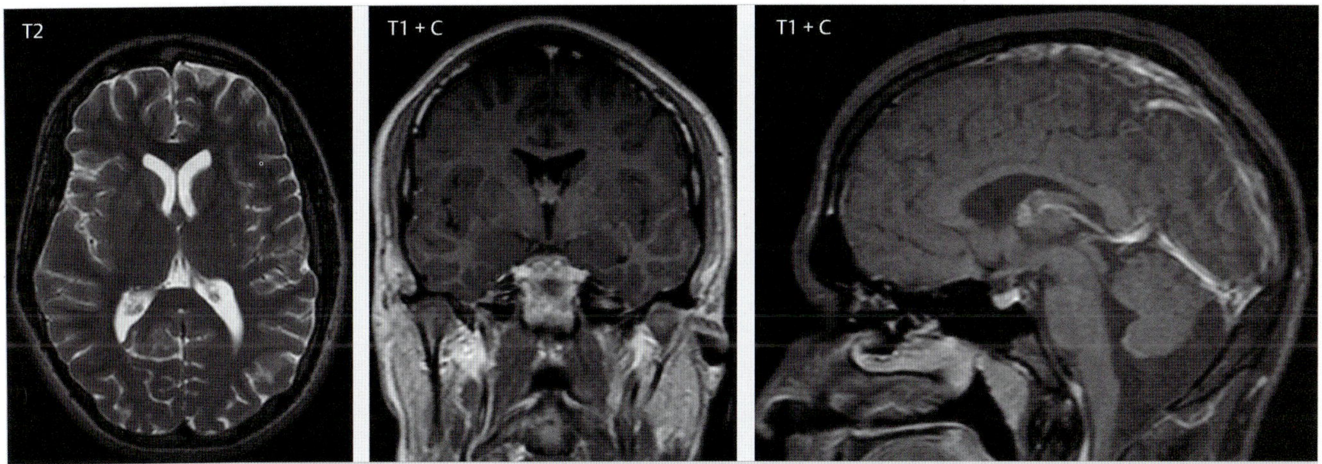


**Fig. 6.10** A 17-year-old male presented with chronic headaches, nausea, and dizziness. Neuroimaging demonstrated a 6-mm colloid cyst, FLAIR hyperintense, Colloid Cyst Risk Score (CCRS) 4.

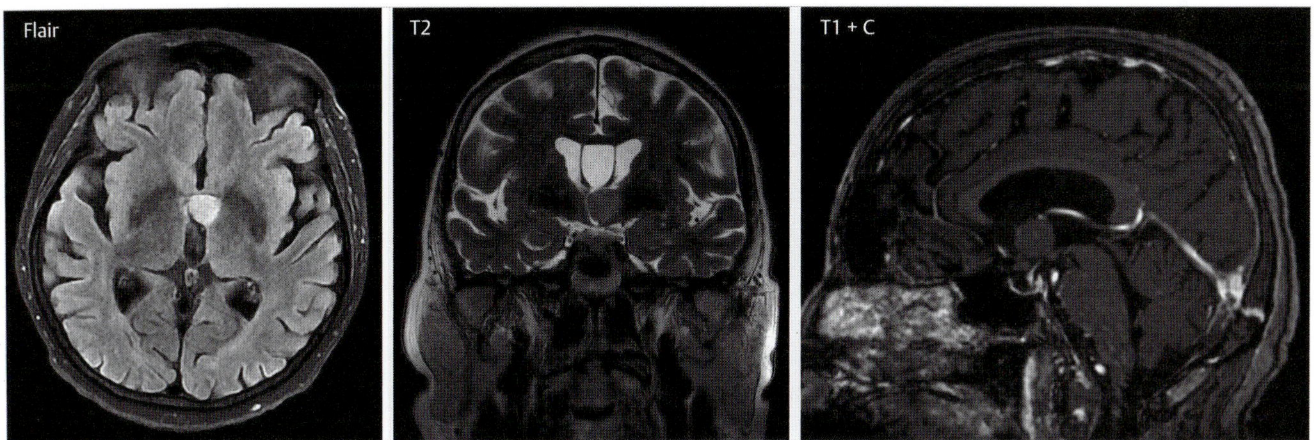


**Fig. 6.11** A 79-year-old Russian-speaking female presented with incidentally discovered 1.6-cm FLAIR-hyperintense colloid cyst, Colloid Cyst Risk Score (CCRS) 3. She had no complaints, was asymptomatic, and neurologically intact. She drives and was fully independent with activities of daily living (ADLs). She lives alone but is in daily contact with family who live nearby.

# References

[1] Boogaarts HD, Decq P, Grotenhuis JA, et al. Long-term results of the neuroendoscopic management of colloid cysts of the third ventricle: a series of 90 cases. Neurosurgery. 2011; 68(1):179–187

[2] Hoffman CE, Savage NJ, Souweidane MM. The significance of cyst remnants after endoscopic colloid cyst resection: a retrospective clinical case series. Neurosurgery. 2013; 73(2):233–237, discussion 237–239

[3] Horn EM, Feiz-Erfan I, Bristol RE, et al. Treatment options for third ventricular colloid cysts: comparison of open microsurgical versus endoscopic resection. Neurosurgery. 2007; 60(4):613–618, discussion 618–620

[4] Isaacs AM, Bezchlibnyk YB, Dronyk J, Urbaneja G, Yong H, Hamilton MG. Long-term outcomes of endoscopic third ventricle colloid cyst resection: case series with a proposed grading system. Oper Neurosurg (Hagerstown). 2020; 19(2): 134–142

[5] Beaumont TL, Limbrick DD, Jr, Rich KM, Wippold FJ, II, Dacey RG, Jr. Natural history of colloid cysts of the third ventricle. J Neurosurg. 2016; 125(6):1420–1430

[6] Zymberg ST, Riechelmann GS, da Costa MDS, Ramalho CO, Cavalheiro S. Third ventricle colloid cysts: an endoscopic case series emphasizing technical variations. Surg Neurol Int. 2021; 12:376

[7] Turillazzi E, Bello S, Neri M, Riezzo I, Fineschi V. Colloid cyst of the third ventricle, hypothalamus, and heart: a dangerous link for sudden death. Diagn Pathol. 2012; 7:144

# Part III

## Open Microsurgical Management of Colloid Cysts



III

# 7 The Microsurgical Resection of Colloid Cysts of Third Ventricle: Transcallosal Approach

*Vinayak Narayan, Simon Hanft, Gaurav Gupta, and Anil Nanda*

**Abstract**

Colloid cyst of third ventricle (CCTV) is a benign tumor, usually seen in the anterior third ventricular region near the foramen of Monro. The gold standard imaging modality to diagnose CCTV is magnetic resonance imaging of the brain. Asymptomatic small CCTV can be managed conservatively with serial neuroimaging to assess for lesion progression. The microsurgery of colloid cyst is challenging due to the deep-seated location, and narrow operative corridor. The main indications of surgery for CCTV are the presence of neurological symptoms, progressive enlargement of cyst, and development of hydrocephalus. Neuronavigation assists the surgeon in defining the extent of craniotomy based on the intraventricular target and helps in following the planned trajectory toward the lesion. The anterior transcallosal approach provides an easier, safer, shorter, and straightforward corridor to expose the third ventricle and foramen of Monro. The complications associated with transcallosal approach include hemiparesis, pericallosal injury, amnesia, seizure, postoperative hydrocephalus, and akinetic mutism. A thorough understanding of the third ventricular anatomy, venous system as well as relevant surrounding structures, careful preoperative planning, and meticulous intraoperative identification of critical structures are the key steps for the safe microsurgical excision of CCTV.

*Keywords:* colloid cyst, third ventricle, approach, surgery, transcallosal

*"This was a highly disappointing procedure thrown in on us when we were just beginning to be confident of exposing third ventricle tumors. Pride goeth before a fall."*

Harvey W. Cushing

## 7.1 Introduction

The microsurgery of intraventricular lesions such as colloid cysts is challenging due to its deep-seated location, narrow operative corridor, and consequent difficult visualization. However, it provides the neurosurgeon an elegant and unique clinical as well as microsurgical experience. Colloid cyst is a benign tumor, usually seen in the anterior third ventricular region near the foramen of Monro. It may vary in size and sometimes may not be diagnosed until it causes rapid decompensation due to the raised intracranial pressure (ICP). The microsurgical approaches for the resection of colloid cyst of third ventricle (CCTV) almost always need the port of entry through the cerebral cortex or corpus callosum—transcortical or interhemispheric transcallosal approaches. Since the first description of the surgery of an intraventricular lesion by Dandy, there has been a constant revolution of the refinements in surgical technique for intraventricular surgery, especially CCTV.[1] The main goals of surgical approach to CCTV include direct trajectory to the cyst in order to avoid damage to eloquent area, minimal retraction of surrounding tissue, optimal corridor space, least cerebrospinal fluid (CSF) contamination, minimal handling of venous structures, possibility to achieve complete excision, and re-establish the CSF flow. In this chapter, we discuss the transcallosal approach for the resection of CCTV with emphasis on the relevant regional anatomy, surgical techniques, and complications and their management, based on the senior author's (Anil Nanda) experience.

## 7.2 Epidemiology and Clinical Features

CCTV is not an uncommon tumor accounting for 0.5 to 2% of all intracranial tumors with an incidence of 3.2 per million per year.[2] It is usually seen in between third and fifth decades with an estimated prevalence of 1 in 8500 people.[3,4] It is usually diagnosed more commonly in males than females.

Multiple previous reports suggest that over 50% of the colloid cysts are symptomatic at presentation; however, incidental diagnosis is also not infrequent.[5,6] It may present with acute, subacute, or chronic hydrocephalus and manifest commonly as headache, vomiting, vision disturbances, gait ataxia, and cognitive impairment while syncope, tinnitus, seizures, incontinence, and psychological symptoms are rare manifestations. Sudden death due to acute hydrocephalus has also been reported in CCTV.[7] The incidental CCTV may progress and rarely undergo contraction and symptom regression.

## 7.3 Clinical Evaluation and Radiological Diagnosis

The clinical picture of raised ICP without any localization or lateralizing signs suggests the possibility of an intraventricular lesion with hydrocephalus. The presence of postural headache, papilledema, and bradycardia without any motor weakness may give a clue regarding the presence of CCTV.

Although computed tomography (CT) of brain is the initial radiological investigation due to the diagnostic ease in surveillance workup, the gold standard investigation for CCTV is magnetic resonance imaging (MRI) of the brain. In CT the lesion appears isodense or hyperdense in the region of foramen of Monro. However, MRI reveals the precise location, size, and extent of the lesion which are the key factors for surgical planning. Apart from routine MRI sequences, diffusion tractography imaging provides more information on the fiber tracts which helps in choosing the least disruptive operative trajectory to approach the lesion.[8] Many surgeons advise for magnetic resonance venography (MRV) to get a clear picture of the draining parasagittal cortical veins and also while considering choroidal dissection to approach the third ventricle.

## 7.4 Surgical Planning and Approach Strategies

The management of CCTV includes both observation and surgery. Asymptomatic small CCTV can be managed conservatively with serial neuroimaging to assess for lesion progression.[2,6] The surgical planning is very crucial in optimizing the surgical goal and reducing patient morbidity. There are various surgical approaches for the resection of CCTV and the main aim of all approaches is the least disruption and minimal displacement of normal anatomy. The basic requirements in any intraventricular approach which helps in complete excision of CCTV with minimal morbidity are adequate brain relaxation, optimum exposure of lesion, and proper visualization while manipulating the deep neural structures. The lateral and third ventricles can be accessed by transcallosal, transcortical, and, in some cases, supracerebellar, subfrontal, pterional, and transtentorial approaches. Additionally, endoscopic techniques are other surgical options for operative management. In this chapter, we focus on the surgical indications, techniques of transcallosal approach and related anatomy of the surgical corridor, tips/pitfalls of the surgical method, and associated potential complications and their management.

## 7.5 Indications for Surgery

The main indications of surgery for CCTV are:

- Presence of neurological symptoms.
- Progressive enlargement of cyst.
- Development of hydrocephalus.

Asymptomatic patients with small cyst and absent hydrocephalus are not an indication for surgery.[2,6,9] In acute deterioration of previously conscious patients, the immediate placement of external ventricular drain or ventriculoperitoneal shunt appears to be a good option prior to definitive surgery as it diverts the CSF flow. However, performing lumbar puncture for draining CSF is contraindicated as it can lead to disastrous herniation.

## 7.6 Surgical Anatomy of Third Ventricle and Technique of Transcallosal Approach

The precise knowledge of the microsurgical anatomy of the third ventricle is very crucial for the complete excision of CCTV. The lateral ventricles communicate with the third ventricle at the foramen of Monro and the latter drains posteriorly into the aqueduct of Sylvius. Approximately one-third part of the third ventricle is located anterior to the foramen of Monro. The anterior wall of third ventricle is formed mainly by the lamina terminalis, which extends from the optic chiasm to the rostrum of the corpus callosum. The columns of fornix and anterior commissure are related to the superolateral and anterosuperior walls, respectively. The lateral wall is constituted posterosuperiorly by the thalamus and inferiorly by the hypothalamus. The thalamic projection, massa intermedia, bridges the third ventricle at the superior–posterior end. The floor of the third ventricle is formed by the optic chiasm in the anterior end, which dips into the infundibular recess before slanting superiorly and posteriorly over the tuber cinereum, the two mammillary bodies, and the posterior perforated substance, located anterior to the cerebral peduncles. The aqueduct is located posterior to peduncles, surrounded by tegmentum of midbrain. The roof of the third ventricle starts anteriorly at the foramen of Monro and ends posteriorly in the suprapineal recess. The roof is separated from the lateral wall by the choroidal fissure. The fornices are attached to the body of fornix in the anterior part of roof and separate into the forniceal crura in the posterior part with an interforniceal white matter connection called the hippocampal commissure. The double-layered trabecular pial tissue covering the fornices and hippocampal commissure is termed as tela choroidea. The internal cerebral veins and medial posterior choroidal arteries traverse through the velum interpositum, which is a space between the layers of tela choroidea. The third ventricular choroid plexus is attached to the roof by the tela choroidea, which communicates through the choroidal fissure with the lateral ventricular tela choroidea. The posterior wall of the third ventricle comprises of the aqueduct, the posterior commissure, the pineal body, the habenular commissure, and the suprapineal recess.[10] The anatomy of the third ventricle is demonstrated in ▶ Fig. 7.1.

Dandy described the transcallosal approach for the first time in 1922 to get access into the ventricular system.[1] The approach to the third ventricle by splitting of the midline forniceal raphe was proposed by Edward Busch in 1944.[11] Anterior transcallosal approach, directed through the corpus callosum, is ideal for reaching the anterosuperior part of the third ventricle while posterior transcallosal approach is best suited to lesions that extend upward from the atrium or third ventricle through the posterior part of the splenium or which arise in the splenium and extend into the atrium and third ventricle.[12] We attempt to describe the anterior transcallosal approach in the chapter. The approach needs a standard parasagittal craniotomy in which the craniotomy is taken across the midline by placing contralateral burr holes and stripping the sagittal sinus prior to passing the craniotome. The placement of lumbar drain may be helpful in interhemispheric approach, if the patient does not have hydrocephalus.

The patient is positioned supine with the sagittal suture in vertical plane and head elevated to 20 to 30 degrees.[13] A right frontal horseshoe or bicoronal incision is preferred. A right frontal parasagittal craniotomy is performed with two-thirds of bone flap anterior and one-third of bone flap posterior to the coronal suture. Neuronavigation assists the surgeon in defining the extent of craniotomy based on the intraventricular target and helps in following the planned trajectory toward the lesion. We have attempted small triangular craniotomy in many anterior CCTV cases. The dura mater is opened based on the superior sagittal sinus, and the draining vein, if any, in front of coronal suture needs to be mobilized for the better lateral retraction of the medial frontal lobe. The arachnoid membrane is identified at the depth of the free edge of falx and opening the membrane exposes corpus callosum and anterior cerebral arteries. The pericallosal arteries must to be identified, and the approach is best directed in between these arteries. The part of the corpus callosum superior to the foramen of Monro is split in the midline. An incision of 1.5 to 2 cm in length provides satisfactory access to both lateral ventricles. The surgical steps to ap-

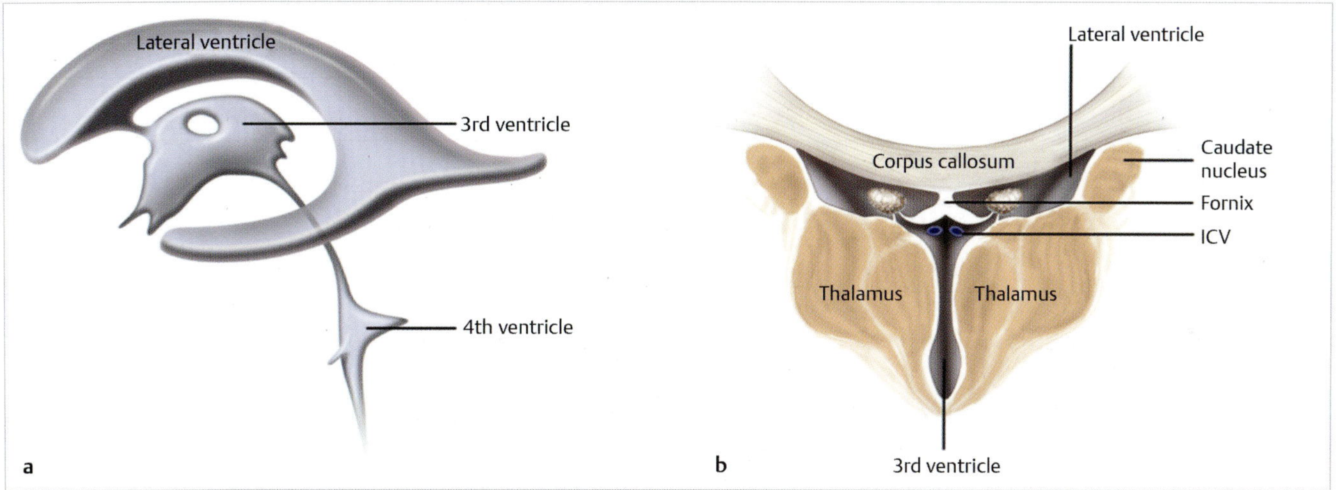


**Fig. 7.1 (a)** Schematic diagram showing the gross anatomy of ventricular system. **(b)** Coronal image showing the anatomy of the third ventricle and related structures. ICV, internal cerebral vein.

proach the third ventricle are demonstrated in ▶ Fig. 7.2. Once the ventricle is opened by the transcallosal approach, the foramen of Monro is identified by tracing the choroid plexus and thalamostriate vein which converge at foramen. There are many methods/approaches to explore the deeper portion of the third ventricle. There are three primary variations of transcallosal approach, namely, transforaminal, interforniceal, and trans/suprachoroidal approaches, of which the former two provide the ability to access and good view of the anterior and middle part of the third ventricle without transecting the fornix.[13] Although the transforaminal approach through the dilated foramen of Monro is the simplest and safest approach, which requires the least manipulation of critical neurovascular structures, and is also ideal for cystic lesions, the interforniceal approach provides the possibility for using combined corridor through foramen of Monro and midline raphae incision. The interforniceal approach is good if the lesion bulges superiorly, displacing the fornices laterally. The trans/suprachoroidal approach is mainly intended for lesions in the middle or posterior third ventricle. If the lesion bulges onto the floor of the lateral ventricle, the subchoroidal approach through the velum interpositum lateral to the internal cerebral veins is a good option.[14]

## 7.7 Advantages, Limitations, and Complications of the Anterior Transcallosal Approach

The anterior transcallosal approach provides an easier, safer, shorter, and straightforward corridor to expose the third ventricle and foramen of Monro than transcortical approach. It does not disrupt the cortex and is rarely associated with postoperative seizures.[15] Also, it is easier to perform than transventricular approach if the ventricles are of normal size or minimally enlarged. The functional consequences are also relatively rare.[16] However, the extent of lateral exposure within the lateral ventricle is quite limited with the approach.

The complications associated with transcallosal approach include hemiparesis due to venous infarct or venous injury or retraction injury, pericallosal vessel injury, amnesia, seizure, postoperative hydrocephalus, and akinetic mutism due to cingulate gyri injury.[17,18] Patients with crossed dominance are generally considered contraindicated for this approach as it may lead to speech and writing defects in such population.[19,20] The preoperative evaluation with MRV, perioperative administration of antiepileptics, careful craniotomy placement for avoiding the damage to parasagittal draining veins, and the meticulous identification of the critical neurovascular structures intraoperatively are the key factors helping in avoiding the major complications.

## 7.8 Illustrated Clinical Case of CCTV—How I Do It?

A 52-year-old male presented in the clinic with history of occasional headache for 1 month. He did not have any significant past medical/surgical history. He was neurologically intact on examination. His cranial nerve and sensory-motor examination appeared normal. He was evaluated with MRI of brain, and it showed a well-circumscribed T1 hyperintense, T2 iso–hyperintense lesion in the anterior third ventricle which was not enhancing on contrast injection which is suggestive of CCTV (▶ Fig. 7.3). The preoperative neuropsychological evaluation appears normal.

## 7.9 Nuances in Clinical Decision-Making and Approach toward Management

The clinical history of headache in the patient without any specific neurologic localization features and MR imaging findings showing anterior third ventricular colloid cyst makes him a candidate for the surgical resection of the cyst. To improve the symptoms caused by a ventricular tumor and to prevent further deterioration, total removal of the ventricular lesion is usually attempted and may be performed as first-line therapy. But in

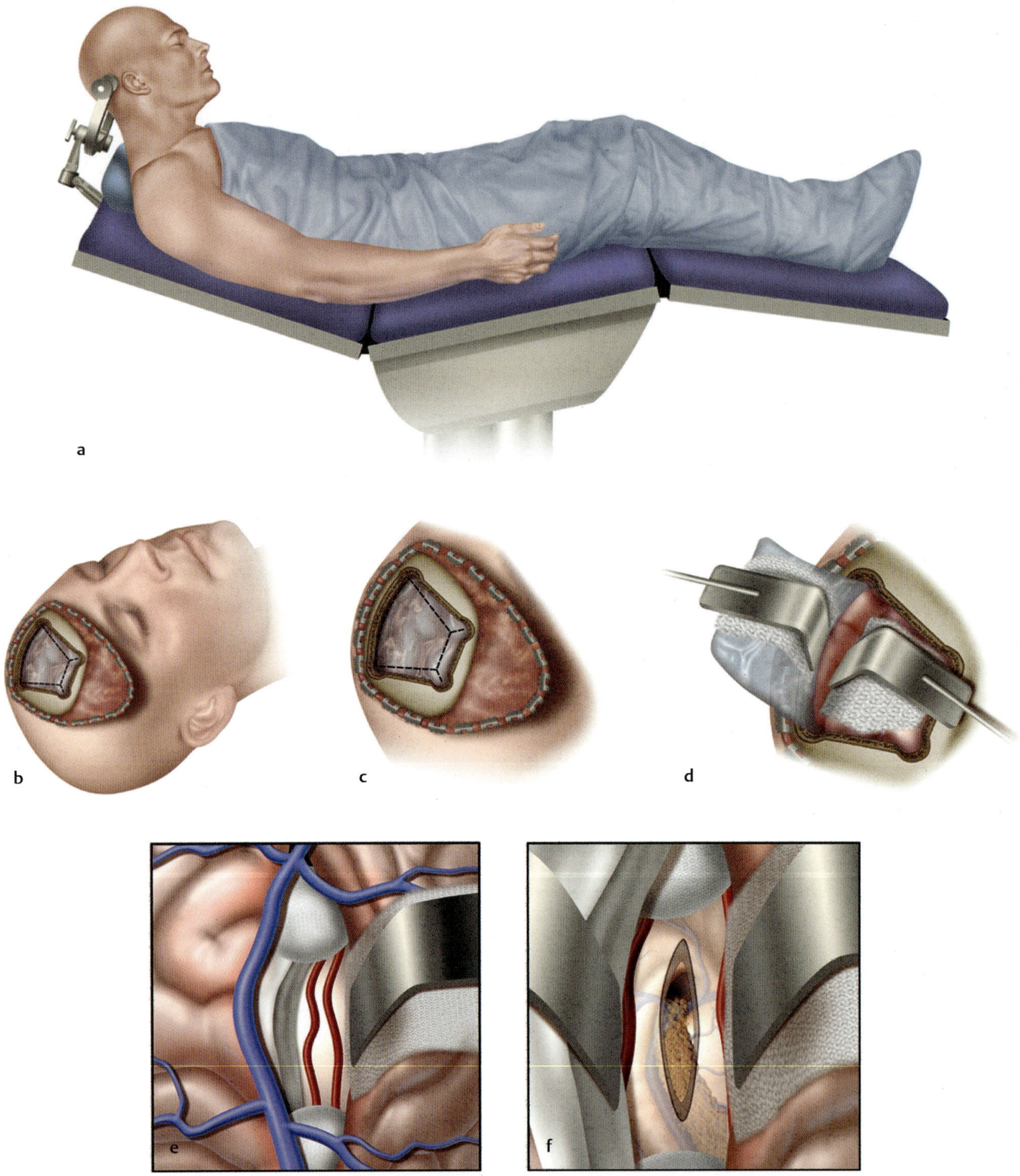

**Fig. 7.2** Schematic representation of the steps of anterior transcallosal approach. **(a)** Positioning of the patient (head in neutral position elevated by 20 to 30 degrees and fixed with Mayfield pins). **(b)** Anatomical orientation of the skin incision and parasagittal craniotomy. **(c)** Magnified view of the burr holes and line of parasagittal craniotomy. **(d)** Developing the microsurgical corridor between the falx (*left*) and frontal lobe (*right*) using brain retractors. **(e)** Exposure of the pericallosal arteries on the surface of corpus callosum with cotton balls on anterior and posterior aspects for providing optimum retraction. **(f)** Separating the pericallosal arteries to either sides and placing 1.5- to 2-cm-long incision on the corpus callosum to access the anterior third ventricular cyst.

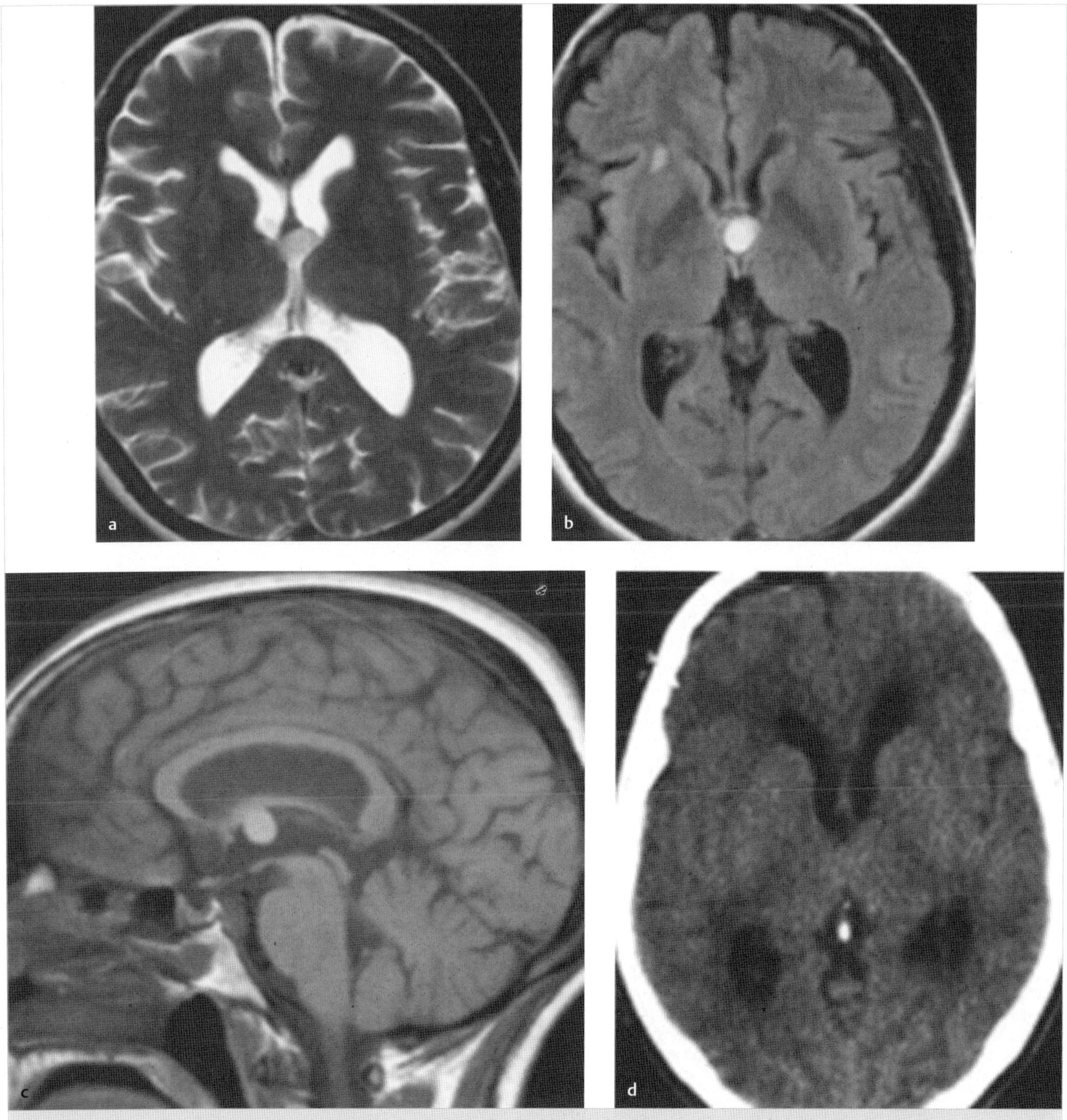

Fig. 7.3 **(a)** Preoperative T2 axial magnetic resonance (MR) image demonstrating the anterior third ventricular colloid cyst. **(b)** Preoperative fluid-attenuated inversion recovery (FLAIR) axial image showing the colloid cyst. **(c)** Preoperative T1 sagittal image showing the colloid cyst. **(d)** Postoperative computed tomography (CT) demonstrating the complete excision of the cyst.

cases where hydrocephalus and the resultant raised ICP are the cause of acute deterioration, re-establishment of CSF circulation by external ventricular drain or ventriculoperitoneal shunt needs to be considered on emergency basis. The aforementioned CSF diversion surgery can be followed by the definitive tumor excision procedure. In this particular case, as the ventricle size appears to be normal and the patient does not have objective signs of raised ICP, the direct surgery for the excision of CCTV by anterior transcallosal approach is considered. The senior author has previously reported the short operating time, acceptable level of complications, and shorter postoperative hospital stay after the microsurgical management of CCTV, which makes this approach of management quite comparable or even better than the endoscopic management.[17]

## 7.10 Surgical Plan and Preparation

The excision of CCTV is a surgical challenge due to its relatively rare occurrence, deep-seated location, proximity to neurovascular structures, and narrow surgical corridor. The technique of right frontoparietal parasagittal craniotomy, anterior transcallosal approach, and excision of the colloid cyst in this patient need careful proper preoperative planning, MR imaging of the brain with MRV, and intraoperative neuronavigation which helps in planning the placement of burr holes to avoid damage not only to the sinus but also to the irregular bridging veins. Also, the intraoperative sensory and motor-evoked potentials monitoring helps in getting a clear picture of retraction pressure on the brain surface. The venous anatomical variations favoring the surgery can be studied from preoperative MR images. A comprehensive neuropsychological evaluation done in this patient consisted of a brief assessment of intellectual, sensorimotor, language, attention, intellectual, and executive skills. A similar comparative examination in the postoperative period may yield more objective outcome assessment which helps in planning further rehabilitation. Also, perioperative antiepileptics administration is crucial to prevent seizures in the postoperative period.

## 7.11 Step-by-Step Techniques in Anterior Transcallosal Approach and Excision of CCTV (▶ Fig. 7.4)

- **Position:** Under general anesthesia with endotracheal intubation, the head was fixed in Mayfield headpins with the patient supine and the head elevated 20 to 30 degrees above the horizontal level. The registration of the neuronavigation device is crucial prior to starting the procedure.
- **Incision:** A horseshoe-shaped skin incision was placed, and the flap was raised. Wound hemostasis was achieved by bipolar cautery.
- **Craniotomy:** Right frontoparietal parasagittal craniotomy with two-thirds of the anteroposterior distance in front of the coronal suture and one-third posterior to the coronal suture. Small triangular craniotomy with the help of neuronavigation as mentioned before is also recommended. The craniotomy should be meticulous to avoid inadvertent injury to the superior sagittal sinus. As the bone flap goes more posterior, the better anterior angulated corridor helps in better access to the anterior third ventricle.
- **Dural opening:** A curvilinear dural opening was made based on superior sagittal sinus, tack-up sutures were placed, and the dura was retracted adequately to prevent ooze from the superior sagittal sinus by creating a tamponade effect.
- **Approach to anterior corpus callosum:** Interhemispheric dissection was done after retracting the medial frontal lobe laterally till corpus callosum was identified. The bridging veins were mobilized adequately, and retraction was minimal to avoid complications. We prefer to use very narrow retractors in such surgeries. The arachnoid membrane over the callosum was opened. This exposed the corpus callosum, and its key identifying features were glistening white color, relative hypovascularity, and the presence of pericallosal arteries on its surface. Once confirmed, it was incised about 1 to 2 cm in length for the optimum accessibility of CCTV. Neuronavigation assists in planning the length of incision. Sometimes cingulate gyrus and callosomarginal arteries may be misidentified as corpus callosum and pericallosal arteries, respectively.
- **Approach to ventricular system:** After callosal opening there are multiple choices for entering into the ventricular system depending on the lesion location and surgeon's expertise. In this case, transforaminal approach was undertaken through the foramen of Monro as it provides a natural corridor to the third ventricle without disturbing the anatomy. In some cases where the foramen is expanded due to the lesion, the excision is easier. Tracing the choroid plexus is the most reliable step to get into the foramen of Monro and the third ventricle. The anatomical orientation can be confirmed by the joining of thalamostriate vein (lateral) and septal vein (medial) to form internal cerebral vein (ICV) at the posterior margin of foramen. The cyst was identified, contents were decompressed completely, and gross total excision of the capsule was performed to avoid recurrence. External ventricular drain under direct visualization was also placed after achieving hemostasis to prevent postoperative hydrocephalus.
- **Closure:** Dural closure was performed in a standard fashion with 4–0 nurolon in watertight fashion to avoid pseudomeningocele. Bone flap was replaced and fixed with titanium miniplates and screws. Galea was closed using interrupted vicryl sutures and skin was stapled.

## 7.12 Postoperative Course and Follow-Up

The patient recovered well from anesthesia and surgery without any complications. He was admitted in neurosurgical intensive unit for observation and monitoring. External ventricular drain was placed at a height of 10 to 15 cm above the external acoustic meatus level till the CSF became clear. Gradual weaning of the drain was done. Postoperative CT imaging done 24 hours after the procedure showed complete excision of the lesion. He did not have any complications like delayed hydrocephalus, pseudomeningocele, or subdural fluid collection. The patient was discharged from the hospital 5 days after surgery. At 6 months follow-up at clinic, he was neurologically intact with complete resolution of the symptoms.

## 7.13 Future Trends

Significant developments have been achieved in the treatment of colloid cyst since the original technique of anterior transcallosal approach was described. The advancements in modern neuroimaging, navigation-guided surgery, and further refinements in microsurgical techniques including flexible endoscope assistance might be the arena of future developments in colloid cyst surgery. The technological innovations along each of these frontiers will result in a better prognostic outcome.

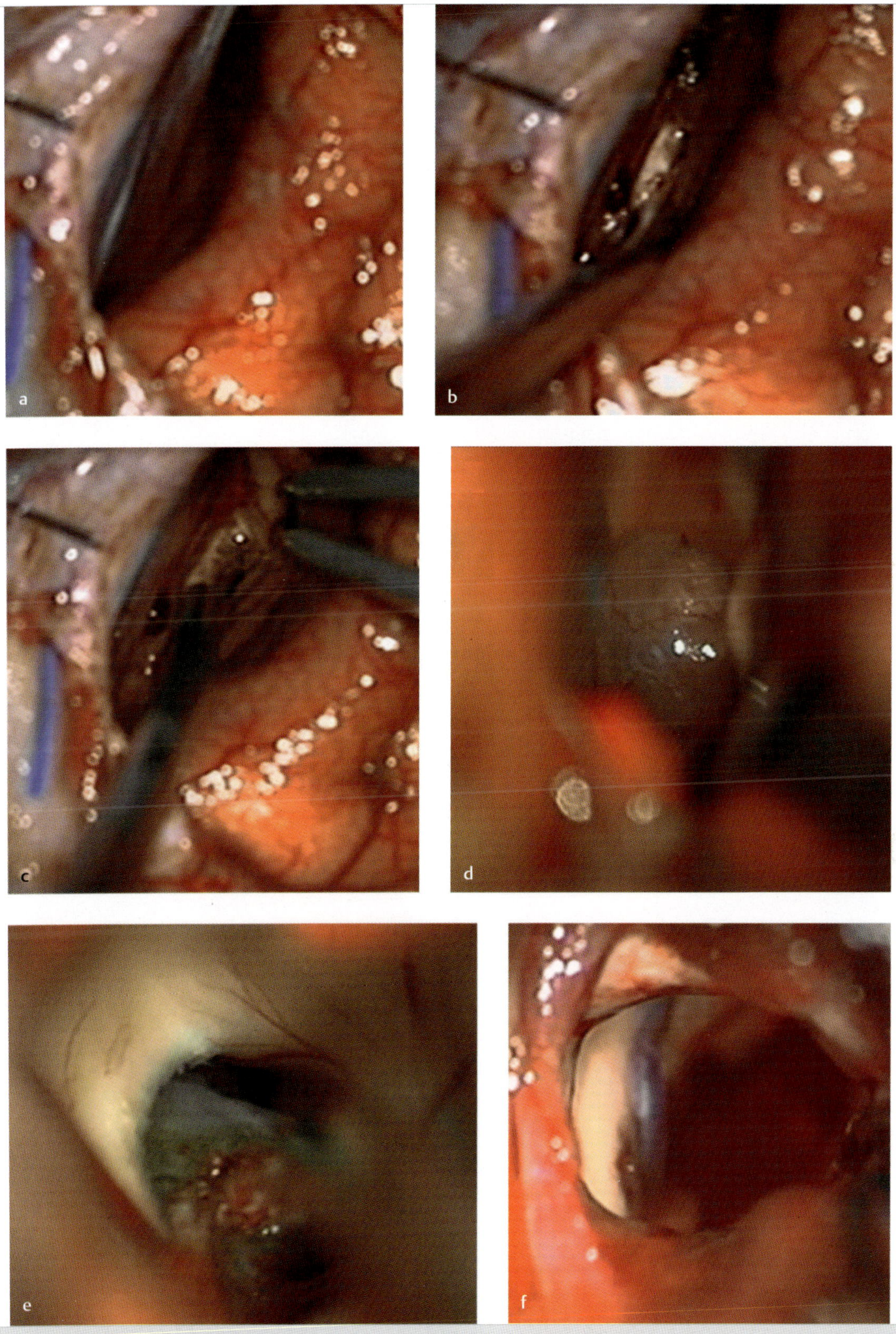

**Fig. 7.4** Intraoperative views of various stages of microsurgical excision of colloid cyst through anterior transcallosal approach. **(a)** The surgical corridor between the falx (*left*) and medial frontal lobe parenchyma (*right*). **(b)** Exposing the corpus callosum (glistening white structure) at the depth of the surgical corridor. **(c)** Opening the corpus callosum for accessing the third ventricle. **(d)** Colloid cyst is visualized at the anterior third ventricular region. **(e)** Excision of the cyst through the transforaminal route. **(f)** Foraminal region after the complete excision of the cyst (septal vein is noted medially, *left*).

## 7.14 Conclusion

Due to the central location and anatomical/functional complexity, the microsurgery of the third ventricle represents in many ways one of the major challenges in intracranial surgery. In addition to the advantages of avoiding cortical incision and providing a set of adequate direct port of entries/trajectories, the anterior transcallosal approach provides natural planes of dissection to the anterior third ventricle. A thorough understanding of the third ventricular anatomy, venous system as well as relevant surrounding structures, careful preoperative planning, and meticulous intraoperative identification of critical structures are the key steps for the safe microsurgical excision of the CCTV.

## Acknowledgments

We thank our graphic designer, Mr. Martinelli Victor Valcin, for the great support in the preparation of the anatomical and surgical illustrations.

## References

[1] Dandy WE. Diagnosis, localization and removal of tumors of the third ventricle. Bull Johns Hopkins Hosp. 1922; 33:188–189

[2] Beaumont TL, Limbrick DD, Jr, Rich KM, Wippold FJ, II, Dacey RG, Jr. Natural history of colloid cysts of the third ventricle. J Neurosurg. 2016; 125(6):1420–1430

[3] de Witt Hamer PC, Verstegen MJT, De Haan RJ, et al. High risk of acute deterioration in patients harboring symptomatic colloid cysts of the third ventricle. J Neurosurg. 2002; 96(6):1041–1045

[4] Gbejuade H, Plaha P, Porter D. Spontaneous regression of a third ventricle colloid cyst. Br J Neurosurg. 2011; 25(5):655–657

[5] Mathiesen T, Grane P, Lindgren L, Lindquist C. Third ventricle colloid cysts: a consecutive 12-year series. J Neurosurg. 1997; 86(1):5–12

[6] Pollock BE, Huston J, III. Natural history of asymptomatic colloid cysts of the third ventricle. J Neurosurg. 1999; 91(3):364–369

[7] Decq P, Le Guerinel C, Brugières P, et al. Endoscopic management of colloid cysts. Neurosurgery. 1998; 42(6):1288–1294, discussion 1294–1296

[8] Yaşargil MG, Abdulrauf SI. Surgery of intraventricular tumors. Neurosurgery. 2008; 62(6) Suppl 3:1029–1040, discussion 1040–1041

[9] Sheikh AB, Mendelson ZS, Liu JK. Endoscopic versus microsurgical resection of colloid cysts: a systematic review and meta-analysis of 1,278 patients. World Neurosurg. 2014; 82(6):1187–1197

[10] Rhoton AL, Jr. The lateral and third ventricles. Neurosurgery. 2002; 51(4) Suppl:S207–S271

[11] Busch E. A new approach for the removal of tumors of the third ventricle. Acta Psychiatr Scand. 1944; 19(1–2):57–60

[12] Lucas TH II, Ellenbogen RG. Microsurgical approaches to the ventricular system. In: Ellenbogen RG, Abdulrauf SI, Sekhar LN, eds. Principles of Neurological Surgery. 3rd ed. Elsevier Saunders; 2012:651–664

[13] Rhoton AL, Jr, Yamamoto I, Peace DA. Microsurgery of the third ventricle: Part 2. Operative approaches. Neurosurgery. 1981; 8(3):357–373

[14] Nair S, Gopalakrishnan CV, Menon G, Easwer HV, Abraham M. Interhemispheric transcallosal transforaminal approach and its variants to colloid cyst of third ventricle: technical issues based on a single institutional experience of 297 cases. Asian J Neurosurg. 2016; 11(3):292–297

[15] Apuzzo ML, Chikovani OK, Gott PS, et al. Transcallosal, interfornicial approaches for lesions affecting the third ventricle: surgical considerations and consequences. Neurosurgery. 1982; 10(5):547–554

[16] Winston KR, Cavazzuti V, Arkins T. Absence of neurological and behavioral abnormalities after anterior transcallosal operation for third ventricular lesions. Neurosurgery. 1979; 4(5):386–393

[17] Sampath R, Vannemreddy P, Nanda A. Microsurgical excision of colloid cyst with favorable cognitive outcomes and short operative time and hospital stay: operative techniques and analyses of outcomes with review of previous studies. Neurosurgery. 2010; 66(2):368–374, discussion 374–375

[18] Apuzzo MJ, Litofsky NS. Surgery in and around the anterior third ventricle. In: Apuzzo MJ, ed. Brain Surgery. New York: Churchill-Livingstone; 1993:541–579

[19] Geschwind N. Disconnexion syndromes in animals and man. I. Brain. 1965; 88 (2):237–294

[20] Heilman KM, Watson RT, Valenstein E. Localization of lesions in neglect. In: Heilman K, Valenstein E, eds. Clinical Neuropsychology. New York: Oxford University Press; 1985:243–293

# 8 The Transcortical Approach

*Hussein A. Zeineddine, David M. Panczykowski, and Arthur Day*

**Abstract**
Colloid cyst can lead to significant life-threatening consequences including hydrocephalus and sudden death. Surgical resection of these lesions should be in the arsenal of all neurosurgeons. This chapter focuses on the principles of surgical management utilizing the transcortical approach.

*Keywords:* colloid cyst, transcortical approach, lateral ventricle, fornix, open surgery

## 8.1 Introduction

The typical colloid cyst (CC) is a midline, histologically benign lesion arising in the roof of the anterior third ventricle, where it has the potential to obstruct cerebrospinal fluid (CSF) flow at the level of the foramen of Monro. In this location, CCs have an intimate anatomic association with the deep venous system (caudate, septal, thalamostriate, and internal cerebral veins), the choroid plexus and its blood supply (the medial posterior choroidal artery [MPChA]), and the fornix, all of which must be protected during any operative manipulation.[1,2,3]

Surgery for those CCs causing hydrocephalus, abrupt onset headaches, or syncope is clearly indicated, but the optimal management strategy for incidentally detected cysts is less clear. All the surgical techniques for the management of CC share three fundamental elements: access to the anterior horn and body of the lateral ventricle, lesion access through the foramen of Monro, and lesion resection. This chapter discusses the technique for transcortical transventricular CC resection, and compares the advantages and disadvantages of this approach over the other choices.[1,2,3]

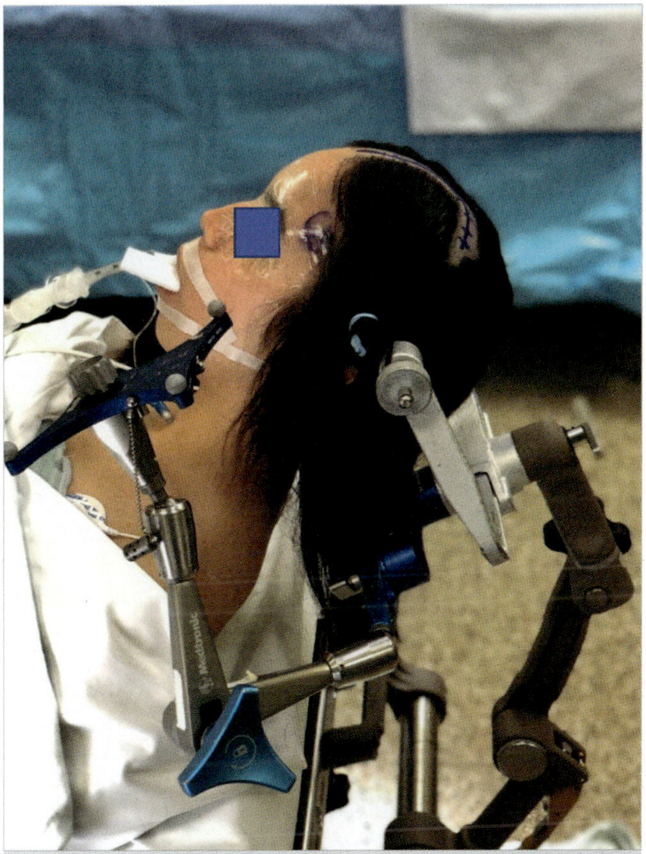

**Fig. 8.1** Operative position (lateral view): The patient is placed in the supine position, with the bed tilted to further elevate the head above the level of the heart. The head is fixated in skull tongs looking straight ahead, but with the ability to rotate the patient as needed to improve the surgeon's hand positions and view. The neck is slightly flexed to allow the operative field to be more horizontal and for the surgeon's hands to rest comfortably.

## 8.2 Surgical Technique

### 8.2.1 Access to the Lateral Ventricle

#### Step 1: Positioning

The patient is placed in the supine position, with the bed tilted to elevate the head above the level of the heart. The neck is maintained in a slightly flexed position to allow the surgeon's hands to be resting comfortably on the head as if flat on a table during the critical portions of the operation (▶ Fig. 8.1).

#### Step 2: Skin Incision

The exposure is always done on the right side unless there is unilateral left ventricular obstruction indicating an eccentric relationship of the cyst at the foramen of Monro. An "L" shaped incision begins at the anterior midline just at the hairline, extends posteriorly on the midline until 2 to 3 cm behind the coronal suture, and then curves 90 degrees toward the right ear approximately 4 cm laterally. A 1-cm strip of hair is removed along this path, with a broader area prepared posteriorly off the midline to allow for placement of a postoperative drain (▶ Fig. 8.2a, b). Raney clips are generally not added for scalp hemostasis, as their use creates a wider zone of hair loss during the healing process. The scalp flap is reflected anteriorly and laterally with low-profile fish-hook retractors creating a flat, unimpeded extracranial working area (▶ Fig. 8.2c).

#### Step 3: Craniotomy/Dural Opening

A 6 × 4 cm rectangular craniotomy is performed, centered just off the midline to the right side, two-third anterior and one-third posterior to the coronal suture (▶ Fig. 8.3a). A "trap-door" dural flap is fashioned based on the superior sagittal sinus, carefully avoiding any injury to veins draining toward the sinus (▶ Fig. 8.3b).

#### Step 4: Corticectomy

A site in the middle frontal gyrus, just at or anterior to the coronal suture and approximately 2 to 3 cm lateral to midline, is

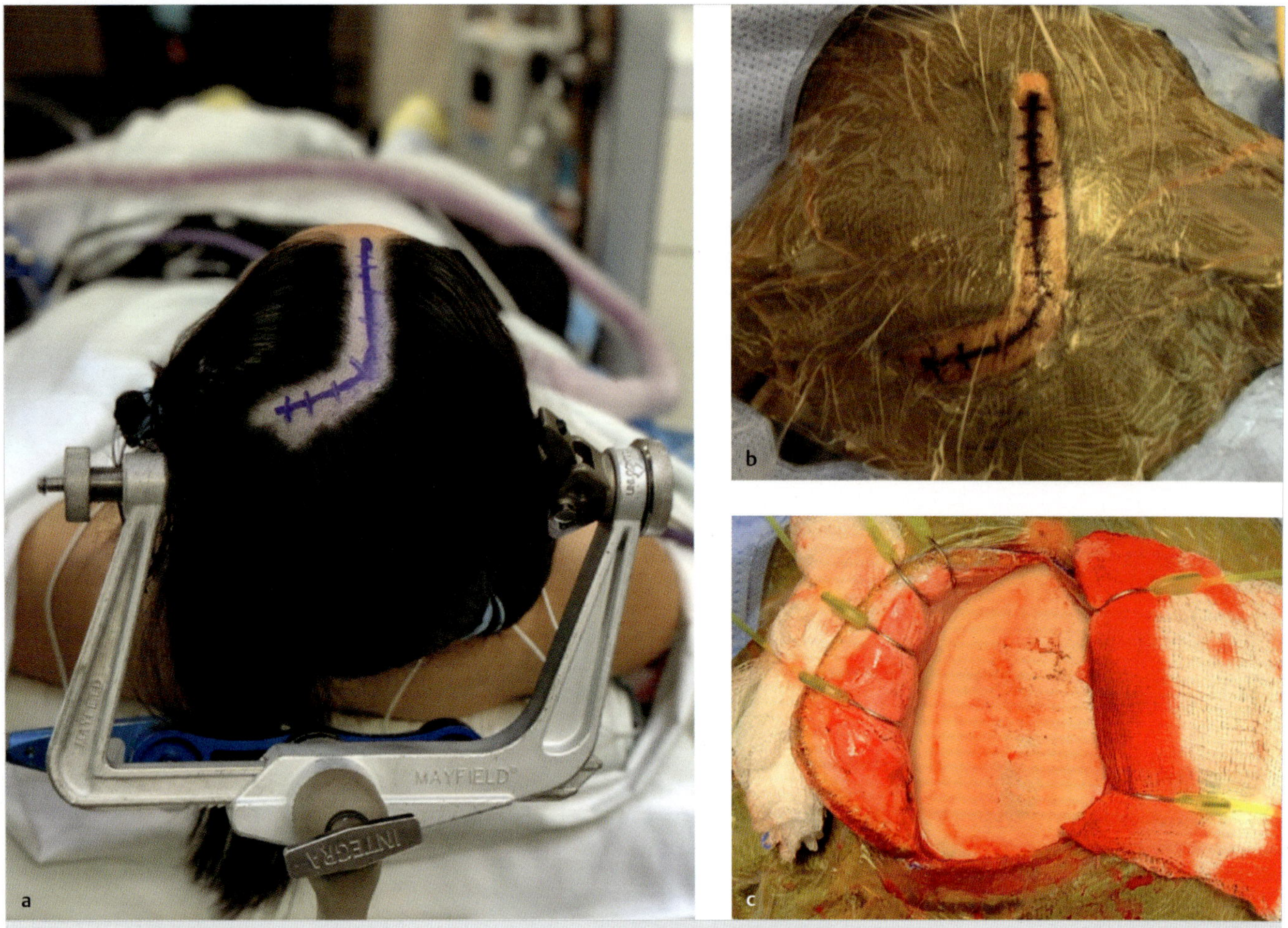


**Fig. 8.2** Incision: **(a)** An "L" shaped pathway is prepared by shaving a thin strip of hair beginning at the anterior midline just at the hairline, extending posteriorly on the midline until 2 to 3 cm behind the coronal suture, and then curving 90 degrees toward the ear approximately 4 cm laterally. **(b)** In almost all cases, a right-sided incision is preferable, but in this case, the patient has a unilaterally obstructed left lateral ventricle, so the planned access is through the left frontal cortex anterior to the coronal suture. **(c)** The scalp flap is reflected anteriorly and laterally with low-profile fish-hook retractors creating a flat, unimpeded working area.

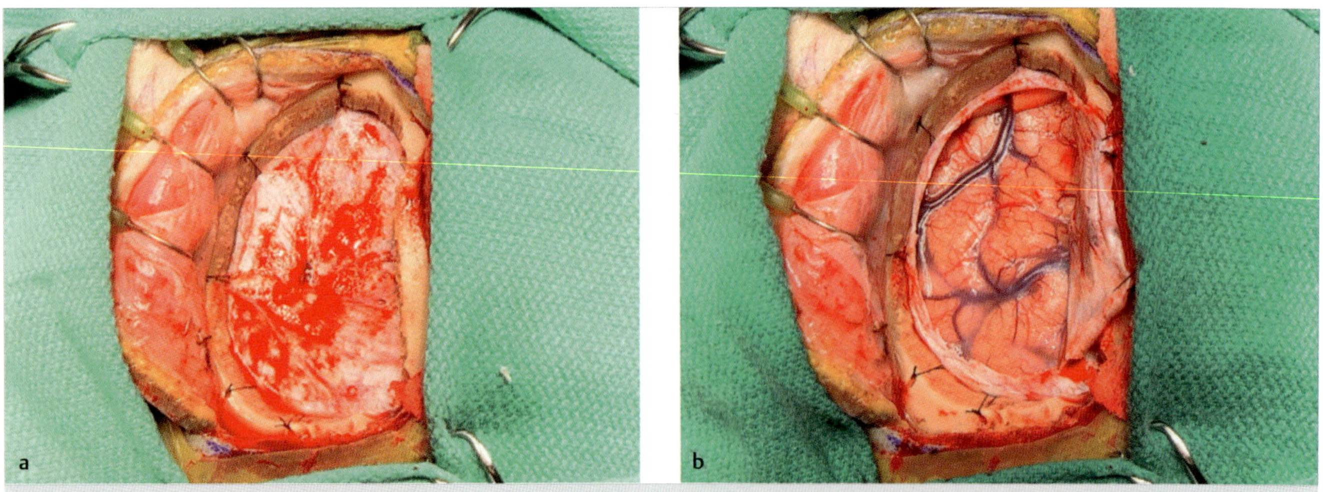

**Fig. 8.3** Craniotomy/dural opening: **(a)** A 6 × 4 cm rectangular craniotomy is performed, centered just off the midline to the right side, two-third anterior and one-third posterior to the coronal suture. **(b)** A "trap-door" dural flap is begun laterally and reflected medially based on the superior sagittal sinus, carefully avoiding any injury to veins draining toward the sinus.

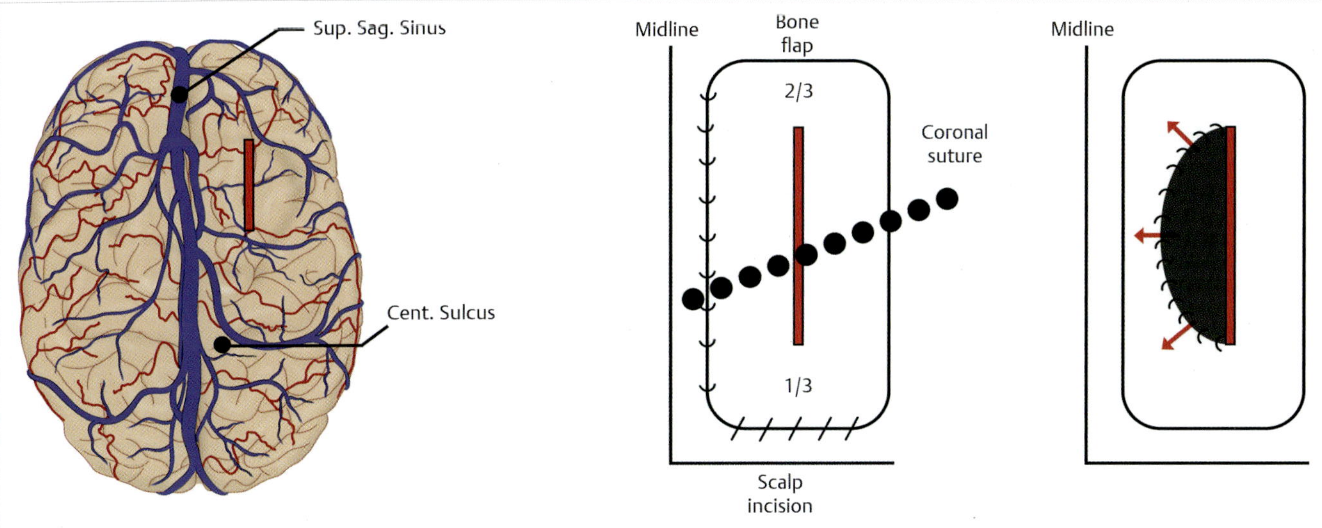


**Fig. 8.4** Corticectomy: **(a)** A 1.5-cm incision (*red line*) is made into the middle frontal gyrus just anterior to the coronal suture and 2 to 3 cm lateral to midline, into an area free of any significant vascular structures. The corticectomy is performed along the long axis of the gyrus, carefully coagulating the region beforehand to avoid any significant subpial or subarachnoid hemorrhage. **(b, c)** After completion of the corticectomy and white matter dissection down to the ventricular surface, a single self-retaining retractor is inserted on the medial side of the incision, with subsequent distraction toward the midline, creating a semi-elliptical view into the ventricular system.

identified as free of any significant vascular structures. A 1.5-cm corticectomy is performed along the long axis of the gyrus, carefully coagulating the region beforehand to avoid any significant subpial or subarachnoid hemorrhage (▶ Fig. 8.4a). The ipsilateral frontal horn is cannulated with a ventricular catheter, using stereotactic guidance if needed. Once the ventricle is encountered, the tube's pathway guides the trajectory of the deeper subcortical white matter dissection (1 cm wide, in the same plane as the corticectomy) down to the ventricular system. After completion down to the ventricular surface, a single self-retaining retractor is inserted on the medial side of the incision, with subsequent distraction toward the midline (▶ Fig. 8.4b, c).

## 8.2.2 Transventricular Access to the Lesion via the Foramen of Monro

Upon entering the lateral ventricle, the choroid plexus is identified and used as an orienting landmark to guide further dissection. Optimal ventricular access exposes the anterior limit of the foramen of Monro and 1 to 2 cm posteriorly to allow wider opening of the choroidal fissure as needed (▶ Fig. 8.5a).

Three variations of access into the third ventricle have been described to achieve adequate exposure of the cyst beyond that available via the foramen of Monro, namely, the transforniceal, interforniceal, and transchoroidal routes (▶ Fig. 8.5b). The most suitable route for an individual lesion is principally determined by its size, location along the third ventricle roof (i.e., anterior, middle, or posterior), and the relationship of the anterior septal (ASV), thalamostriate (TSV), and internal cerebral (ICV) veins with the foramen of Monro. The typical CC arises in the anterior roof of the third ventricle, and its anterior border is visible through the foramen of Monro.

In some cases, the lesion can be removed entirely through a *transforaminal* route. When more space is needed, a *transforniceal* approach may be undertaken with sectioning of the ipsilateral fornix at the foramen of Monro. However, this is an unfavorable option in the modern microsurgical era, as the risk of significant memory impairment is substantial. Most cysts originate from and/or are attached to structures posterior to the foramen of Monro, making the *transchoroidal* route preferable. The base of the choroid plexus in the lateral ventricle is anchored to the fornix and thalamus via the taenia fornix and taenia choroidea, respectively (▶ Fig. 8.5c). The choroid plexus is coagulated and then distracted laterally, and the taenia fornix on the medial side of the choroid plexus is sharply sectioned parallel to the adjacent fornix (▶ Fig. 8.5d). The surgeon can then view the vascular structures (ICV, MPChA) that run in the roof of the anterior third ventricle. Separating and working between the medial surfaces of the two ICVs, the TSV and other thalamic veins bridging from the ICV to the thalamus are easily displaced laterally. Continuing this approach exposes the underlying MPChA and its branches and their attachments to the posterior wall of the cyst, making the final detachment much more directly visible and controllable.

Lesions arising in the posterior one-third of the third ventricle require an *interforniceal* approach to adequately access the cyst wall and its attachments. In this approach, the two leaflets of the septum pellucidum are opened posterior to the foramen of Monro, and a midline plane between the fornices is defined. The fornices are separated longitudinally until the third ventricle roof with its blood vessels (ICV, MPChA) is exposed and handled as previously described.

## 8.2.3 Lesion Resection

The turgor of the cyst wall facilitates the separation of the cyst wall from the displaced vasculature and choroid plexus. Once the lesion's posterior extension is clarified sufficiently, the cyst is punctured and decompressed, avoiding spillage of the cyst

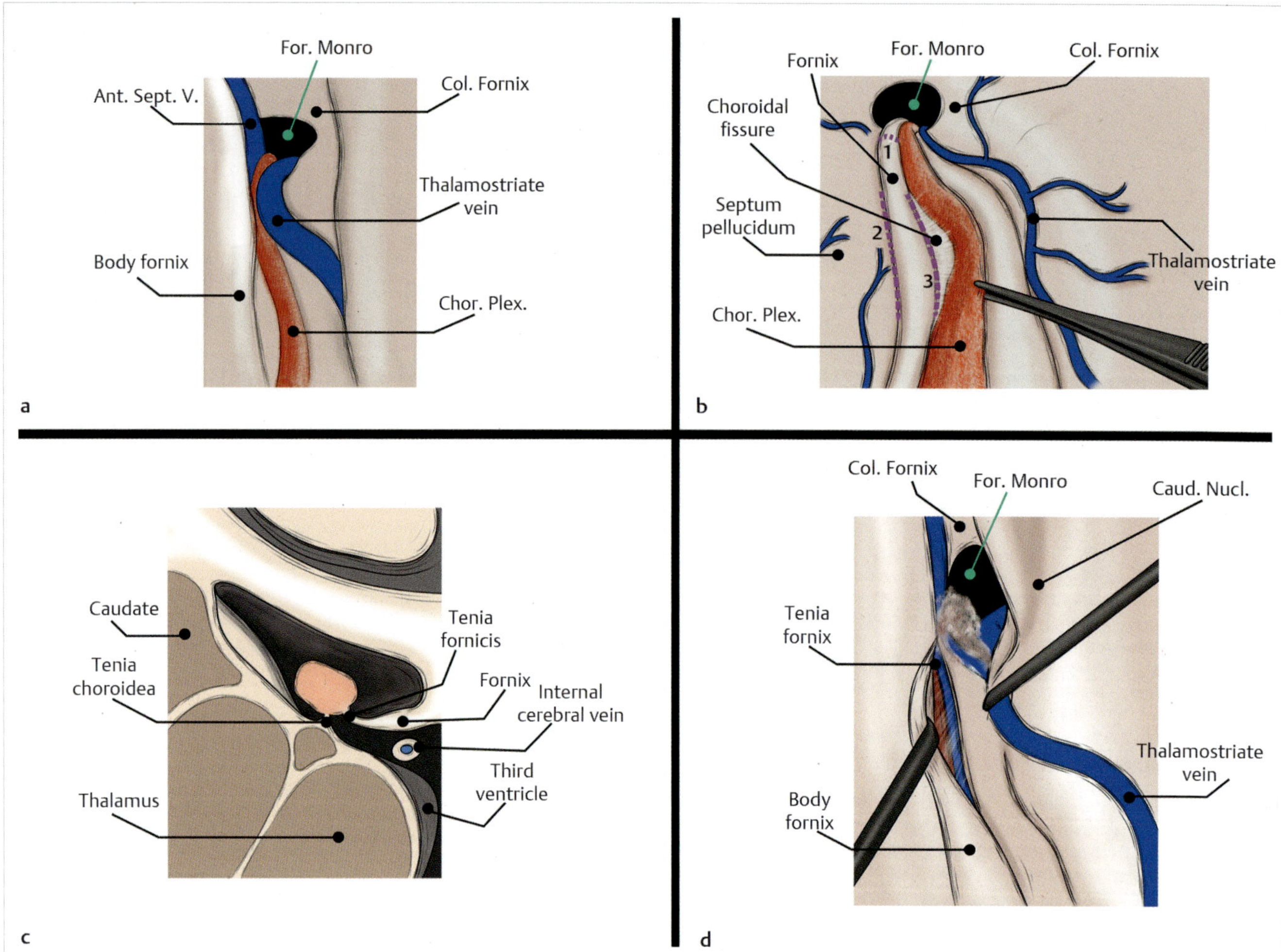


**Fig. 8.5** Transventricular access to the lesion via the foramen of Monro. **(a)** Upon entering the lateral ventricle, the choroid plexus is identified and used as an orienting landmark to guide further dissection. Optimal ventricular access exposes the anterior limit of the foramen of Monro and 1 to 2 cm posteriorly to allow wider opening of the choroidal fissure as needed. **(b)** Three variations of access into the third ventricle have been described to increase exposure of the cyst beyond that available via the foramen of Monro, namely, the transfornicial (*dashed line 1*), interforniceal (*dashed line 2*), and transchoroidal (*dashed line 3*) routes. (Editorial comment: We do not recommend the transfornicial approach because it is associated with an increased risk of postoperative memory impairment.) **(c)** The base of the choroid plexus in the lateral ventricle is anchored to the fornix and thalamus via the taenia fornix and taenia choroidea, respectively. **(d)** The transchoroidal approach: The choroid plexus is carefully coagulated just posterior to the foramen, making sure not to injure any venous structures. The choroid is then distracted laterally, and the taenia fornix on the medial side of the choroid plexus is sharply sectioned parallel to the adjacent fornix.

contents into the deep ventricular system. The posterior extent of the cyst is then further clarified, following which the cyst wall is carefully dissected circumferentially away from the ICVs and TSVs. Small branches from the MPChAs draping over the cyst and supplying the choroid plexus of the third ventricle are coagulated and divided, after which the specimen can be removed safely without vascular or forniceal injury.

### 8.2.4 Closure and Postoperative Care

A subdural drain laid over the surface of the cortex is brought out through a separate stab-incision posteriorly and connected to a gravity drainage system. The drain is left in place until the next day, at which time the CSF outflow is assessed. Continued high output should prompt a CT scan prior to its removal. Prophylactic antiepileptics, typically levetiracetam, are administered and kept in place at least until the first postoperative outpatient visit in 2 weeks. The patient is admitted to the neurointensive care unit postoperatively for the first night and is typically discharged home on postoperative day 2 or 3.

## 8.3 Rationale and Advantages

Methods for the surgical treatment of CCs include coaxial techniques (stereotactic aspiration and working-channel endoscopy) and open microsurgical (bimanual) intervention via transcortical or transcallosal routes.

The coaxial techniques share frontal transcortical access to the lateral ventricle, albeit through a smaller channel than that required for open techniques, and have been employed by some in an effort reduce tissue disruption. Stereotactic aspiration alone is associated with higher risks of neural and vascular injury, difficulty in puncturing small or thick-walled lesions, and difficulty in aspirating viscous cystic contents. This technique also has a substantially higher recurrence rates compared to open surgical series.[4,5]

Working-channel endoscopy sacrifices bimanual dissection for separating the lesion from its attachments, and is generally limited to lesions immediately accessible through the foramen of Monro. A meta-analysis of literature published between 1994 and 2014 comparing CC resection techniques indicates that at most centers, endoscopic techniques have been associated with significantly lower incidence of complete resection (58 vs. 97%) and higher rates of recurrence (4 vs. 1.5%) and reoperation (3 vs. 0.4%).[6] (Note that during the two decades covered in the meta-analysis, the endoscopic technique has evolved significantly. Thus, the data contained within the cited study represent the entire learning curve and not the state of the art.)

The transcallosal approach, preferred by many surgeons in patients who have small ventricles, permits bimanual microdissection without the need for cortical resection. The incidence of postoperative seizures may be less than that associated with a transcortical entry point. This approach, however, requires significant lateral mobilization of the frontal lobe away from the midline, placing the ipsilateral supplementary motor area and midline bridging veins at serious risk of injury and increasing the risk of venous infarction and/or hemorrhage. The deeper midline dissection places both the cingulate gyri and the pericallosal arteries at risk of injury with resultant deficits.[2,5] The transcallosal approach accesses the ventricle along a midline trajectory, forcing greater distraction of the fornix to reach the third ventricle or necessitating interforniceal dissection.

The principal advantages of the transcortical approach as described herein include ease of access (particularly when accompanied by hydrocephalus), a more direct trajectory of visualization to and through the foramen of Monro, and adaptability to individual anatomy and pathology. The transcortical approach is performed through a minimal 1.5-cm linear corticectomy in a functionally silent area of frontal cortex, not much bigger and in the same region as that used for the coaxial working-channel techniques. Unlike the transcallosal approach, it does not require dissection of large arterial branches or mobilizing bridging veins.[7,8]

## 8.4 Conclusion

Microsurgical resection through a transcortical approach provides optimal visualization and maneuverability for safe and complete lesion resection. This approach may be applied regardless of ventricular size, cyst consistency, or cyst position, and allows the surgeon to choose between a transforaminal, interforniceal, and transchoroidal pathways to the lesion, based on cyst size, location, and consistency. Particularly when using the transchoroidal approach, the experienced surgeon can see and dissect the walls of the cyst completely with greatly reduced risks of injury to the fornix or adjacent vasculature.

## References

[1] Beaumont TL, Limbrick DD, Jr, Rich KM, Wippold FJ, II, Dacey RG, Jr. Natural history of colloid cysts of the third ventricle. J Neurosurg. 2016; 125(6): 1420–1430

[2] Horn EM, Feiz-Erfan I, Bristol RE, et al. Treatment options for third ventricular colloid cysts: comparison of open microsurgical versus endoscopic resection. Neurosurgery. 2008; 62(6) Suppl 3:1076–1083

[3] Desai KI, Nadkarni TD, Muzumdar DP, Goel AH. Surgical management of colloid cyst of the third ventricle—a study of 105 cases. Surg Neurol. 2002; 57(5): 295–302, discussion 302–304

[4] Hoffman CE, Savage NJ, Souweidane MM. The significance of cyst remnants after endoscopic colloid cyst resection: a retrospective clinical case series. Neurosurgery. 2013; 73(2):233–237, discussion 237–239

[5] Mathiesen T, Grane P, Lindgren L, Lindquist C. Third ventricle colloid cysts: a consecutive 12-year series. J Neurosurg. 1997; 86(1):5–12

[6] Sheikh AB, Mendelson ZS, Liu JK. Endoscopic versus microsurgical resection of colloid cysts: a systematic review and meta-analysis of 1,278 patients. World Neurosurg. 2014; 82(6):1187–1197

[7] Nair S, Gopalakrishnan CV, Menon G, Easwer HV, Abraham M. Interhemispheric transcallosal transforaminal approach and its variants to colloid cyst of third ventricle: technical issues based on a single institutional experience of 297 cases. Asian J Neurosurg. 2016; 11(3):292–297

[8] Hernesniemi J, Leivo S. Management outcome in third ventricular colloid cysts in a defined population: a series of 40 patients treated mainly by transcallosal microsurgery. Surg Neurol. 1996; 45(1):2–14

# 9 Transcortical Transventricular Approach for Colloid Cysts and Salvage Approaches by Converting to Open Resection

*Jacob S. Young, Roberto Rodriguez Rubio, and Michael W. McDermott*

**Abstract**

The optimal approach for surgical removal of colloid cysts is controversial. Proponents of the endoscopic approach tout its minimally invasive nature and reports of shorter length of stay and operating times. Alternatively, open microsurgical approaches have been shown to yield more complete resections and, in most experienced centers, have comparable morbidity profiles to the endoscopic approach. The transcortical transventricular approach is favored by our group given it has a much lower seizure risk than the transcallosal approach and provides an ideal line of site for safe resection of cyst contents. Here, we describe the relevant cranial, cortical, and white matter anatomy during the operative approach and highlight the literature comparing the various approach strategies. Moreover, when an endoscopic approach is felt to be unsafe for complete resection, we propose a workflow for safe conversion to the open microsurgical technique with the same incision and craniotomy. Given the published data, a transcortical transventricular approach may be best for younger symptomatic patients with colloid cysts.

*Keywords:* colloid cyst, transcortical/transventricular approach, endoscopic approach, conversion to open surgery

## 9.1 Introduction

To this day, the surgical treatment of colloid cysts remains a topic of discussion and debate in neurosurgery. Nevertheless, the available data provides a foundation for the appropriate management of these benign lesions. First, not all colloid cysts identified with imaging require surgical removal. There have been reports of spontaneous cyst regression.[1,2] Although there are data suggesting poor outcomes can occur in symptomatic patients,[3] asymptomatic cysts can be safely observed when discovered incidentally. Pollock and Huston previously reported on the natural history of 168 patients managed over 25 years at the Mayo Clinic.[4] In this series, 68 patients were asymptomatic with a mean age of 57 years and a mean cyst diameter of 8 mm. Out of these 68 asymptomatic patients, 58 (85%) were followed for a mean period of 79 months. During this follow-up period, there were no cases of sudden death and the percentage of patients that became symptomatic was 0, 0, and 8% at 2, 5, and 10 years, respectively. Only 3% of these cysts enlarged and only 3% of patients developed hydrocephalus. The authors concluded that it was safe to observe patients who were asymptomatic with interval imaging. In a follow-up paper, the same group analyzed factors associated with symptomatic versus asymptomatic patients. They found that younger age (44 vs. 57 years), larger cyst size (13 vs. 8 mm), increased ventricular size (83 vs. 31%), and increased T2 signal on magnetic resonance imaging (MRI) (44 vs. 8%) were associated with a greater likelihood of the patient being symptomatic.[5] Increased ventricular size was the most important factor in the development of symptoms.

More recently, Beaumont et al created a Colloid Cyst Risk Score (CCRS) based on factors that may be associated with a higher risk of being symptomatic or developing hydrocephalus.[6] Of the 163 patients included in the study, over half were found incidentally. Of these, 58% were followed for an average of 5.1 years. Five patients (8.8%) progressed and underwent surgery. None of the patients with asymptomatic cysts experienced acute obstructive hydrocephalus or sudden deterioration in the absence of trauma. They used the clinical and radiographic traits of the patients in this cohort to develop a five-point risk score stratification of patients based on age, presence of headaches, cyst size, fluid-attenuated inversion recovery (FLAIR) hyperintensity on MRI, and location within Zone I of the third ventricle (anterior third ventricle from the lamina terminalis to a vertical line through the mid-mamillary body tangential to the massa intermedia). The total score was predictive of symptomatic clinical status and a subset of patients presenting with symptomatic obstructive hydrocephalus. They concluded that patients with risk factor score of $\geq 4$ should be considered for surgical treatment.

More support for intervention in large colloid cysts with hydrocephalus comes from Singh et al who reported that patient deaths were significantly higher in the cohort of patients who did not undergo surgical resection compared to the cohort who had a procedure.[7] Additionally, neurocognition improved in patients who underwent surgical resection, although this may be from improvement in hydrocephalus.[8] Kone et al found that patients with headaches and colloid cysts who underwent surgical resection had less headache disability and self-reported a better quality of life than patients who did not undergo surgery.[9]

In the following sections, we have described the relevant anatomy and the senior author's technique for a transcortical, transventricular (TC/TV) approach for symptomatic colloid cysts.

## 9.2 Anatomy

The dorsal portion of the right frontal lobe of the cerebrum is the preferred site for entry with this approach. It is critical to have a clear understanding of the topographical correlation of cranial, cortical, and white matter structures to plan the best trajectory and corridor to access a lesion in the ventricle.[10] From coronal perspective, two cranial landmarks are helpful for surgical planning. The first is the bregma—formed by the junction of coronal and sagittal sutures—which lies at the same coronal plane as the foramen of Monro (FoM), and serves to plan the skin incision and position of the craniotomy according to the zone in which the colloid cyst resides. The second is the postcoronal point (i.e., 3 cm lateral and 1.5 cm posterior to bregma), a cranial landmark for the junction of the precentral sulcus and the superior frontal sulcus, which helps to identify a safe posterior limit of the transcortical exposure without disrupting the sensorimotor strip (▶ Fig. 9.1). This incision is planned with the assistance of intraoperative navigation. The entry point is within the supplementary motor area well in front of the primary motor cortex. The middle frontal gyrus is preferred for a better angle to the roof of the third ventricle, which has its inferior limit at the stephanion, the cranial landmark formed by the junction of superior temporal line and the coronal suture.

The subcortical white matter along the path of entry into the ventricle contains associative fibers found within the middle frontal gyrus consisting of the superior longitudinal fasciculus (SLF) II, dorsal segment of the arcuate fasciculus (AF, posterior part of the gyrus), and the inferior fronto-occipital fasciculus (IFOF, mid part of the gyrus) (▶ Fig. 9.2). These fibers lie superficial to the rest of the tracts within the middle frontal gyrus, whereas the associative fibers found within the superior frontal lobe (i.e., SLF I and frontal aslant tracts) are deeper to the projection and commissural fibers.[11]

After transecting the commissural fibers covering the ependyma, the ventricle is entered through the roof of the frontal horn and orientation is obtained by recognizing the choroid plexus (▶ Fig. 9.3), the caudate vein, the septal vein, the thalamostriate vein, and the FoM, usually filled with the colloid cyst. We previously described surgical zones for access to the third ventricle as they relate to positions of the junction of the septal vein with the internal cerebral vein (ICV) anteriorly and the medial atrial vein (MAV) posteriorly (refer to Osorio et al,[12] ▶ Fig. 9.4). Zone I describes that portion of the third ventricle anterior to the junction of the septal vein with the ICV. This insertion site is variable with respect to the position of the choroid plexus looping into the roof of the third ventricle, which is typically used to define the posterior limit of the FoM. However, the tinea fornicea can be opened back to this junction behind the choroid plexus without division of the septal vein, providing increased exposure and a working corridor to the superior cyst wall attachments. Zone II is the portion of the third ventricle behind the junction of the septal vein with the ICV back to the MAV, the latter crossing the posterior floor of the lateral ventricle and roof of the third ventricle to join the ICV. The MAV drains the pulvinar of the thalamus, and like the thalamostriate vein, cannot be divided without unacceptable risk of venous infarction. Zone III is the posterior portion of the third ventricle behind the MAV (see ▶ Fig. 9.10b), which can only be seen from anteriorly and above.

The point of attachment of colloid cysts is the roof of the third ventricle where the capsule of the cyst receives blood supply from the posterior medial choroidal (PMCh) arteries. The PMCh

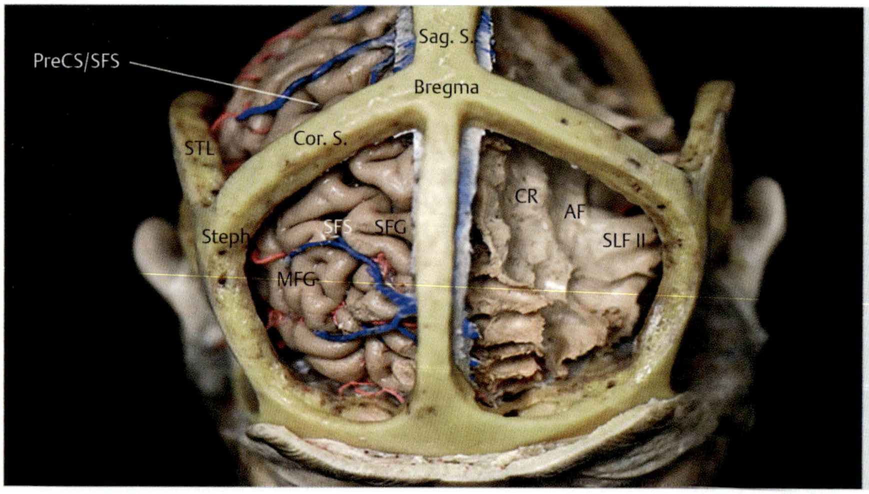


**Fig. 9.1** Anatomical dissection demonstrating the cranial surface, cortical gyrus, and underlying white matter with relevant landmarks for a transcortical transventricular approach to the third ventricle. (AF, arcuate fascicles; Cor. S., coronal suture; CR, corona radiata; MFG, middle frontal gyrus; Sag. S., sagittal suture; SFG, superior frontal gyrus; SFS, superior frontal sulcus; SLF, superior longitudinal fasciculus II; Steph., Stephanion; STL, superior temporal line.)

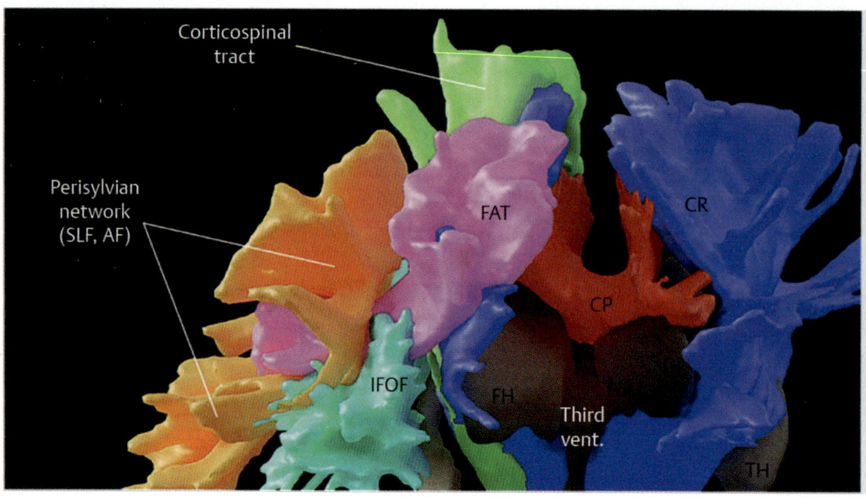


**Fig. 9.2** Tractography of the white matter projections from the cortical surface down to the third ventricle. (AF, arcuate fascicles; CP, callosal projections; CR, corona radiata; FAT, frontal aslant tract; FH, frontal horn; FoM, foramen of Monro; IFOF, inferior frontal occipital fasciculus; SLF, superior longitudinal fasciculus II; TH, temporal horn; Third vent., third ventricle.)

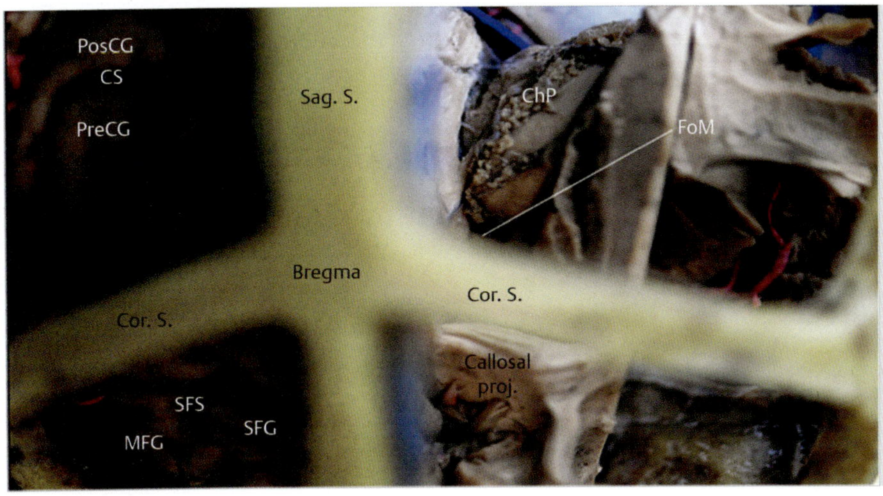


**Fig. 9.3** Anatomical dissection demonstrating the relationship between the cranial surface, cortical gyri, white matter tracts, and foramen of Monro. (Callosal proj., callosal projections; CG, central gyrus; ChP, choroid plexus; Cor. S., coronal suture; CS, central sulcus; FoM, foramen of Monro; MFG, middle frontal gyrus; PosCG, postcentral gyrus; PreCG, precentral gyrus; Sag. S., sagittal suture; SFG, superior frontal gyrus; SFS, superior frontal sulcus.)

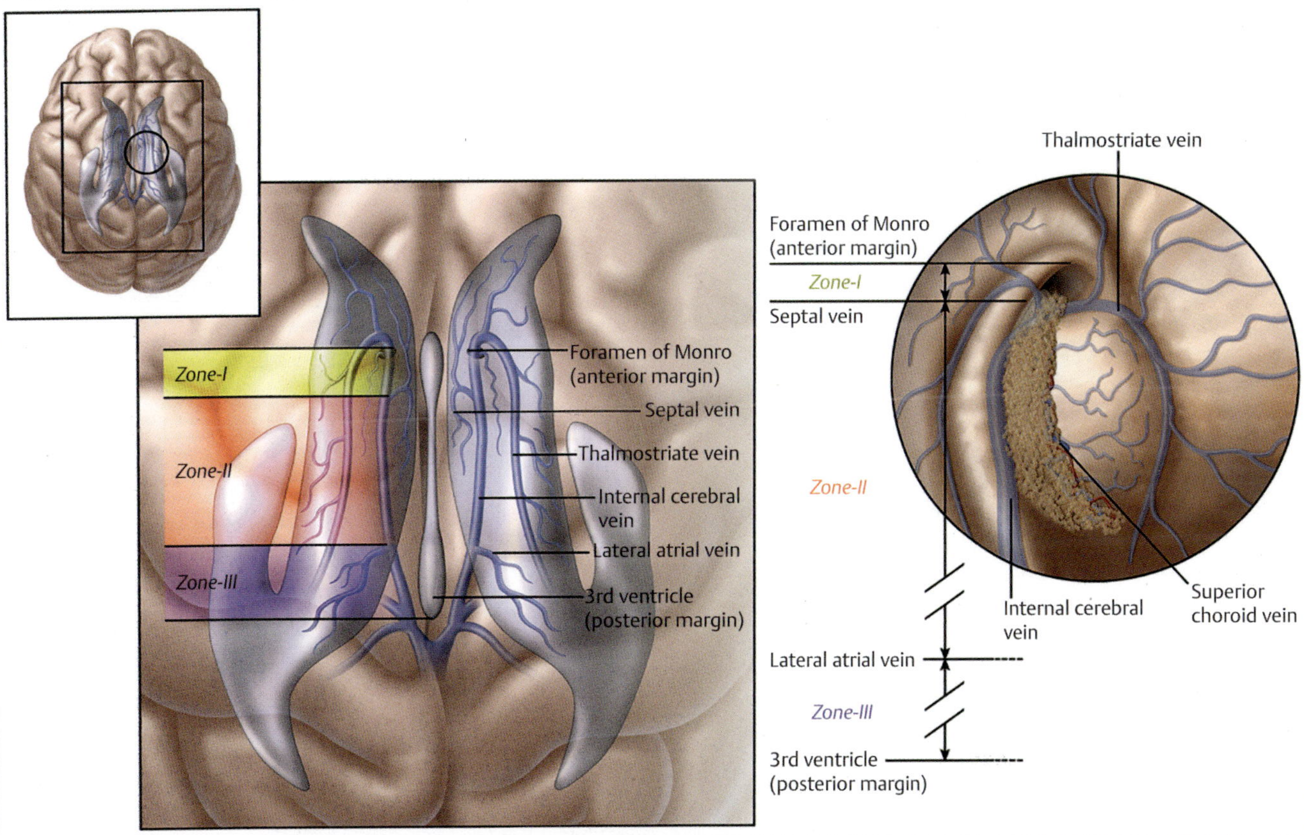


**Fig. 9.4** An illustration of the operative zones of the third ventricle based on relationships defined by the anterior column of the fornix, the septal vein, and the middle atrial vein. Zone I extends from the anterior column of the fornix to the anterior margin of the septal vein. (Used with permission from Dr. Michael W. McDermott.)

arteries lie within the velum interpositum medial to the ICVs. In larger cysts small branches from the PMCh arteries come from the roof of the third ventricle all the way along the wall of the cyst. It is for this reason that the cyst wall cannot be grasped and pulled out as arterial hemorrhage will result. Careful opening of the roof of the third ventricle allows one to identify the blood supply to the cyst wall, coagulate the vessels, and divide them sharply allowing for safe dissection of cyst capsule from the roof and lateral walls of the third ventricle.

## 9.3 Surgical Techniques

After induction of general anesthesia, the patient is positioned supine with the head of the bed slightly elevated, the neck extended on the chest, and the head slightly flexed on the neck. The head is placed in Mayfield pins and the registration of image guidance to physical space is completed. After confirming the accuracy of the registration, an entry point is selected on the scalp that provides a trajectory through the middle frontal gyrus to the FoM just anterior to the coronal suture. A coronal scalp incision is used and a bone flap two-third in front of the coronal suture and one-third behind the coronal suture is marked out. The medial margin of the bone flap is 1 cm from midline to maintain a safe distance from the superior sagittal sinus. The dura is opened in a U-shaped fashion and an image-guided stylet is used to insert an external ventricular drain (EVD) into the frontal horn of the lateral ventricle; the proximal end is closed with bone wax (▶ Fig. 9.5a). The operating room microscope is brought into position and a linear 2 cm corticectomy is made on the middle frontal gyrus (▶ Fig. 9.5b). Following the EVD catheter, a straight Rhoton #4 micro-dissector is used to sweep in an anterior–posterior direction to separate the white matter fibers. The bipolar or suction should not be used to remove white matter to create the tract as this may prevent co-apting of the walls of the tract and formation of subdural hygromas. As the roof of the ventricle is opened, subependymal veins will need to be coagulated and divided. The ventricle is entered, and retractors or tubes placed and the venous anatomy and location of the FoM confirmed (▶ Fig. 9.6a–c).

Colloid cysts are never swinging from the roof of the third ventricle like a grape on the vine, but rather are always adherent to the body and column of the fornix, the roof of the third ventricle, and choroid plexus of the lateral ventricle as it turns

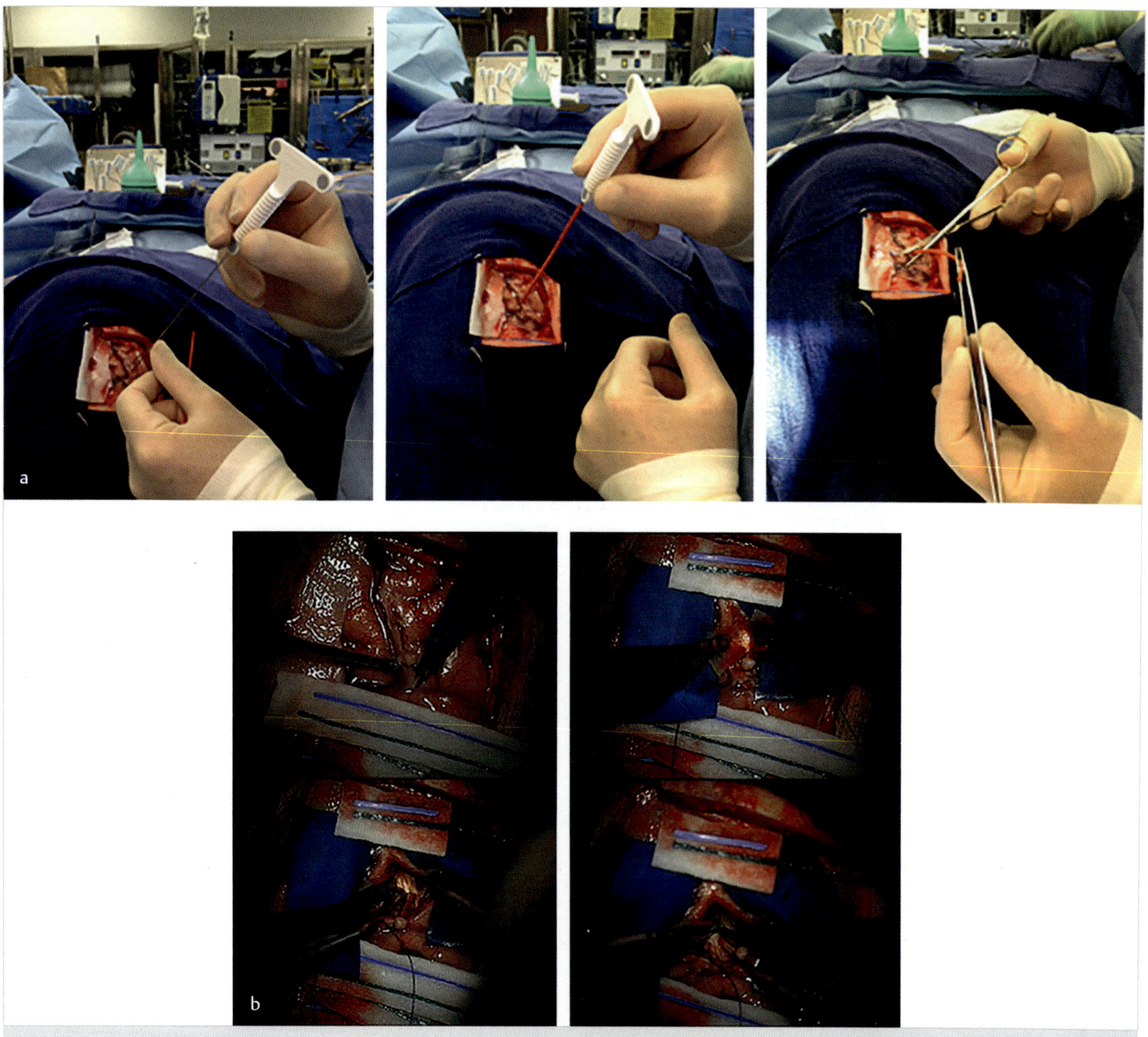

Fig. 9.5 (a) Utilization of an image-guided stylet to insert an external ventricular drain (EVD) into the frontal horn of the lateral ventricle. (b) Creation of a linear 2 cm corticectomy in the middle frontal gyrus with use of the operating microscope.

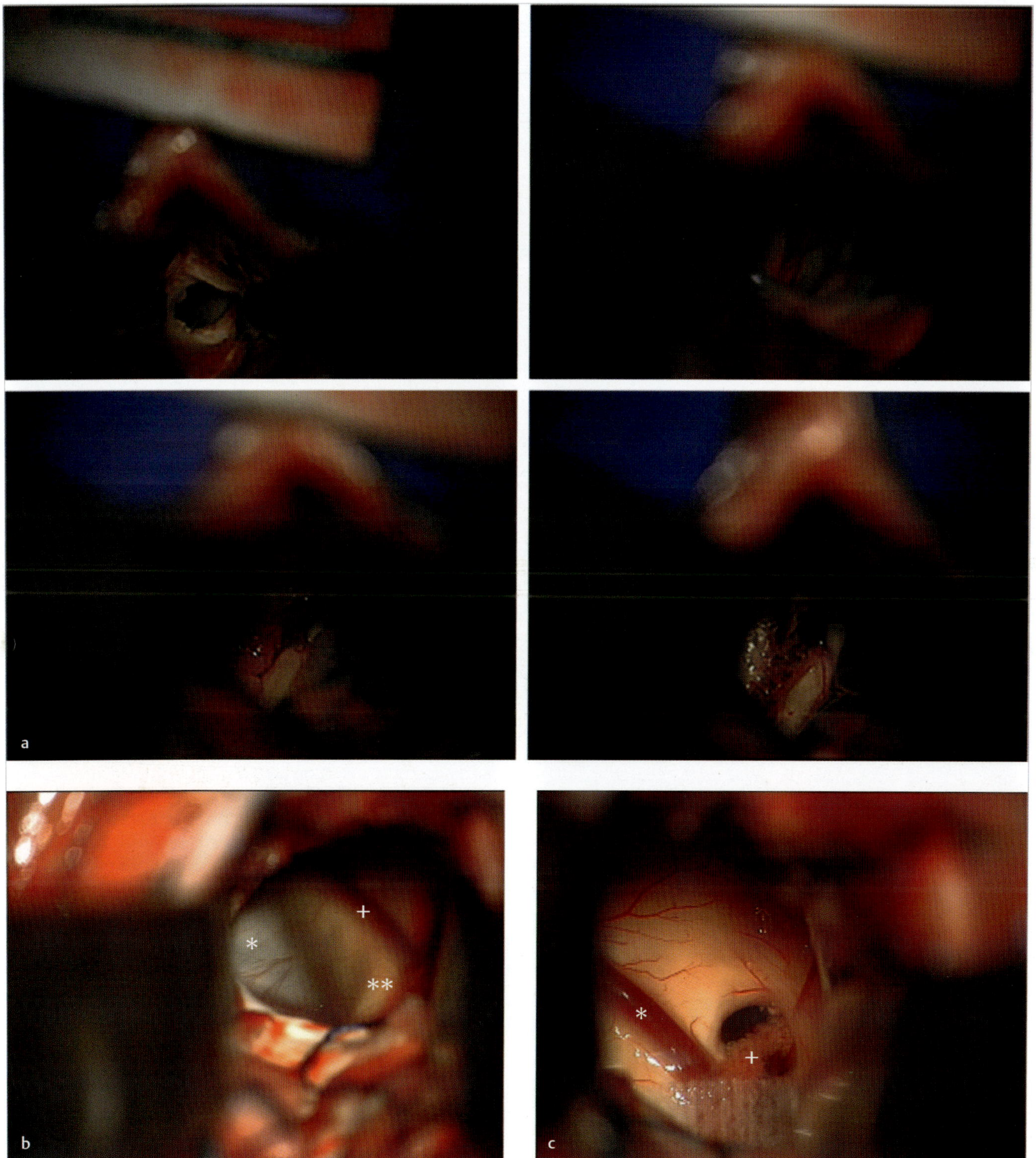

**Fig. 9.6** **(a)** Introduction of tubular retractors to safely identify venous anatomy and create corridor into the right lateral ventricle. **(b)** Initial exposure into ventricle; blue membrane is septum pellucidum (*) which was opened; vein crossing below is septal vein (+); behind that is fornix (**). **(c)** Initial view of foramen of Munroe after opening the septum; septal vein on left (*) and choroid plexus (+) entering front part of the foramen with cyst wall visible in upper quadrant of the foramen. Note how small the foramen appears as most of the cyst is high up in the roof of the third ventricle.

the corner to the roof of the third ventricle. After coagulation and removal of choroid plexus, the tinea fornicea can be opened back to the entry of the septal vein into the ICV (▶ Fig. 9.7). Next, the cyst wall is opened and colloidal material sucked out with collapse of the cyst wall (▶ Fig. 9.8a, b). The cyst capsule can now be detached from the roof of the third ventricle and be completely excised with minimal ischemic injury to surrounding structures (▶ Fig. 9.9).

For larger cysts, dissection of the tinea fornicea can be done safely all the way back to the MAV. The first step is to dissect the septal vein from the body of the fornix, and then coagulate and divide it. The senior author has never seen any consequence of dividing the septal vein. Sharp dissection of the velum interpositum allows identification of the choroid, posterior medial chorodial artery (PMCHr), and ICV, which can be displaced laterally (▶ Fig. 9.10a–c). The cyst wall will be adherent to both ICVs, and this is when the more lateral approach via the middle frontal gyrus is critical to provide the necessary line of sight and working angle to facilitate removal. This dissection is the only way to guarantee safe, complete removal of large cysts.

After cyst removal, an EVD is left in place for several days until the cerebrospinal fluid (CSF) clears. The tract to the ventricle can be temporarily filled with hemostatic agents and then irrigated for removal (▶ Fig. 9.11). It is possible to bring together the pia at the top of the gyrus. Typically, the assistant using two nontoothed forceps holds the pia together, and the surgeon can place one or two absorbable sutures to close the tract. Using this technique, the author has not encountered development of symptomatic subdural hygroma yet.

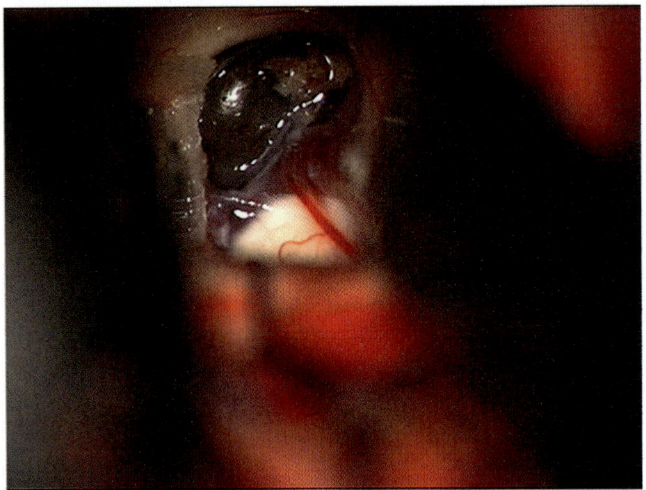

**Fig. 9.7** Foramen opened wider after coagulating and cutting choroid, dissecting wall of cyst from fornix, and opening membrane at the junction of septal, caudate, and thalamostriate veins.

## 9.4 Review of the Literature for Colloid Cyst Resection: Comparison of Endoscopic, Transcallosal, and Transcortical/ Transventricular Approaches

Majority of the published literature has focused on either endoscopic, transcallosal, or transcortical/transventricular resection of colloid cysts. Importantly, most of the literature only compares two of these approaches, rather than all three, and often the open microsurgical group only includes one of the above approaches, necessitating a careful review of the patient cohort when interpreting the data.

In a comparison of the endoscopic and microsurgical approaches to colloid cyst resection, Grondin et al found that while both approaches were capable of removing the cyst contents, the endoscopic approach was much less likely to result in complete resection of the cyst wall (12 vs. 100% respectively).[13] In their review of the literature, Grondin et al found that an endoscopic approach was more likely to result in a recurrence (likely due to lower rates of gross total resection), but the open microsurgical approach had higher rates of complication and shunt dependence. Other authors have replicated this finding that endoscopic resection can reliably result in aspiration of cyst contents and coagulation of the cyst wall; however, nearly half of the patients will be left with some residual cyst wall in this approach.[14] A retrospective case series of colloid cysts resected endoscopically found a recurrence rate of 6.3% over a

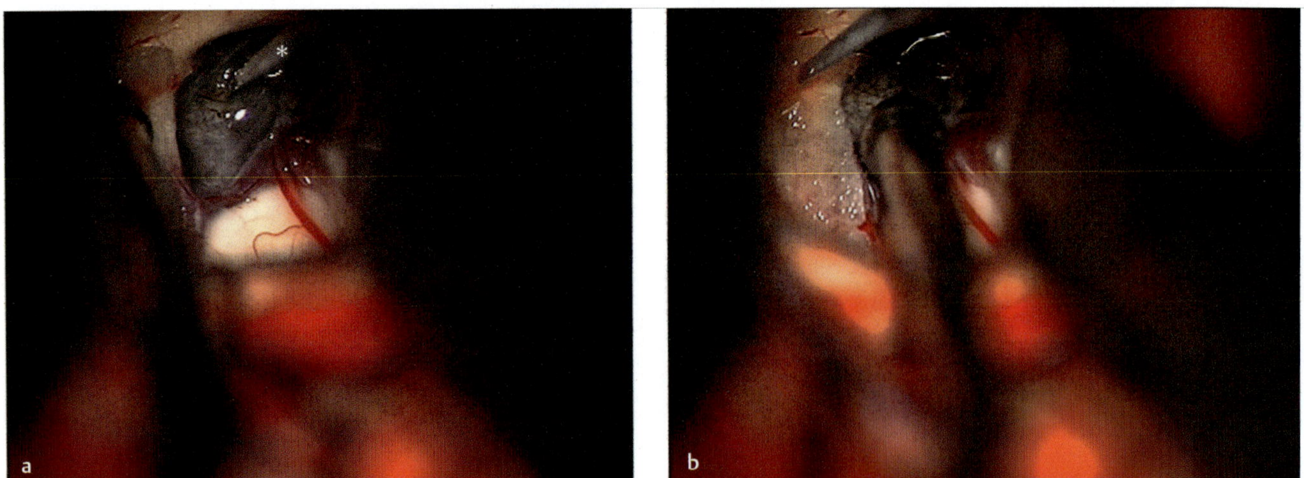

**Fig. 9.8** **(a)** Incision in wall of cyst with ophthalmic blade (*); note foramen is kept open by gentle countertraction on column of fornix covered by sponge using suction (finger off hole). **(b)** Aspirating cyst to decompress and allow for further dissection and excision; cyst contents are often partly liquid and partly semi-solid.

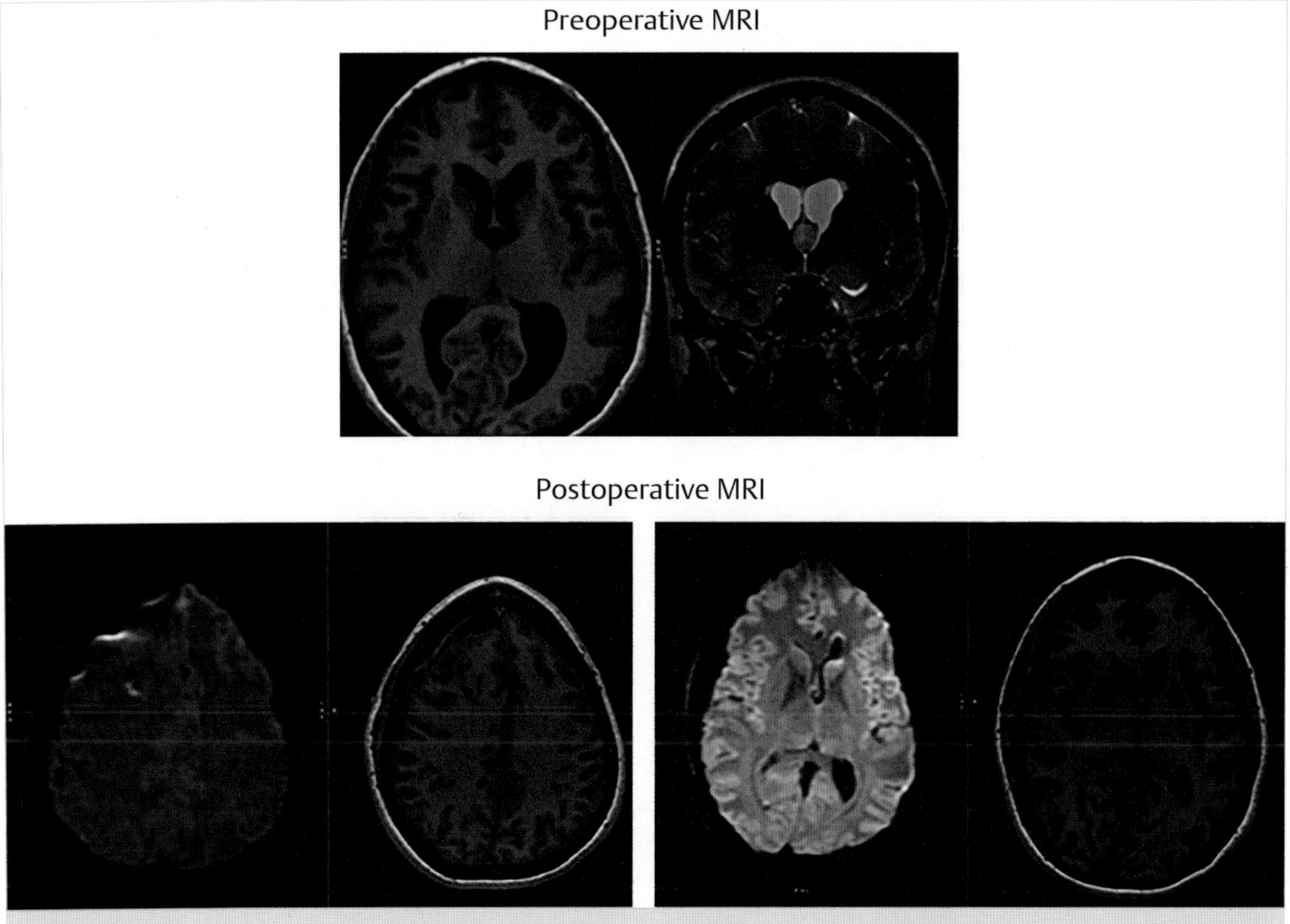


**Fig. 9.9** Preoperative axial T1 and coronal T2 image of colloid cyst. Postoperative diffusion-weighted imaging (DWI) and axial T1 images of a resected cyst showing limited restricted diffusion around the collapsed entry tract and the resected cyst.

51-month follow-up with a 13.9% morbidity rate, demonstrating the significance of residual colloid cyst remnants.[15]

Although there appears to be a higher rate of subtotal resection and subsequent cyst recurrence with the endoscopic approach, one benefit of the endoscopic approach is that some authors have found it to be associated with shorter operating times and hospital lengths of stay.[16] However, a retrospective analysis of the University of California, San Francisco colloid cyst patient cohort found that patients who had an open transcortical approach had the same operating room time and length of stay as those who underwent endoscopic resection.[12] Moreover, in a review of patients who underwent the transcallosal approach (mean cyst size 1.6 cm), average operating room time was 124 minutes (18 minutes from cyst visualization to removal) and hospital length of stay was 3.5 days, which were both similar to the endoscopic resection group.[17]

In support of open approaches yielding more complete resections, a study from the Barrow Neurosurgical Institute compared the endoscopic approach with the transcallosal approach and found the transcallosal approach to achieve a gross total resection more often (94 vs. 47%, respectively), with similar rates of shunting and length of stay for the two groups.[16]

In an important retrospective study, Milligan and Meyer reviewed 127 patients who had either a transcortical or transcallosal approach to intraventricular lesions and found that the transcallosal approach carried a 4.4-fold increased risk of seizure.[18] More recent work has found even lower rates of seizure in the transcortical patient population.[19] Increased morbidity of the transcallosal approach may be related to veins taken during the approach to facilitate operative exposure, as shown by Hassaneen et al.[20] In addition to seizures, the most common neurological morbidity of the transcallosal approach is hemiplegia, and there was a 4.4% recurrence rate.[21]

As the health care climate shifts to focus more on costs of the procedure and the cost of readmissions, more work is needed to address which approach is superior in this regard. Some studies have found a higher rate of readmissions with microsurgical resection, which contributed to a significantly higher cost of the procedure.[22] Furthermore, as technology continues to improve, novel techniques that make the open resection more minimally invasive, such as tubular retractors, may provide a better safety profile while still offering ideal working space to completely resect the lesion, as reported by Eichberg et al.[23]

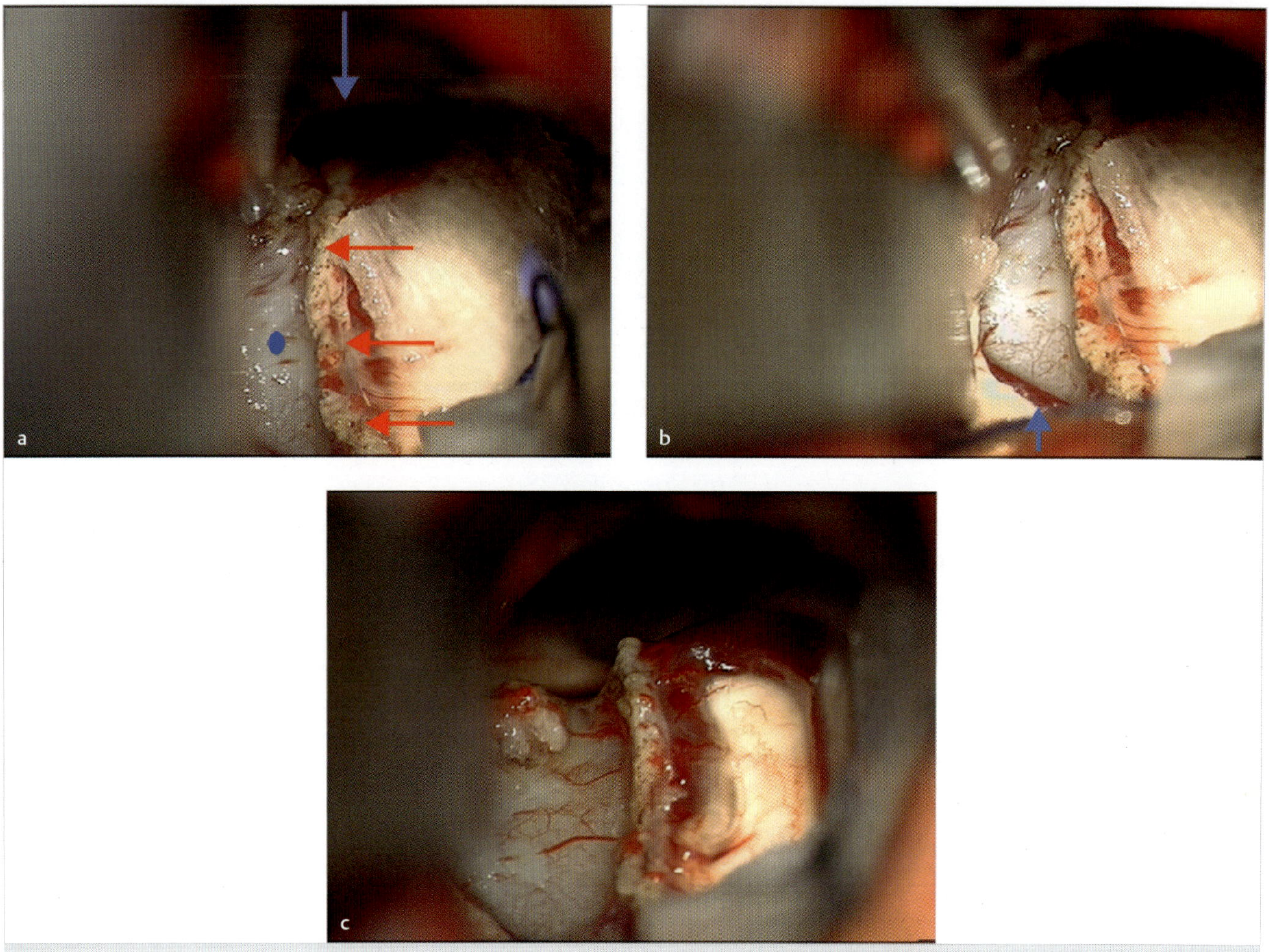


**Fig. 9.10** **(a)** Image showing foramen of Monro (*blue arrow*), medial edge of choroid plexus (*red arrows*) seen with tinea forniceal approach, and colloid cyst capsule in Zone II (*blue circle*). **(b)** Medial atrial vein (*short blue arrow*) defining the posterior limit of Zone II. **(c)** Anterior view into the anterior third ventricle with thalamostriate vein laterally along the floor of the lateral ventricle and the vascular superior wall of large colloid cyst occupying Zones II and III of the third ventricle.

## 9.5 Conversion from Endoscopic to Open Resection

Rarely, endoscopic approaches may need to be safely converted to open microsurgical resection to salvage the operation in an attempt to not leave significant residual cyst behind.[24] In recent retrospective reports, this occurred in between 5 and 17% of cases, usually due to adhesions between the cyst and fornix.[25,26] Preservation of the fornix is critical as damage during surgery has been shown to impact day-to-day memory and mamillary body volume,[27] and therefore we feel that conversion to an open approach offers the patient less morbidity than aggressive endoscopic dissection of a cyst adhered to the forniceal structures. Once the transcortical–transventricular approach is performed along the same path as was used for the peel-away sheath for the endoscope, by utilizing a mini-craniotomy during the opening for the endoscope, the surgeon obtains the exact same incision and exposure needed for a salvage microsurgical approach.[12] Our philosophy is that if the endoscopic operation has been underway for more than 1 hour, and the surgeon is unable to completely excise the cyst capsule after more than an hour of effort, the surgeon can make the decision to convert to a transcortical–transventricular microsurgical approach. When converting from an endoscopic approach to the transcortical–transventricular approach, the peel-away sheath used for the endoscope must be removed and the corticectomy enlarged. Self-retaining retractors are inserted, and the transcortical–transventricular approach followed as described in the section above.

## 9.6 Conclusion

Not all colloid cysts require resection, but for symptomatic patients there are multiple approaches that provide access to the third ventricle for resection of colloid cyst. The endoscopic approach is associated with a higher likelihood of leaving a cyst remnant. Among the open approaches, the transcallosal approach has a higher rate of postoperative seizure than the

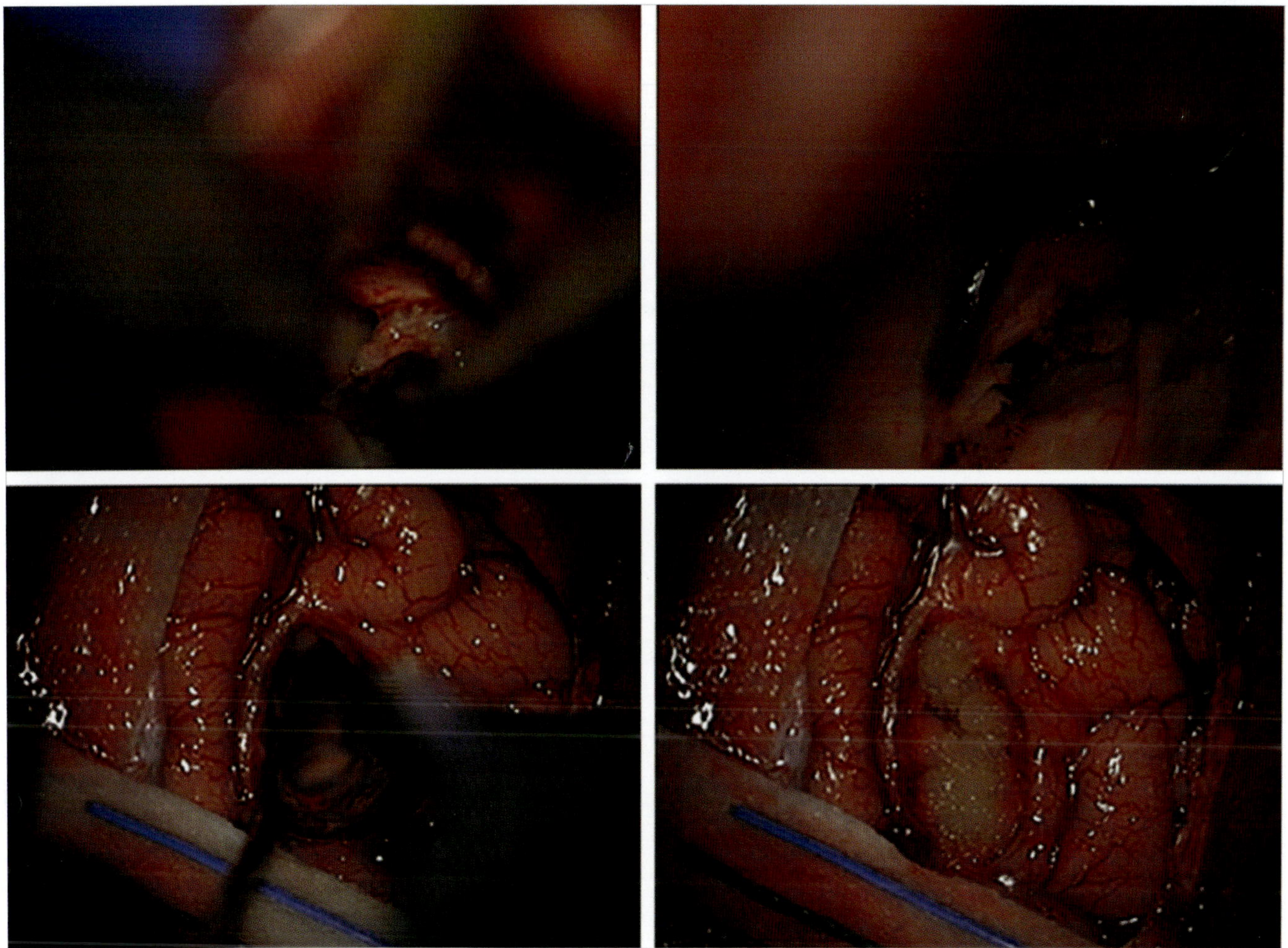

**Fig. 9.11** Filling the tract to the ventricle with hemostatic agents before irrigating out the hemostatic material.

transcortical–transventricular approach. For this reason, for young symptomatic patients with Zone II and III cysts, the authors prefer an open transcortical/transventricular approach with image guidance. Younger patients with Zone I cysts are appropriate for either endoscopic or open transcortical/ transventricular resection. For older patients, regardless of the zone of the cyst, an endoscopic approach is utilized but the operating room is prepared for the possibility of converting to an open microsurgical approach. By having the microscope ready in the operating room, a failed endoscopic approach can be salvaged by converting to an open microscopic resection.

# References


[1] Peeters SM, Daou B, Jabbour P, Ladoux A, Abi Lahoud G. Spontaneous regression of a third ventricle colloid cyst. World Neurosurg. 2016; 90:704.e19–704.e22

[2] Turel M, Kucharczyk W, Gentili F. Spontaneous resolution of colloid cyst of the third ventricle: implications for management. Asian J Neurosurg. 2017; 12(2): 203–206

[3] Mathiesen T, Grane P, Lindgren L, Lindquist C. Third ventricle colloid cysts: a consecutive 12-year series. J Neurosurg. 1997; 86(1):5–12

[4] Pollock BE, Huston J. Natural history of asymptomatic colloid cysts of the third ventricle. J Neurosurg. 1999; 91(3):364–369

[5] Pollock BE, Schreiner SA, Huston J, III. A theory on the natural history of colloid cysts of the third ventricle. Neurosurgery. 2000; 46(5):1077–1081, discussion 1081–1083

[6] Beaumont TL, Limbrick DD, Jr, Rich KM, Wippold FJ, II, Dacey RG, Jr. Natural history of colloid cysts of the third ventricle. J Neurosurg. 2016; 125(6): 1420–1430

[7] Singh H, Burhan Janjua M, Ahmed M, et al. Factors influencing outcome in patients with colloid cysts who present with acute neurological deterioration. J Clin Neurosci. 2018; 54:88–95

[8] Roth J, Sela G, Andelman F, Nossek E, Elran H, Ram Z. The impact of colloid cyst treatment on neurocognition. World Neurosurg. 2019; 125:e372–e377

[9] Kone L, Chaichana KL, Rincon-Torroella J, Snyman C, Moghekar A, Quiñones-Hinojosa A. The impact of surgical resection on headache disability and quality of life in patients with colloid cyst. Cephalalgia. 2017; 37(5):442–451

[10] Ribas GC. Applied Cranial-Cerebral Anatomy: Brain Architecture and Anatomically Oriented Microneurosurgery. Cambridge University Press; 2018

[11] Yagmurlu K, Vlasak AL, Rhoton AL, Jr. Three-dimensional topographic fiber tract anatomy of the cerebrum. Neurosurgery. 2015; 11(2) Suppl 2:274–305, discussion 305

[12] Osorio JA, Clark AJ, Safaee M, et al. Intraoperative conversion from endoscopic to open transcortical-transventricular removal of colloid cysts as a salvage procedure. Cureus. 2015; 7(2):e247

[13] Grondin RT, Hader W, MacRae ME, Hamilton MG. Endoscopic versus microsurgical resection of third ventricle colloid cysts. Can J Neurol Sci. 2007; 34(2): 197–207

[14] Longatti P, Godano U, Gangemi M, et al. Italian neuroendoscopy group. Cooperative study by the Italian neuroendoscopy group on the treatment of 61 colloid cysts. Childs Nerv Syst. 2006; 22(10):1263–1267

[15] Hoffman CE, Savage NJ, Souweidane MM. The significance of cyst remnants after endoscopic colloid cyst resection: a retrospective clinical case series. Neurosurgery. 2013; 73(2):233–237, discussion 237–239

[16] Horn EM, Feiz-Erfan I, Bristol RE, et al. Treatment options for third ventricular colloid cysts: comparison of open microsurgical versus endoscopic resection. Neurosurgery. 2007; 60(4):613–618, discussion 618–620

[17] Sampath R, Vannemreddy P, Nanda A. Microsurgical excision of colloid cyst with favorable cognitive outcomes and short operative time and hospital stay: operative techniques and analyses of outcomes with review of previous studies. Neurosurgery. 2010; 66(2):368–374, discussion 374–375

[18] Milligan BD, Meyer FB. Morbidity of transcallosal and transcortical approaches to lesions in and around the lateral and third ventricles: a single-institution experience. Neurosurgery. 2010; 67(6):1483–1496, discussion 1496

[19] Eichberg DG, Sedighim S, Buttrick S, Komotar RJ. Postoperative seizure rate after transcortical resection of subcortical brain tumors and colloid cysts: a single surgeon's experience. Cureus. 2018; 10(1):e2115

[20] Hassaneen W, Suki D, Salaskar AL, et al. Immediate morbidity and mortality associated with transcallosal resection of tumors of the third ventricle. J Clin Neurosci. 2010; 17(7):830–836

[21] Nair S, Gopalakrishnan CV, Menon G, Easwer HV, Abraham M. Interhemispheric transcallosal transforaminal approach and its variants to colloid cyst of third ventricle: technical issues based on a single institutional experience of 297 cases. Asian J Neurosurg. 2016; 11(3):292–297

[22] Connolly ID, Johnson E, Lamsam L, Veeravagu A, Ratliff J, Li G. Microsurgical vs. Endoscopic excision of colloid cysts: an analysis of complications and costs using a longitudinal administrative database. Front Neurol. 2017; 8: 259

[23] Eichberg DG, Buttrick SS, Sharaf JM, et al. Use of tubular retractor for resection of colloid cysts: single surgeon experience and review of the literature. Oper Neurosurg (Hagerstown) 2019;16(5):571–579

[24] da C F Pinto PH, Nigri F, Gobbi GN, Caparelli-Daquer EM. Conversion technique from neuroendoscopy to microsurgery in ventricular tumors: technical note. Surg Neurol Int. 2016; 7 Suppl 31:S785–S789

[25] Vorbau C, Baldauf J, Oertel J, Gaab MR, Schroeder HWS. Long-term results after endoscopic resection of colloid cysts. World Neurosurg. 2019; 122: e176–e185

[26] Greenlee JDW, Teo C, Ghahreman A, Kwok B. Purely endoscopic resection of colloid cysts. Neurosurgery. 2008; 62(3) Suppl 1:51–55, discussion 55–56

[27] Denby CE, Vann SD, Tsivilis D, et al. The frequency and extent of mammillary body atrophy associated with surgical removal of a colloid cyst. AJNR Am J Neuroradiol. 2009; 30(4):736–743

# Part IV

## Endoscopic Management of Colloid Cysts



IV

# 10 The Endoscopic Resection of Colloid Cysts

*Sascha Marx and Henry W.S. Schroeder*

**Abstract**
This chapter describes our endoscopic technique for the gross total resection of colloid cysts via a ventriculoscope emphasizing the bimanual sharp dissection and hemostasis techniques.

*Keywords:* colloid cyst, endoscopic resection, small chamber irrigation technique, dryfield technique, bimanual sharp dissection, neuronavigation

## 10.1 The Evolution of Neuroendoscopy in Colloid Cyst Removal

The neuroendoscopic approach to colloid cysts of the third ventricle underwent a rapid evolution over the course of the last 30 years, leading to a procedure with equal efficacy and reduced invasiveness when compared to microsurgical procedures. The first reports of neuroendoscopic management of colloid cyst need to be seen as experimental attempts. In 1988, Auer et al included one colloid cyst within their experience of 133 neuroendoscopic procedures for various pathologies. However, they could not fenestrate the outer colloid cyst membrane and had to switch to a microsurgical approach.[1] In 1983, 5 years before this, Powell et al reported a series of neuroendoscopic procedures for colloid cysts with the goal of fenestrating the membrane and aspirating the cyst content.[2] The techniques reported between 1980 and the early 1990s were mainly restricted to endoscopic colloid cyst fenestration, aspiration of the cyst content, and coagulation of the cyst capsule. Not unexpectedly, a certain percentage of cyst recurrences were reported after neuroendoscopic treatment of colloid cysts.[1,2,3,4]

A meta-analysis involving 1,278 patients, comparing neuroendoscopic and microsurgical approaches to colloid cysts, found that the microsurgical resection is associated with a higher rate of gross total resections (GTRs) (96.8 vs. 58.2%), lower rate of recurrence (1.5 vs. 3.9%), and fewer reoperations than with endoscopic procedures (0.4 vs. 3.9%).[5] However, the meta-analysis is biased in a way that most of those pilot studies from the early years of neuroendoscopic colloid cyst removal were included. The endoscopic approach to colloid cysts has some advantages over microsurgery, such as reduced complication rate and faster recovery.[6,7,8,9] A recent review, including only studies after 2000, shows the beginning of a bimanual dissection technique through a channel ventriculoscope.[9] With several modifications of the surgical technique which we implemented over the years, a safer and more radical cyst resection could be achieved.

## 10.2 Anterolateral Entry Point

A total removal of colloid cysts in combination with a minimal risk of traumatizing important neurovascular structures can be achieved most easily with an optimal entry point.[10] With that background the position of the burr hole underwent an evolution in two directions: from medial to lateral and from precoronal to anterior. The burr hole location in many studies during the first decade of neuroendoscopic colloid cyst removal was just precoronal and 2.5 cm lateral, reflecting more or less the traditional Kocher's point.[3,4,6,11,12,13,14,15] However, this burr hole location has several disadvantages: the cyst attachment cannot be reached without violating the fornix because it is approached from above. The access to the foramen of Monro is tangential instead of perpendicular. The convex distension of the roof of the third ventricle created by the cyst growth is more difficult to approach.[11,16]

In recent years, more and more studies advocate a burr hole placed far more anterolaterally.[10,16,17,18,19,20,21,22] In a study by Rangel-Castilla et al, a trajectory was drawn on the magnetic resonance (MR) images of 39 patients to get the optimal entry point. It was found to be around 4 cm lateral to the midline and 4.5 cm anterior to the coronal suture, depending on the ventricular size.[10] Wilson et al described the optimal entry point as approximately 5 cm precoronal and 5 to 7 cm lateral, depending on the ventricle size/configuration.[16] In our experience, the optimal entry point should be as far lateral as possible without damaging the head of the caudate nucleus (▶ Fig. 10.1). Thus, neuronavigational guidance is mandatory to localize the optimal entry point and to access the lateral ventricle.[23] Due to cosmetic reasons the skin incision should be behind the hairline or in a wrinkle in the forehead in bald patients. Some authors advocate a medial but far anterior entry point to have a better bleeding control and to inspect the aqueduct.[24,25] However, usually this approach leads to entering the frontal sinus and should not be done from our point of view. Neuroendoscopic approaches to colloid cysts should be on the right side, except if the right hemisphere is dominant, the cyst bulges much more into the left lateral ventricle, and if a significant ventricular asymmetry exists favoring the left lateral ventricle.[3,6,13,14,15,16,17,20,21,22] A port technique using endoscopic visualization and bimanual dissection via two burr holes or by craniotomy is proposed by some authors.[14,26] However, that is not necessary in most of the patients in our experience. Referring to the concept of minimal invasiveness, there is a broad agreement that colloid cysts should be accessed via a single burr hole.

## 10.3 Cyst Evacuation

GTR should be the aim of colloid cyst surgeries because a subtotal resection increases the risk of cyst recurrence. Cyst aspiration alone without cyst wall resection led to a high rate of recurrence in early endoscopic series.[6] Therefore, most authors agree today that a simple cyst aspiration as done by stereotactic evacuation or earlier neuroendoscopic techniques is not sufficient.[12] The cyst opening should be done with scissors after coagulation of the cyst wall. Thereafter, the cyst content should be aspirated. It is of utmost importance to use an endoscope with a large working channel which allows the application of a large caliber suction tube. Due to the highly viscous content, the aspiration would otherwise be ineffective. Our ventriculoscope has a 2.9 mm working channel which allows us to use a 2.7 mm endotracheal suction catheter, which in most cases leads to a successful aspiration of the cyst content.

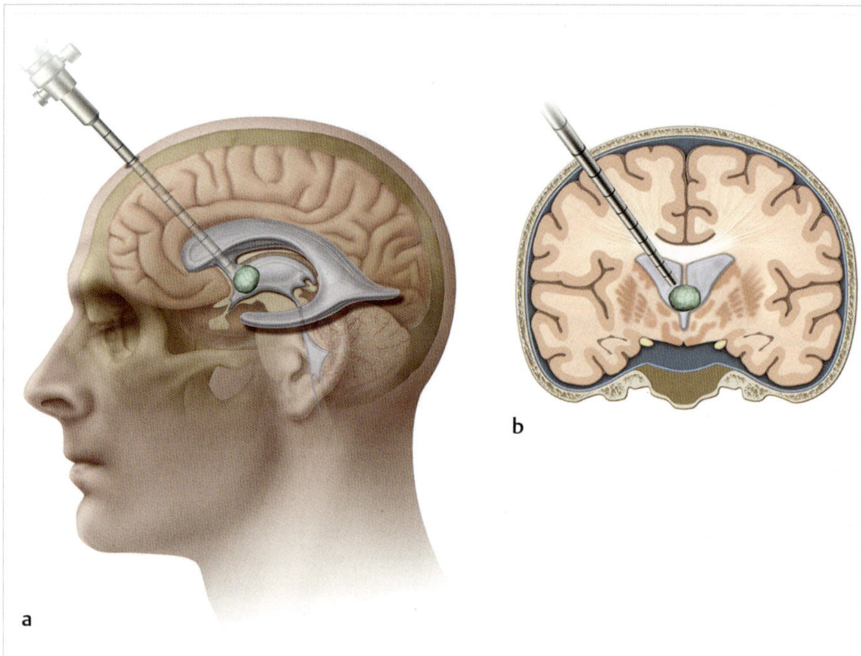


**Fig. 10.1 (a,b)** Schematic drawing showing the anterolateral approach trajectory to a colloid cyst of the third ventricle.

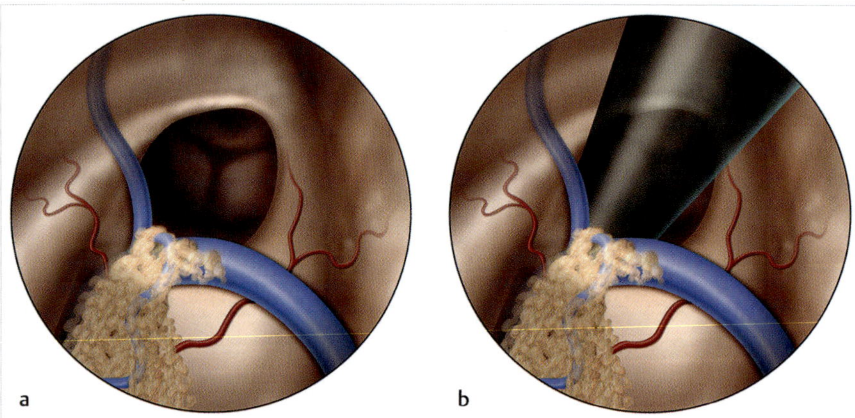


**Fig. 10.2 (a,b)** The endoscopic sheath can be used to retract the fornix a little bit upward to enable access to the vessels at the tela choroidea.

## 10.4 Bimanual Sharp Dissection

Colloid cysts are usually attached to the tela choroidea via a vascularized pedicle. That fact and the close vicinity to the internal cerebral veins make the disconnection of the cyst from the tela choroidea the most critical step of the cyst removal. To get a safe resection it is mandatory to deal with the vessels inside the pedicle and the choroid plexus. Some groups describe removing this part of the cyst by pulling.[4,6,13,18,19] Gentle traction can lead to a total cyst removal without causing hemorrhage in some cases, but those are rare based on our experience. Simply pulling usually leads to hemorrhage with blurring of the view and should be avoided. All adhesions should be visualized, coagulated, and then cut with scissors. Scissors with only one mobile blade are safer to use close to vulnerable neurovascular structures. The fixed blade can be easily guided underneath the structure to be cut and then the other blade is closed. Although that step is important, a couple of authors do not mention this in their approach to deal with the attachment of the cyst to neurovascular structures.[24,27,28]

The inability to perform a two-handed (bimanual) dissection was considered as the major limitation of the endoscopic versus the microsurgical technique. With a one-handed technique the neurosurgeon can only pull, coagulate, or cut. However, the cyst falls down to the foramen when no traction is applied with consecutive obscured vision and blocked access to the cyst pedicle. A bimanual resection technique is possible and has been described several times with the aid of multichannel endoscopes.[12,16,17,20,21,22,29] The cyst wall is put under tension with the aid of a grasping forceps. Then the vessels inside the pedicle are coagulated with the bipolar diathermy probe and cut with scissors thereafter.

## 10.5 Use of the Endoscopic Sheath

The endoscopic sheath can be used as a retractor to get better access to the tela choroidea and cyst pedicle. For a foramen of Monro of adequate size, we use the endoscopic sheath to retract the fornix a little bit upwards to gain access to the vessels originating from the tela choroidea (▶ Fig. 10.2). If the cyst pedicle after mobilizing the cyst into the lateral ventricle is long enough to allow cyst displacement, the cyst is pushed upwards over the fornix along the septum pellucidum with the endoscopic sheath. By this movement the pedicle is placed under tension which enables safe cutting under very good visual control.

## 10.6 Gross Total Resection

GTR should be the goal in every colloid cyst removal. However, if the cyst cannot be resected completely, small remnants need to be left in place and devitalized by bipolar coagulation.[3,11,12,15,18,19,29] Although those remnants may not lead to recurrences in the short term, late recurrences are possible.[12,16,30] Overall, the correlation of cyst remnant and recurrence is difficult to assess because often the authors do not describe how much of the cyst was left behind.[29] In our opinion, a near-total resection with minor capsule remnant may be desirable in elderly patients because the life-time chance of a clinically relevant recurrence is comparatively low. If there is a major problem in achieving a GTR, a switch to microscopic removal is indicated.

## 10.7 Small Chamber Irrigation Technique and Dry Field Technique for Hemostasis

When a significant hemorrhage which cannot be easily managed by irrigation alone occurs, the following small chamber irrigation technique is applied[31]: The endoscope is retracted approximately 4 mm into the sheath, creating a small chamber in front of the lens within the sheath. This small space can easily be cleared of bloody cerebrospinal fluid (CSF) by forced irrigation, enabling a good view. The endoscope is then used to carefully approach the bleeding vessel, and coagulation under direct visualization is performed. If this hemostasis technique fails, the dry field technique is applied[32]: The CSF is aspirated with the aid of a pediatric endotracheal suction tube and a 20-mL syringe. The bleeding usually stops spontaneously without any coagulation after some CSF has been removed. The ventricles are filled up with lactated Ringer solution after hemostasis has been achieved in order to prevent a ventricle collapse. Then the dissection can be continued.

## 10.8 Technique of Colloid Cyst Resection

The basic steps of colloid cyst resection are shown in ▶ Fig. 10.3. At first the cyst is inspected in the foramen of Monro, and the fornix, choroid plexus, thalamostriate vein, and septal vein are identified (▶ Fig. 10.3a). Then the choroid plexus and capsule vessels are coagulated (▶ Fig. 10.3b). Next, the cyst is opened with scissors (▶ Fig. 10.3c) and the cyst content is aspirated with a suction tube (▶ Fig. 10.3d). Thereafter, the cyst is carefully mobilized into the lateral ventricle (▶ Fig. 10.3e). Then the procedure is continued using the bimanual dissection technique. A flexible grasping forceps is introduced via the side channel and a bipolar electrode or scissors are inserted via the main working channel (▶ Fig. 10.3f). The cyst is carefully pulled upwards which exposes the pedicle of the cyst. The vessels within the pedicle are coagulated (▶ Fig. 10.3g) and the pedicle is cut with scissors (▶ Fig. 10.3h). The cyst should be removed only after sharp dissection of all adhesions to the choroid plexus and tela choroidea. Blunt dissection and simply pulling should be avoided whenever possible to prevent venous hemorrhage. Septostomy is indicated if one foramen of Monro remains occluded. This has never occurred in our experience. Furthermore, there is no indication for a third ventriculostomy. Finally, the ipsilateral foramen of Monro is inspected to rule out forniceal damage (▶ Fig. 10.3i). The roof with the tela choroidea is visualized with a 45-degree endoscope in order to confirm that total cyst resection has been achieved and the ventriculoscope and endoscopic sheath are removed from the ventricle. The burr hole is covered with a titanium plate. Galea and skin are sutured.

## 10.9 Selection of the Best Approach Tailored to Each Individual Patient

The endoscopic approach to colloid cyst is not a one-size-fits-all concept because there are patients with MR image appearances unsuitable for an endoscopic cyst removal. Slit ventricles after shunting are a contraindication for an endoscopic approach in our opinion, and we would not externalize the shunt in order to increase the ventricular size. A transcallosal microsurgical resection is the procedure of choice under these circumstances because it is less traumatic to the fornix in very narrow ventricles compared to an endoscopic approach. When the foramen of Monro is very small (1 to 2 mm), the cyst large, and the cyst content most probably firm, as indicated by a black signal in T2-weighted images, we prefer a microsurgical technique. In some patients, we made an endoscopic inspection to confirm the MR imaging findings and then used the endoscopic puncture channel to insert a translucent tube and performed a transcortical microsurgical cyst resection. In more posteriorly located cyst under the roof of the third ventricle or in case of a small foramen of Monro, a purely transforaminal endoscopic approach would lead to contusion of the fornix and should be avoided.[3,14,19] An endoscopic opening of the choroidal fissure to enlarge the foramen of Monro has been reported.[13,33] We agree that an endoscopic transforaminal approach can be extended by opening of the choroidal fissure under certain circumstances, when the foramen is dilated by the lesion and the overlying tela is stretched and the veins are separated. However, usually a microsurgical dissection is far less traumatic to the fornices when using a bimanual sharp dissection technique in which soft micropatties are used to gently separate the fornix from the thalamus. In case a cavum septi pellucidi is present, a medial burr hole at Kocher's point is preferred in order to achieve an interforniceal approach to the cyst.[22] Of course, the distance of the fornices needs to be of adequate length for this approach. We think that the approach should be individually tailored according to the anatomical conditions of the patients.

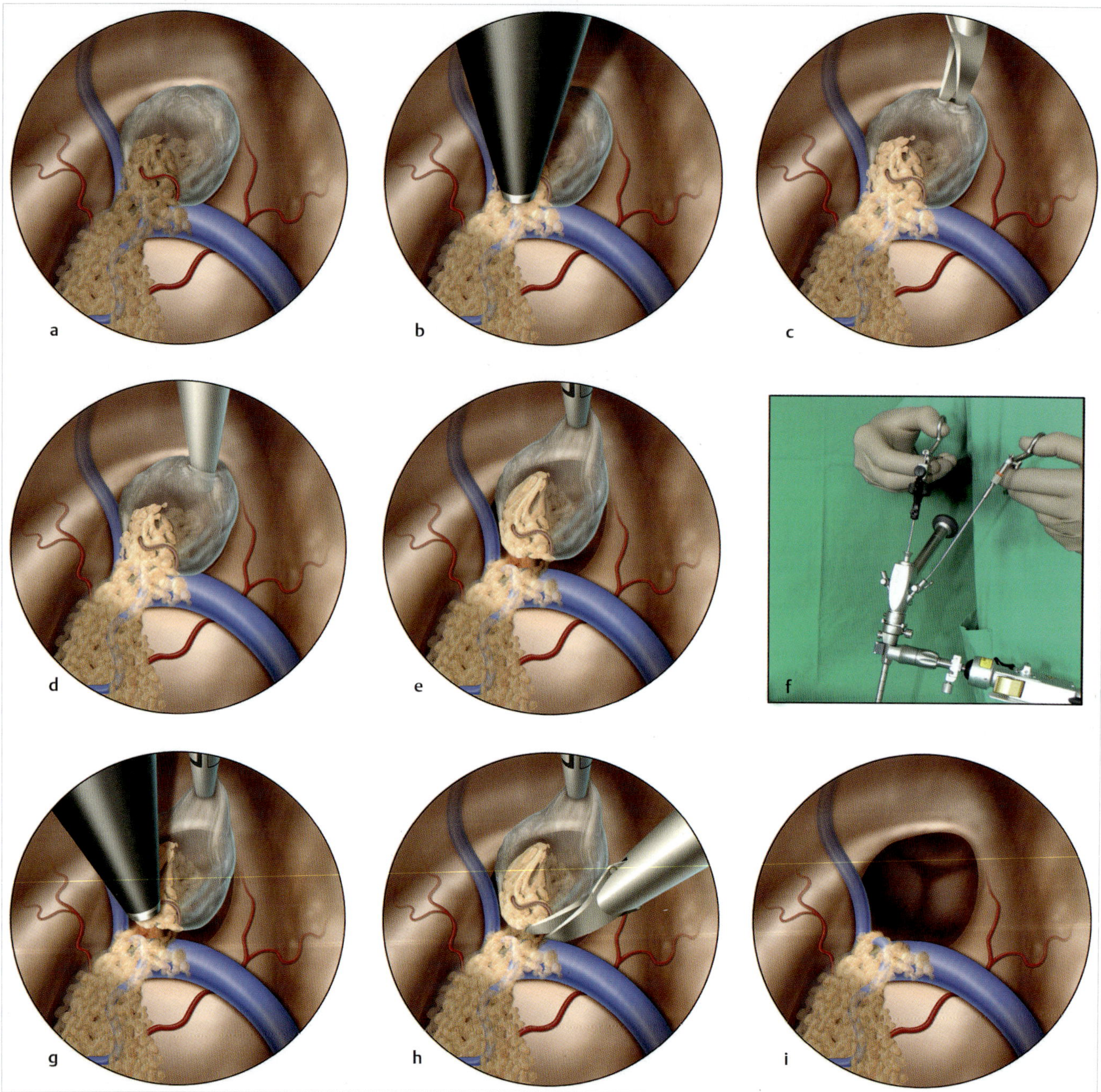


**Fig. 10.3** Illustration showing the surgical steps of colloid cyst removal. **(a)** Inspection of the foramen of Monro with fornix (F), choroid plexus (CP), septal vein (SV), and thalamostriatic (T) vein. The foramen is occluded by a colloid cyst (C). **(b)** Coagulation of the choroid plexus with the bipolar diathermy probe. **(c)** Incision of the cyst capsule with scissors. **(d)** Aspiration of the cyst content with a suction tube. **(e)** Mobilization of the cyst into the lateral ventricle. **(f)** Bimanual dissection technique to expose the cyst pedicle. A flexible grasping forceps is inserted via the left side channel. The other instrument is introduced via the 2.9-mm straight main working channel. **(g)** Coagulation of the cyst pedicle with the bipolar diathermia probe using the bimanual technique. **(h)** Cutting of the cyst pedicle with scissors using the bimanual technique. **(i)** Inspection of the foramen of Monro after cyst removal.

## 10.10 Case Presentation: "How I Do It"

### 10.10.1 Clinical Presentation, Nuances of Clinical Decision-Making, and Endoscopic Management

We present a 36-year-old female patient who complained of headache, nausea, and vomiting. The case is shown in ▸ Video 10.1. MR imaging revealed a colloid cyst of the third ventricle, which appears hyperintense in the T1-weighted images and isointense in the T2-weighted images, predicting a cyst content which can be aspirated (▸ Fig. 10.4). There was unilateral hydrocephalus with dilation of the left lateral ventricle. Because of this dilation and the large foramen of Monro on the left side, a left frontal approach was chosen. The optimal anterolateral entry point is selected with the aid of neuronavigation. The endoscopic surgery attempted GTR of the cyst.

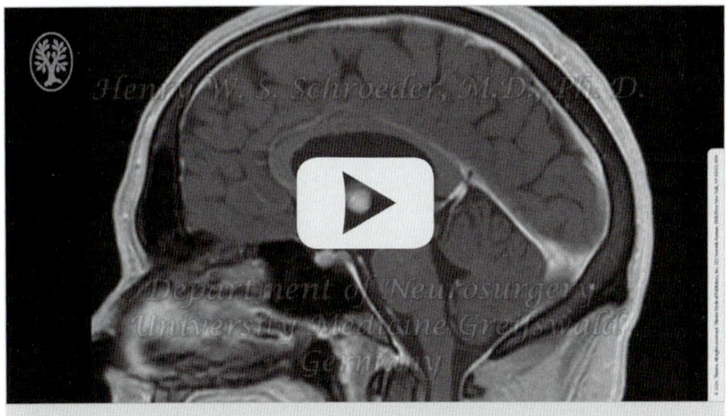

**Video 10.1** Endoscopic resection of a colloid cyst of the third ventricle using a sharp bimanual dissection technique.

## 10.10.2 Surgical Procedure

A navigated, single portal, transcortical, transventricular, transforaminal approach is used which was planned according to MR imaging. The operating room (OR) setup can be seen in ▶ Fig. 10.5. General anesthesia is induced. Thereafter, the patient is placed supine with the head in a three-point fixation. The neck is in a slight anteflexion. For antibiotic prophylaxis 1.5 g cefuroxime is administered intravenously as a single shot. Neuronavigation (Kolibri, BrainLab, Munich, Germany) is registered and accuracy is verified. Based on that the ideal entry point is selected (▶ Fig. 10.6a). The burr hole is placed 5 cm anteriorly to the coronal suture and 4.5 cm laterally to the midline (▶ Fig. 10.7a). Skin incision is made behind the hairline for cosmetic reasons (▶ Fig. 10.7b). Since only the left ventricle is

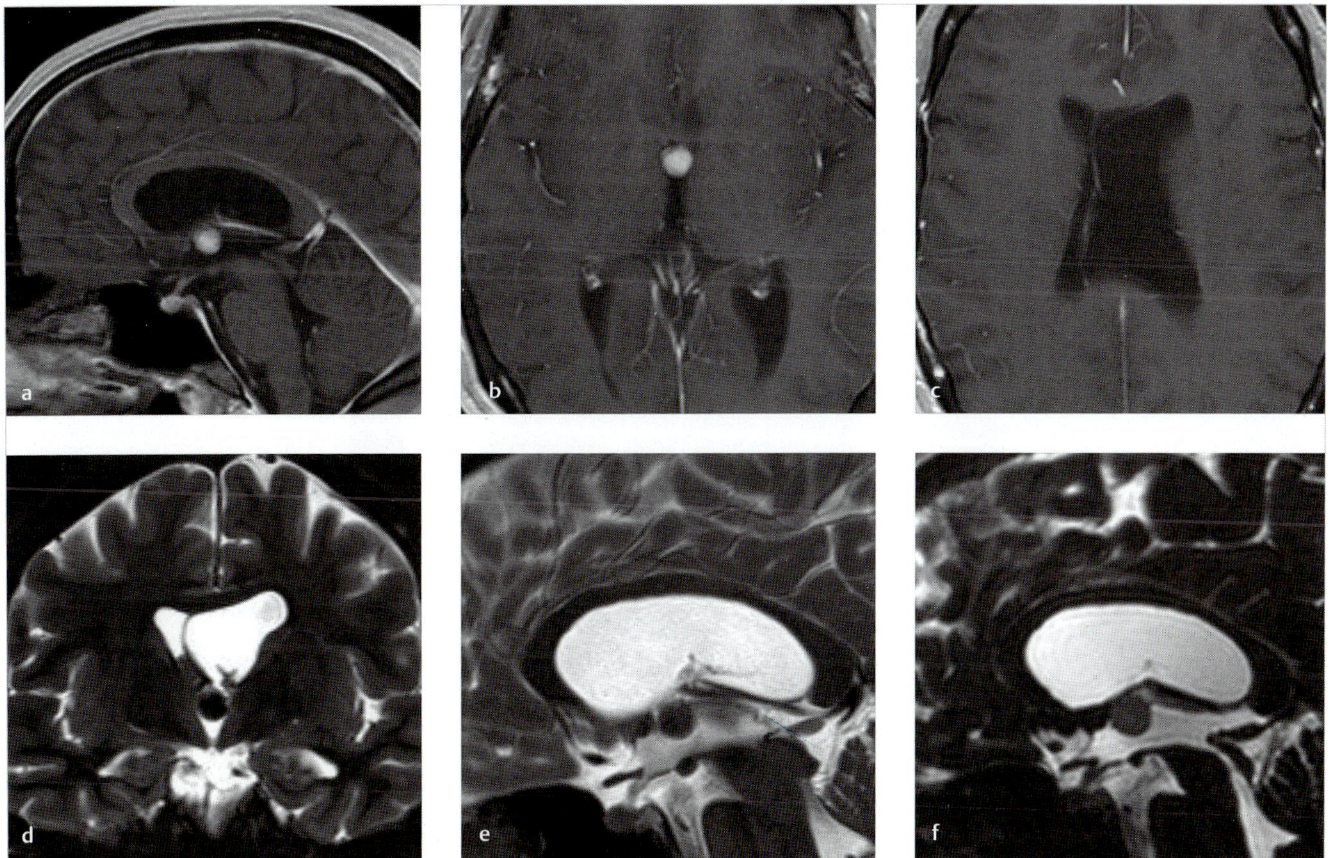

**Fig. 10.4** A 36-year-old female presented with headache, nausea, and vomiting. **(a–f)** Magnetic resonance (MR) imaging shows a colloid cyst within the third ventricle which is hyperintense on T1- and isointense on T2-weighted images causing univentricular hydrocephalus with ventricular dilation of the left lateral ventricle.

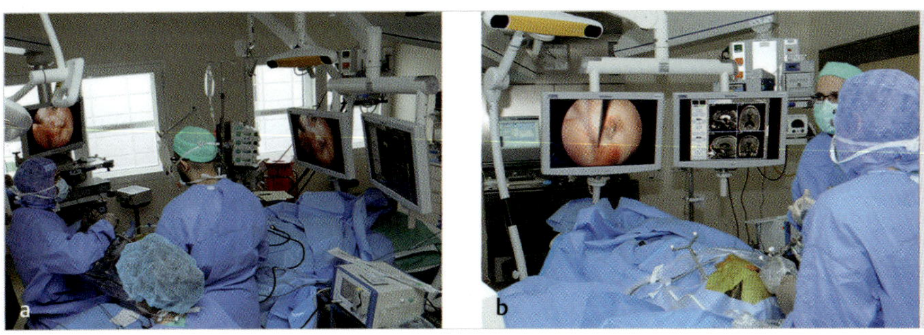

**Fig. 10.5** **(a,b)** Neuroendoscopic setup in the operating room.

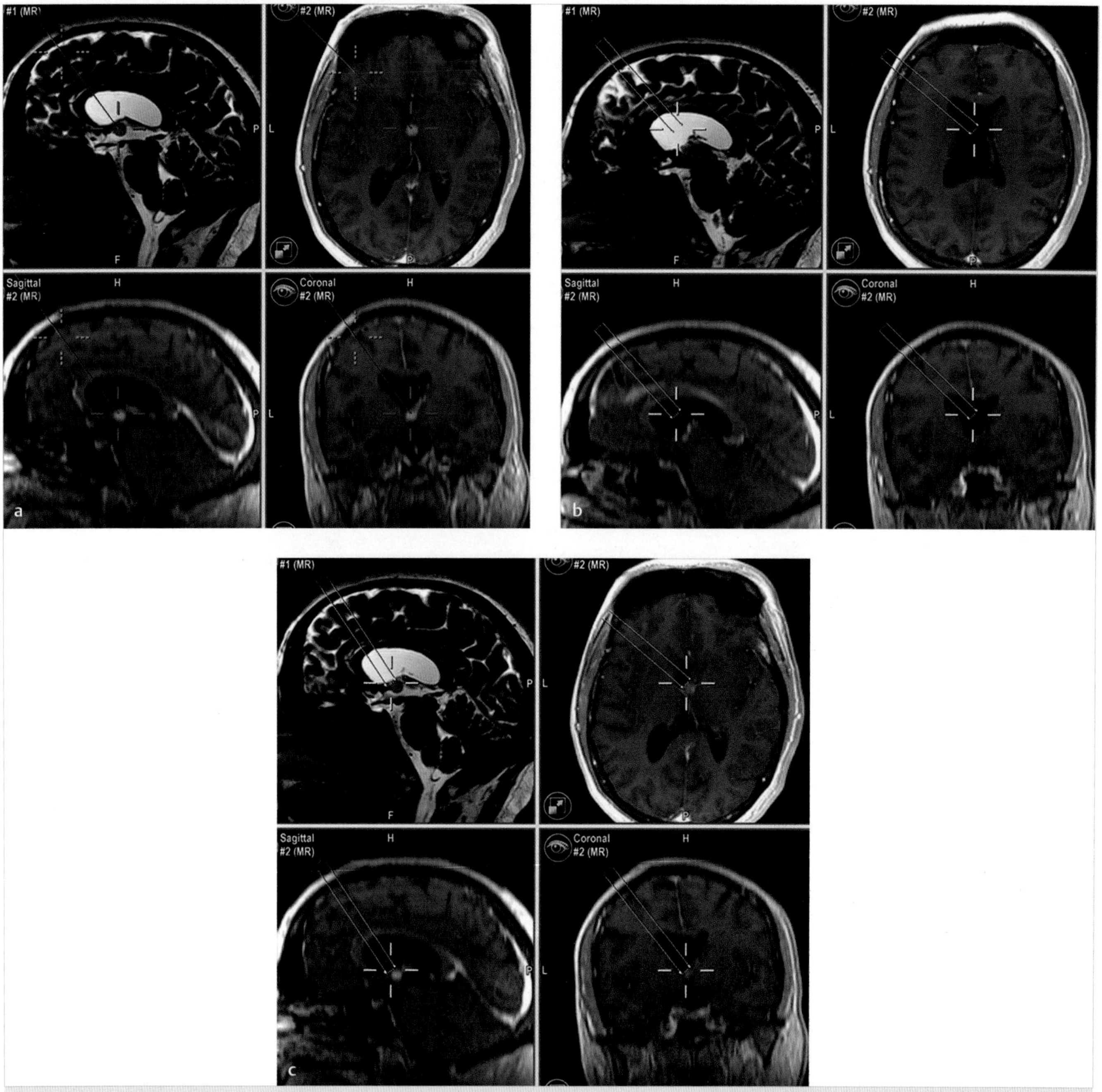

Fig. 10.6 Screenshots of the approach planning and insertion of the endoscope into the lateral ventricle. (a) Planning of the approach with determination of the anterolateral entry point. The trajectory slides just over the head of the caudate nucleus. The approach is from the left side because the cyst is more apparent within the left foramen of Monro. (b) Initial puncture direction is more medial and cranial to avoid damage to the caudate nucleus. (c) Final optimal position of the endoscope after slight retraction of the head of the caudate nucleus.

dilated and the left foramen of Monro is larger, a left approach is chosen. Disinfection and draping of the surgical area are followed by a 3-cm skin incision and placement of a 1-cm burr hole. The dura is opened in a cruciate fashion. The cortex is coagulated. Thereafter, the endoscopic sheath of the LOTTA ventriculoscope with trocar inside is introduced under navigational guidance into the frontal horn of the lateral ventricle.[34] When the lateral ventricle is punctured, the trajectory is more medial and cranial than the true trajectory to the cyst location (▶ Fig. 10.6b). Once the ventricle is reached, the head of the caudate nucleus is gently pushed laterally with the endoscopic sheath to get the optimal trajectory to the cyst (▶ Fig. 10.6c). This procedure leads to the most lateral trajectory to the cyst without injuring the caudate nucleus. After removal of the trocar, the ventricle is inspected with the ventriculoscope.

The first landmarks that have to be identified are caudate nucleus, choroid plexus, fornix, thalamostriate vein, and septal vein (► Fig. 10.8a). A colloid cyst obstructing the foramen of Monro is seen (► Fig. 10.8b). At first the choroid plexus covering the cyst and capsule vessels is coagulated (► Fig. 10.8c). The cyst capsule is incised with scissors (► Fig. 10.8d). The yellow colloid content of the cyst is spontaneously escaping out of the cyst (► Fig. 10.8e). The content is aspirated with a pediatric 2.7-mm endotracheal suction tube and a syringe (► Fig. 10.8f). Subsequently, the cyst membrane is grasped, and the cyst is carefully mobilized into the lateral ventricle (► Fig. 10.8g). The contralateral choroid plexus is adherent to the cyst (► Fig. 10.8h) and should not be disrupted, but coagulated and cut. A vascularized pedicle connects the cyst to the tela choroidea. A bimanual dissection technique is used to allow a proper control of that pedicle. Via the left side

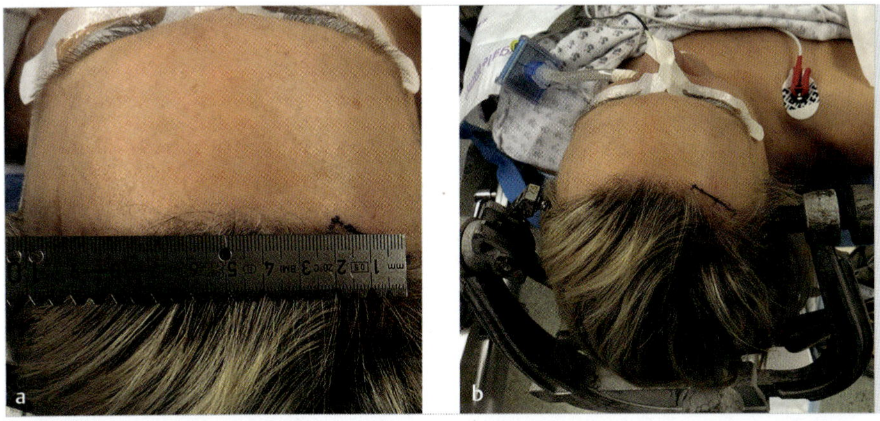

**Fig. 10.7 (a)** The optimal entry point is 4.5 cm lateral to the midline. **(b)** The patient is positioned supine with sharp head fixation in a Mayfield clamp. The head is in neutral position and slightly anteflexed. For cosmetic reasons, the skin incision is just behind the hairline.

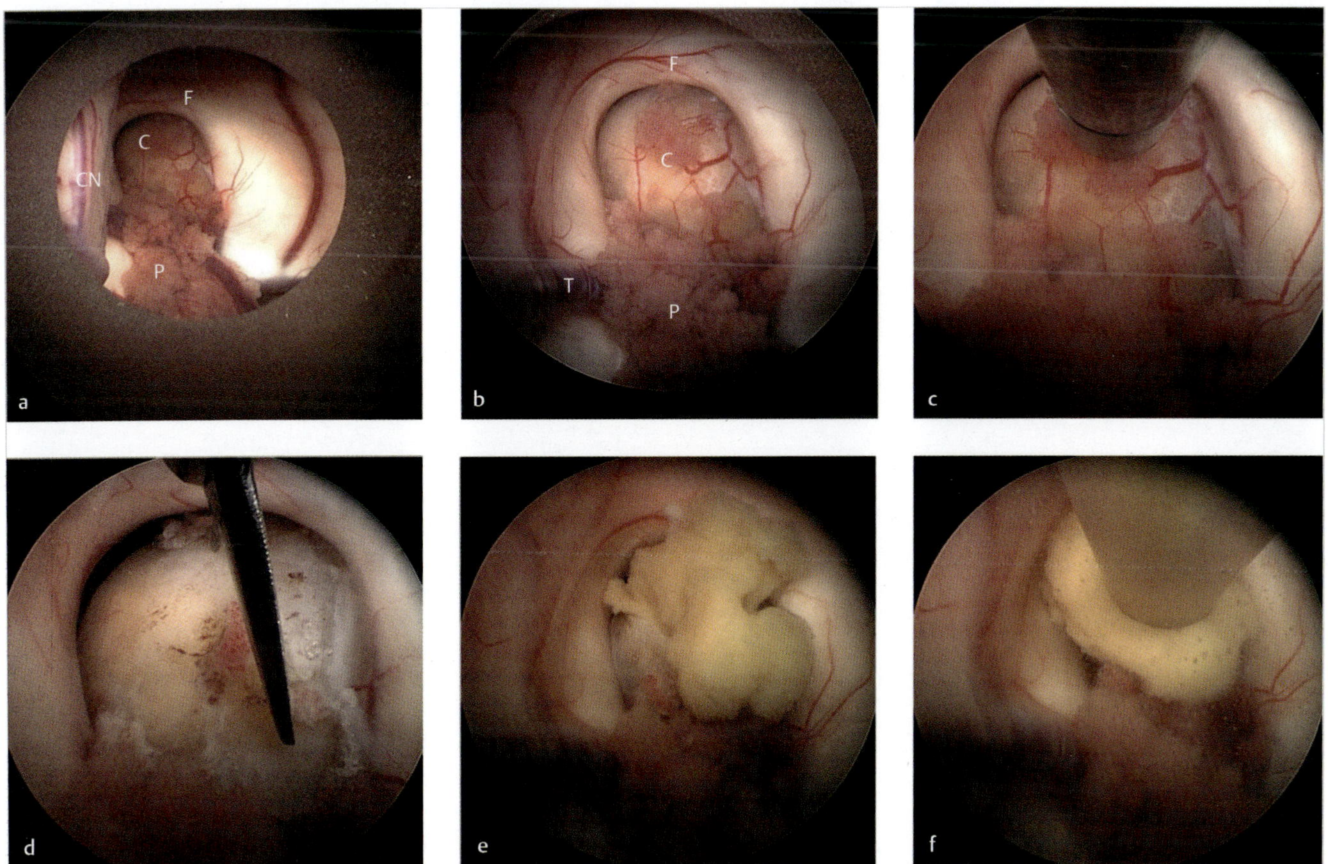


**Fig. 10.8** Endoscopic images showing the surgical steps of colloid cyst removal. **(a)** View after entering the left lateral ventricle showing that the approach trajectory is just sliding over the head of the caudate nucleus. The foramen of Monro with cyst, fornix, and choroid plexus is seen. **(b)** Colloid cyst occluding the foramen of Monro with fornix, choroid plexus, and thalamostriate vein. **(c)** Coagulation of the choroid plexus and cyst capsule with a bipolar diathermy probe. **(d)** Incision of the cyst capsule with scissors. **(e)** Yellow cyst content escaping from the cyst. **(f)** Aspiration of the cyst content with a suction tube.

*(Continued)*

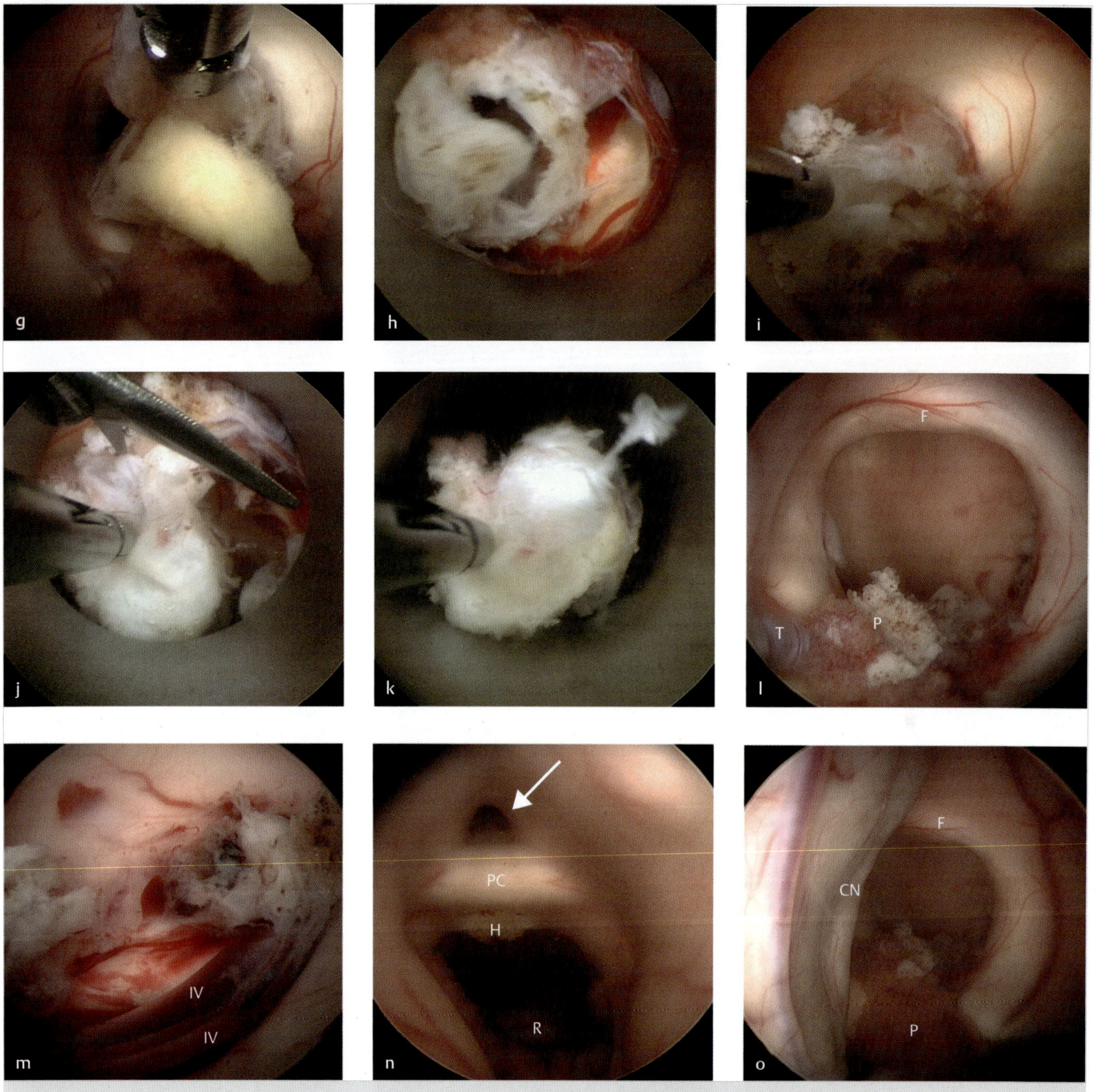


**Fig. 10.8** (*Continued*) **(g)** Mobilization of the cyst into the lateral ventricle with a biopsy forceps. **(h)** Evacuated colloid cyst with contralateral choroid plexus. **(i)** Bimanual dissection technique to detach the cyst from the tela choroidea. A flexible grasping forceps is inserted via the left side channel. **(j)** Scissors are introduced via the main straight working channel and the pedicle is cut. **(k)** Removal of the cyst together with the endoscope via the endoscopic sheath. **(l)** Inspection of the foramen of Monro after cyst removal showing an intact fornix and vein. **(m)** Inspection of the roof of the third ventricle with a 45-degree endoscope showing the tela choroidea and internal cerebral veins, but no residual cyst. **(n)** View of the posterior third ventricle showing the patent aqueduct. **(o)** The caudate nucleus showing a slight indentation caused by the retraction with the endoscopic sheath, but no structural damage. (*Arrow* shows entrance of the aqueduct; C, cyst; CN, caudate nucleus; F, fornix; H, habenular commissure; IV, internal cerebral vein; P, choroid plexus; PC, posterior commissure; R, roof; T, tela choroidea.)

channel of the ventriculoscope a small flexible grasping forceps is inserted. With gentle traction the cyst capsule is held up, allowing visualization of the cyst pedicle (▶ Fig. 10.8i). Only the thin cyst capsule should be grasped and not the tela choroidea or the choroid plexus. Via the main working channel, a bipolar diathermy probe is introduced, and the vessels are coagulated. Finally, the pedicle is cut with microscissors (▶ Fig. 10.8j). Since the cyst is too large to be removed via the working channel, the ventriculoscope is withdrawn from the endoscopic sheath together with the forceps holding the cyst (▶ Fig. 10.8k). A vigorous irrigation of the ventricles is done next to remove spilled cyst content. The inspection shows

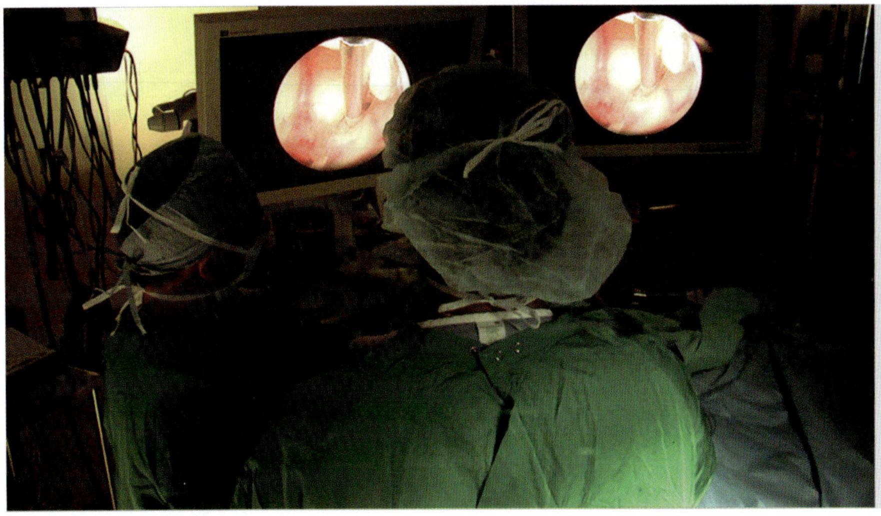

**Fig. 11.3** Illustration of high-definition monitors placed on the patient's left side, directly in front of the surgery team, standing on the right side of the operating room table.

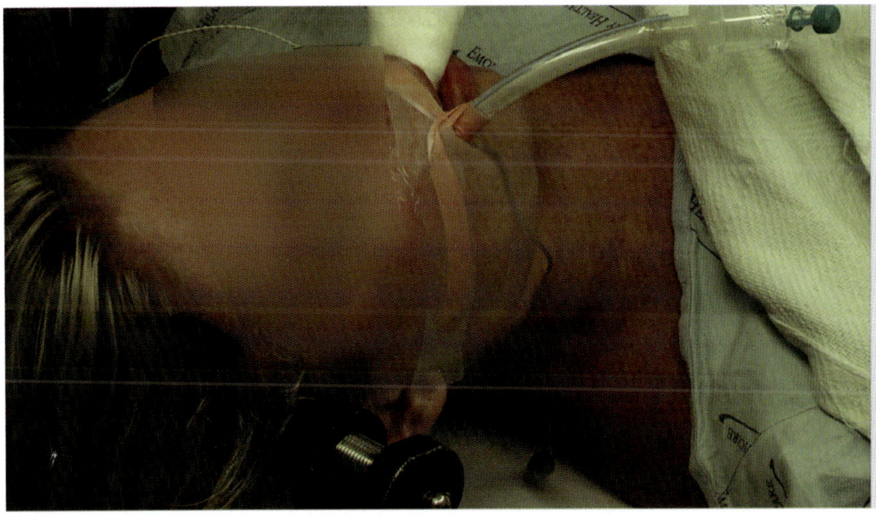

**Fig. 11.4** The 2-cm incision used for the anterolateral endoscopic approach, placed 8 cm posterior to the nasion and 5 cm to the right of midline.

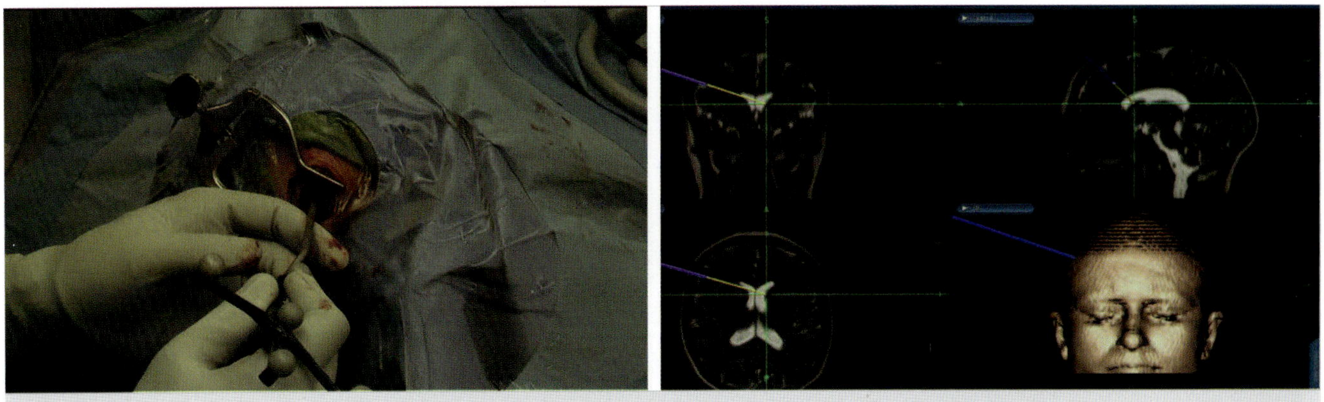

**Fig. 11.5** Intraoperative neuronavigation depicting the correct trajectory of the endoscope toward the anterior horn of the lateral ventricle while avoiding the caudate nucleus.

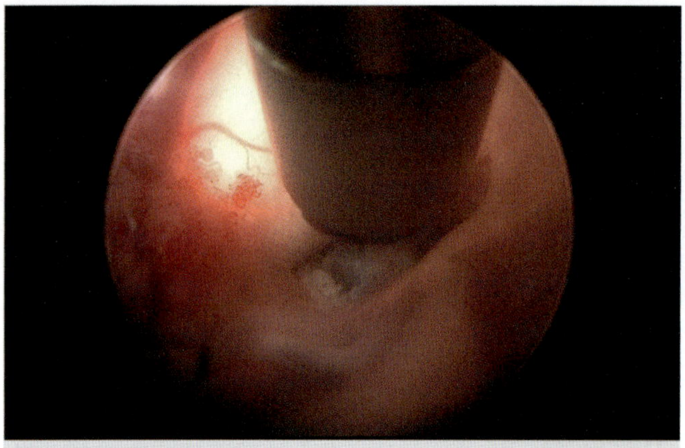

**Fig. 11.6** A picture showcasing endoscopic electrocautery of the colloid cyst capsule.

bipolar device, thus allowing for communication between the two ventricles, being careful to avoid the septal vein and fornix. An external ventricular drain (EVD) catheter is subsequently placed in order to allow for drainage of any additional blood during the postoperative period for 24 to 48 hours.

## 11.5 Clinical Outcomes

Multiple studies have demonstrated excellent clinical outcomes for patients treated with this approach. In an investigation of 483 patients undergoing colloid cyst resection via microsurgery or endoscopic excision, Connolly et al concluded that although both the groups had similar comorbidity profiles, patients treated with an endoscopic approach experienced decreased rates of postoperative seizures.[24] In addition, patients undergoing microsurgical resection had significantly greater incidence of re-admission and associated costs. Similarly, a systematic review and meta-analysis by Sheikh et al revealed that patients undergoing endoscopic resection experienced less morbidity than those treated with endoscopy.[25] However, microsurgical resection was associated with greater rates of complete resection and decreased recurrence.

## 11.6 Illustrative Example: Endoscopic Approach for Resection of a Recurrent Colloid Cyst in the Foramen of Monro

### 11.6.1 History of Present Illness, Physical Examination, and Imaging

The patient is a 50-year-old female with a past medical history significant for a colloid cyst (with two prior microsurgical resections) who was referred to our clinic with a chief complaint of headache and evidence of recurrence on imaging. The patient was initially diagnosed with a colloid cyst 12 years prior, when she presented with obstructive hydrocephalus and unresponsiveness. She underwent an emergent craniotomy at that time

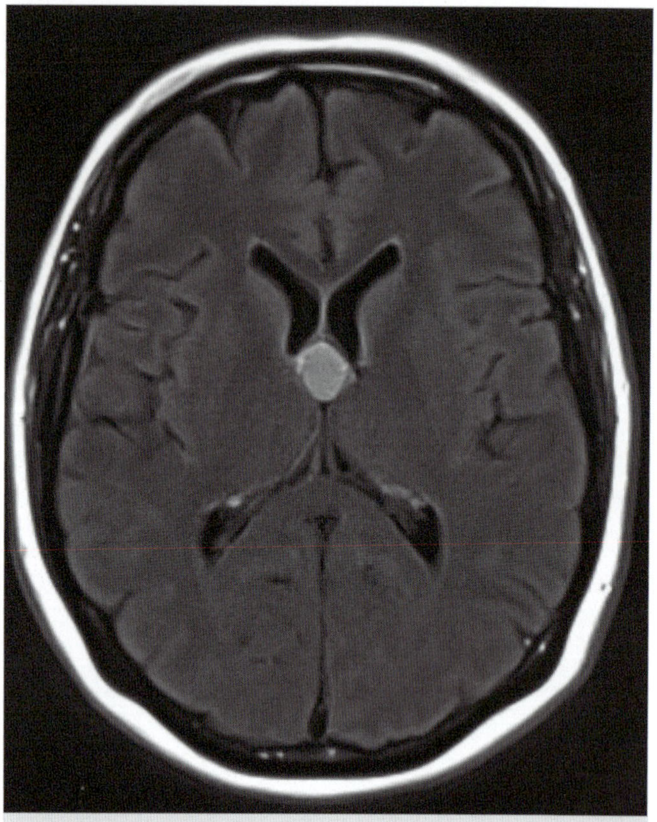

**Fig. 11.7** Axial T2-weighted–fluid-attenuated inversion recovery (T2-FLAIR) magnetic resonance imaging (MRI) demonstrating a 1.5-cm colloid cyst in the interventricular foramen of Monro.

for her colloid cyst via a right, transcortical transfrontal approach. She developed recurrence 4 years later, which necessitated an additional resection via the same approach. Postoperative magnetic resonance imaging (MRI) revealed a residual colloid cyst present following the second operation, and it has been gradually enlarging each year. At present, the patient complains of severe, 7/10 right-frontal, nonradiating headaches, which have been increasing in frequency and intensity over the past several months. In addition, the patient reports dizziness upon standing, which resolves spontaneously after several minutes as well as increased difficulties with her memory. However, she denies any paresthesias, seizures, nausea/vomiting, changes in her vision or hearing, loss of consciousness, or weakness.

Physical examination, including a musculoskeletal and neurological examination, was unremarkable. A healed, right-frontal incision, with evidence of prior craniotomy, was observed.

MRI revealed a large recurrence of her colloid cyst, now measuring 1.3 cm (▶ Fig. 11.7). The ventricles were slightly enlarged but unchanged from MRI obtained 6 months prior. A right transfrontal tract was visible.

### 11.6.2 Clinical Decision-Making

Given that the patient had experienced recurrence and continuous enlargement of her colloid cyst, in addition to being symptomatic, additional intervention was warranted. Endoscopic resection was discussed with the patient and family. The risks and benefits of surgery were discussed, and the patient expressed her desire to proceed with the endoscopic resection.

### 11.6.3 Operative Setup and Preparation

The patient was taken to the operating room where she underwent endotracheal intubation. A Foley catheter was placed to monitor urinary output as well as several intravenous (IV) lines and an arterial line. The patient was placed supine on the operating table. The patient's head was subsequently maintained in the neutral position using a three-pin Mayfield fixation device. At this point, the Medtronic Stealth image guidance system was registered using surface matching. A 2-cm incision was then marked on the right anterior lateral portion of the forehead measuring approximately 8 cm posterior to the nasion and 5 to 7 cm to the right of midline. The hair was clipped slightly in this region in order to allow for entry of the EVD catheter at the end of the case. At this point, the incision was prepped and draped in a sterile fashion.

### 11.6.4 Burr Hole Placement and Ventricular Entry

The 30-degree working channel endoscope was confirmed to be working properly prior to placement of the skin incision. The camera and light source were connected to the neuroendoscope to allow for a brilliant display visualized on multiple monitors directly in front of the surgeon. At this point, the incision was made in the right anterolateral frontal position. The Bovie electrocautery was used to cauterize the dermis and subcutaneous layers, reaching the right frontal skull. A self-retaining retractor was placed in the wound. The burr hole was then created with a Medtronic high-speed burr, thereby allowing for exposure of the underlying dura. The dura was opened in a cruciate fashion, exposing the underlying right frontal lobe. At this point, using image guidance, a 19.5-French sheath trocar was inserted transcortically into the frontal horn of the right lateral ventricle. The trocar was then removed, confirming CSF flow. The sheath was peeled down to the level of the scalp and stapled into position.

At this point, the working channel endoscope was inserted through the sheath into the anterior horn of the right lateral ventricle for visualization of the intraventricular anatomy. As noted before, the patient had two prior craniotomies for resection of her colloid cyst, each through a transfrontal approach on the right hand side. There appeared to be a significant amount of scar tissue at the level of the foramen of Monro. Using the tip of the working channel endoscope, the opening into the third ventricle was enlarged and care was taken not to stretch the forniceal bundle. An image depicting the salient anatomy, including the fornix, choroid plexus, and colloid cyst obstructing the foramen of Monro, is presented in ▶ Fig. 11.8.

### 11.6.5 Choroid Plexus and Cyst Cauterization

Endoscopic bipolar cautery through the working channel was then used to cauterize the choroid plexus overlying the colloid cyst. This colloid cyst was intimately associated with the right septal vein in addition to the right thalamostriate vein. Using cautery with the working channel endoscope, the colloid cyst capsule was cauterized away from the deep venous system. This represents a critical portion of the procedure and is depicted in ▶ Video 11.1. Adequate cauterization of the cyst is crucial to achieve safe dissection while minimizing procedural complications such as hemorrhage. The contents of the colloid cyst were aspirated after it was punctured in order to allow for mobilization of the colloid cyst capsule wall.

### 11.6.6 Cyst Removal

Sharp scissors and blunt forceps were subsequently passed through the working channel and used to dissect the colloid cyst capsule off the surrounding internal cerebral veins, bilaterally. This allowed for complete resection of the colloid cyst capsule en bloc without damaging the underlying vasculature. Careful inspection of the third ventricle was performed multiple times to assess for any residual colloid cyst capsule. Furthermore, there was no damage to any components of the venous system that the colloid cyst capsule was intimately associated

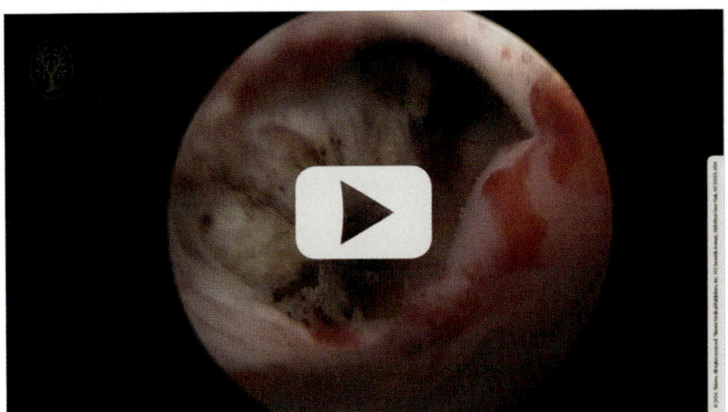

**Video 11.1** Decompression of the colloid cyst using bipolar cautery via the working channel endoscope.

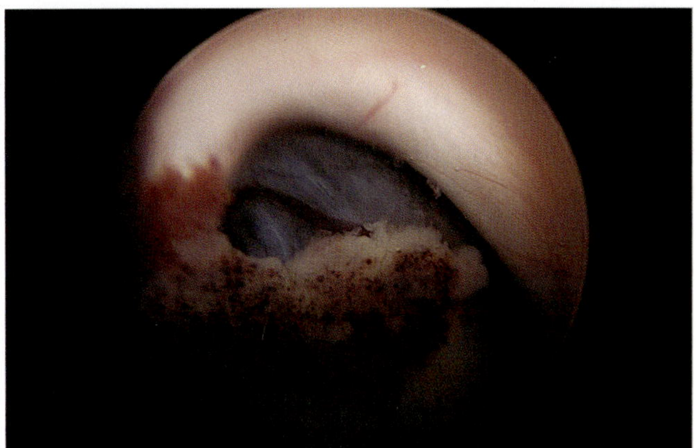

**Fig. 11.8** Endoscopic photograph showcasing the relevant third ventricle anatomy, including the fornix as well as the choroid plexus lying in front of the colloid cyst in the foramen of Monro.

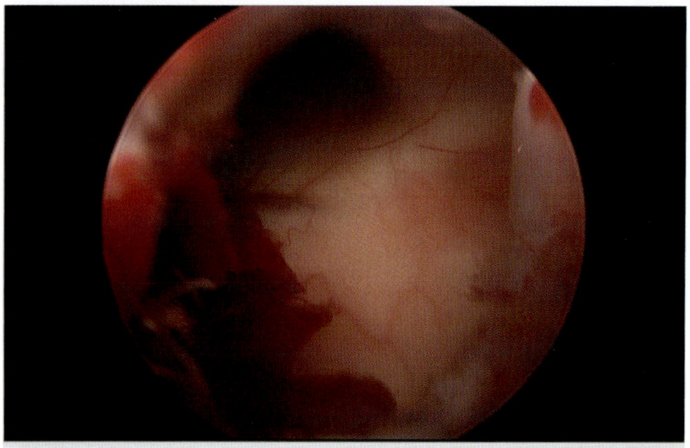

**Fig. 11.9** Photograph depicting a small, residual bleed following en bloc removal of the colloid cyst.

with, and the forniceal bundles remained intact. There was no need for placement of septostomy due to the existence of natural septations secondary to the patient's prior hydrocephalus. At this point, copious amounts of irrigation were used to flush out the ventricular system. Endoscopic bipolar cautery and bulb irrigation were employed to address any residual bleeding in the ventricle (▶ Fig. 11.9). The EVD catheter was left in the ventricular system at a depth of 6.5 cm. This was tunneled up posteriorly through the scalp and held in position with a skin stitch.

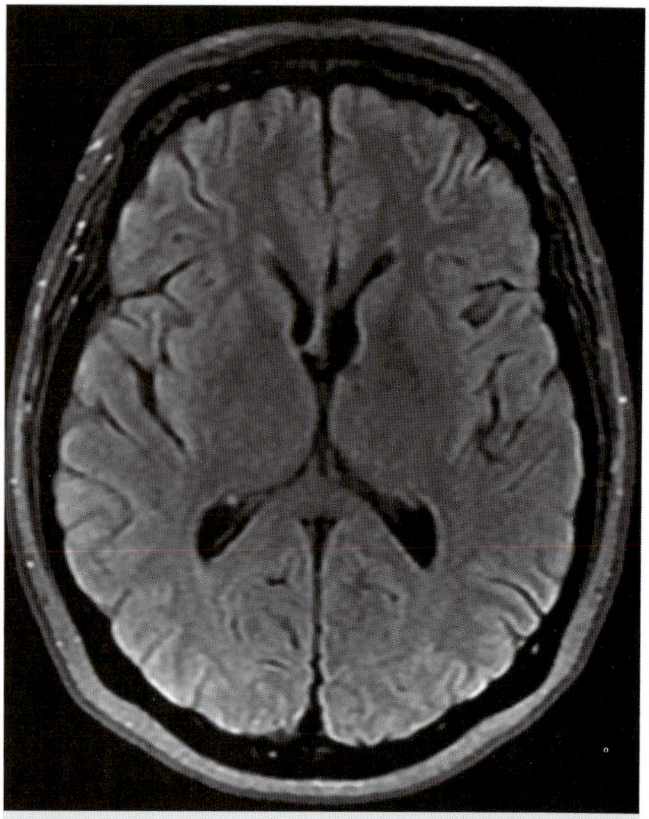

**Fig. 11.10** Axial T2-weighted–fluid-attenuated inversion recovery (T2-FLAIR) magnetic resonance imaging (MRI) at 1-year follow-up with no evidence of intracranial colloid cyst.

### 11.6.7 Closure and Follow-Up

Gelfoam was used to cover the burr hole and a titanium cover was screwed into position, allowing for entry of the EVD catheter. Copious irrigation was used to wash out the incision, which was then re-approximated via multiple 3–0 Vicryl sutures and a running 3–0 chromic gut stitch.

At 1-year follow-up, the patient reports feeling well. She denies any headaches, visual symptoms, or dizziness. Her short-term memory is improving. No evidence of colloid cyst is seen on follow-up T2-FLAIR MRI (▶ Fig. 11.10).

## References

[1] Little JR, MacCarty CS. Colloid cysts of the third ventricle. J Neurosurg. 1974; 40(2):230–235

[2] Desai KI, Nadkarni TD, Muzumdar DP, Goel AH. Surgical management of colloid cyst of the third ventricle—a study of 105 cases. Surg Neurol. 2002; 57(5): 295–302, discussion 302–304

[3] Armao D, Castillo M, Chen H, Kwock L. Colloid cyst of the third ventricle: imaging-pathologic correlation. AJNR Am J Neuroradiol. 2000; 21(8):1470–1477

[4] Turillazzi E, Bello S, Neri M, Riezzo I, Fineschi V. Colloid cyst of the third ventricle, hypothalamus, and heart: a dangerous link for sudden death. Diagn Pathol. 2012; 7:144

[5] Carrasco R, Pascual JM, Medina-López D, Burdaspal-Moratilla A. Acute hemorrhage in a colloid cyst of the third ventricle: a rare cause of sudden deterioration. Surg Neurol Int. 2012; 3:24

[6] Silva D, Matis G, Chrysou O, et al. Sudden death in a patient with a third ventricle colloid cyst. Arq Neuropsiquiatr. 2012; 70(4):311

[7] Shapiro S, Rodgers R, Shah M, Fulkerson D, Campbell RL. Interhemispheric transcallosal subchoroidal fornix-sparing craniotomy for total resection of colloid cysts of the third ventricle. J Neurosurg. 2009; 110(1):112–115

[8] Nair S, Gopalakrishnan CV, Menon G, Easwer HV, Abraham M. Interhemispheric transcallosal transforaminal approach and its variants to colloid cyst of third ventricle: technical issues based on a single institutional experience of 297 cases. Asian J Neurosurg. 2016; 11(3):292–297

[9] Horn EM, Feiz-Erfan I, Bristol RE, et al. Treatment options for third ventricular colloid cysts: comparison of open microsurgical versus endoscopic resection. Neurosurgery. 2007; 60(4):613–618, discussion 618–620

[10] Eichberg DG, Sedighim S, Buttrick S, Komotar RJ. Postoperative seizure rate after transcortical resection of subcortical brain tumors and colloid cysts: a single surgeon's experience. Curcus. 2018; 10(1):e2115

[11] Sabanci PA, Aras Y, Ali A, et al. Transcortical removal of third ventricular colloid cysts: comparison of conventional, guided microsurgical and endoscopic approaches and review of the literature. Turk Neurosurg. 2017; 27(4):546–557

[12] Powell MP, Torrens MJ, Thomson JL, Horgan JG. Isodense colloid cysts of the third ventricle: a diagnostic and therapeutic problem resolved by ventriculoscopy. Neurosurgery. 1983; 13(3):234–237

[13] Caemaert J, Abdullah J. Endoscopic management of colloid cysts. Tech Neurosurg. 1996; 1:185–200

[14] Decq P, Le Guerinel C, Brugières P, et al. Endoscopic management of colloid cysts. Neurosurgery. 1998; 42(6):1288–1294, discussion 1294–1296

[15] Gaab MR, Schroeder HW. Neuroendoscopic approach to intraventricular lesions. J Neurosurg. 1998; 88(3):496–505

[16] Lewis AI, Crone KR, Taha J, van Loveren HR, Yeh HS, Tew JM, Jr. Surgical resection of third ventricle colloid cysts. Preliminary results comparing transcallosal microsurgery with endoscopy. J Neurosurg. 1994; 81(2):174–178

[17] Margetis K, Christos PJ, Souweidane M. Endoscopic resection of incidental colloid cysts. J Neurosurg. 2014; 120(6):1259–1267

[18] Wilson DA, Fusco DJ, Wait SD, Nakaji P. Endoscopic resection of colloid cysts: use of a dual-instrument technique and an anterolateral approach. World Neurosurg. 2013; 80(5):576–583

[19] Greenlee JDW, Teo C, Ghahreman A, Kwok B. Purely endoscopic resection of colloid cysts. Neurosurgery. 2008; 62(3) Suppl 1:51–55, discussion 55–56

[20] Levine NB, Miller MN, Crone KR. Endoscopic resection of colloid cysts: indications, technique, and results during a 13-year period. Minim Invasive Neurosurg. 2007; 50(6):313–317

[21] Boogaarts HD, Decq P, Grotenhuis JA, et al. Long-term results of the neuroendoscopic management of colloid cysts of the third ventricle: a series of 90 cases. Neurosurgery. 2011; 68(1):179–187

[22] Longatti P, Godano U, Gangemi M, et al. Italian neuroendoscopy group. Cooperative study by the Italian neuroendoscopy group on the treatment of 61 colloid cysts. Childs Nerv Syst. 2006; 22(10):1263–1267

[23] Vorbau C, Baldauf J, Oertel J, Gaab MR, Schroeder HWS. Long-term results after endoscopic resection of colloid cysts. World Neurosurg. 2019; 122:e176–e185

[24] Connolly ID, Johnson E, Lamsam L, Veeravagu A, Ratliff J, Li G. Microsurgical vs. endoscopic excision of colloid cysts: an analysis of complications and costs using a longitudinal administrative database. Front Neurol. 2017; 8:259

[25] Sheikh AB, Mendelson ZS, Liu JK. Endoscopic versus microsurgical resection of colloid cysts: a systematic review and meta-analysis of 1,278 patients. World Neurosurg. 2014; 82(6):1187–1197

# 12 Endoscopic Resection of Colloid Cysts of the Third Ventricle: 20 Years at Washington University

*Thomas L. Beaumont, Keith M. Rich, and Ralph G. Dacey, Jr.*

**Abstract**

Colloid cysts of the third ventricle are histologically benign lesions that can cause obstructive hydrocephalus and death. Historically, colloid cysts have been removed by open microsurgical approaches, most commonly the interhemispheric-transcallosal (IHTC) approach. More recently, minimally invasive endoscopic and port-based techniques have offered decreased complications, reduced length of stay (LOS) and improved patient satisfaction. We performed a retrospective analysis of patients with colloid cysts who underwent surgery at the Washington University over nearly two decades, with the primary goal of comparing outcomes associated with open microsurgical approaches versus the more recently implemented neuroendoscopic approach. The primary endpoint was rate of perioperative complications. The study included patients with colloid cysts who underwent microsurgical resection (MR) by craniotomy with either an IHTC or transcortical-transventricular (TCTV) approach, or by single burr hole endoscopic approach. Endoscopic resection (ER) optimized nearly all procedure-related variables compared to MR and reduced total inpatient cost by more than 50%. While coagulated residual cyst wall remnants were more common after ER, this was not associated with a significantly increased rate of reoperation for recurrence. Taken together, for neurosurgeons with endoscopic expertise, neuroendoscopy is a safe and effective minimally invasive approach for resection of colloid cysts of the third ventricle.

*Keywords:* colloid cyst, endoscopic, hydrocephalus, neuroendoscopy, third ventricle

## 12.1 Introduction

Colloid cysts of the third ventricle are rare, histologically benign lesions that occur in the region of the foramen of Monro where they can cause obstructive hydrocephalus, clinical deterioration, and death. Their incidence has been estimated at 3.2 cases per million per year, accounting for approximately 2% of all intracranial tumors.[1] Approximately half of patients with colloid cysts are symptomatic at diagnosis and require neurosurgical intervention.[2,3,4] Colloid cysts can be a formidable neurosurgical challenge due to their location deep within the brain, intimately associated with the fornix and critical deep draining veins to which they are commonly adherent (▶ Fig. 12.1). Historically, colloid cysts have been removed with transcranial microsurgery by an interhemispheric transcallosal (IHTC) or transcortical transventricular (TCTV) approach. Open microsurgical approaches have a relatively high rate of complications in reported series, ranging from 3.5 to 33%, with an average rate of at least 20%.[5,6,7] Over the past two decades, neuroendoscopic techniques have offered increasingly favorable results with significantly decreased complication rates, typically < 5%, along with optimal procedure-related variables and improved patient satisfaction.[8,9,10,11,12]

Early case series comparing endoscopic resection (ER) to microsurgical resection (MR) consistently demonstrated decreased operative time, decreased perioperative complications, and reduced length of stay (LOS).[5,6,13,14] Nonetheless, these studies also demonstrated an increased rate of residual cyst wall remnants and cyst recurrence following ER, which was confirmed in several subsequent case series.[14,15,16,17] As the endoscopic technique has continued to evolve, more recent series have reported rates of gross total resection (GTR) and recurrence similar to that achieved by microsurgical techniques.[11,12,18] Nonetheless, it remains unclear how the presence of coagulated cyst wall remnants after ER relates to radiographic recurrence and the need for reoperation, and this is particularly the case when the remnant is small and thoroughly coagulated. Reported colloid cyst recurrence rates in the setting of coagulated cyst wall remnants range widely from 11.1 to 33.3%, although the latter

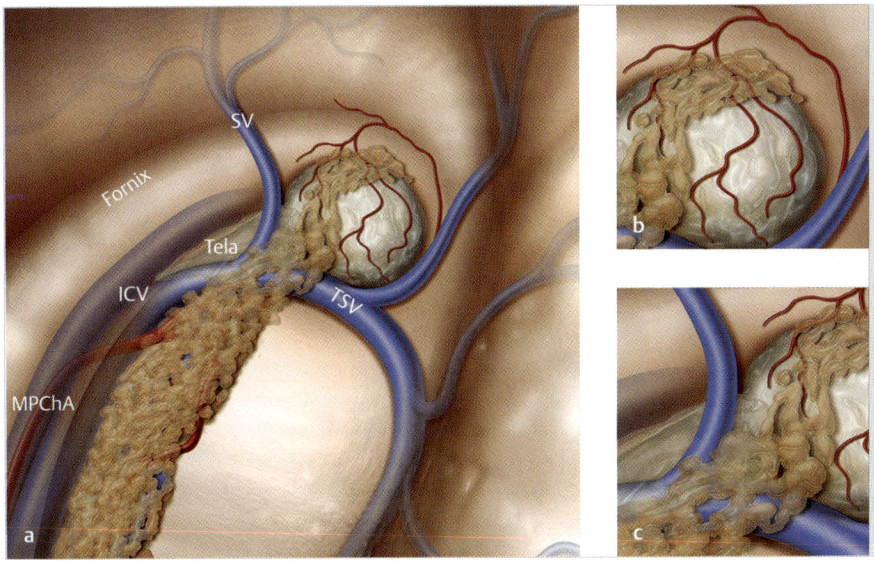


**Fig. 12.1** Critical neurovascular anatomy and potential attachment points for colloid cysts of the third ventricle. **(a)** Critical structures include the fornix, internal cerebral veins (ICV), septal veins (SV), thalamostriate vein (TV), tela choroidia (Tela), and choroid plexus. The medial posterior choroidal artery (MPChA) extends anteriorly and must be identified, particularly during resection of posteriorly positioned cysts. **(b)** The cyst is commonly invested with choroid plexus and intimately associated with the fornix, although nonadherent. A small penetrating artery extending from the fornix to the cyst can be present. **(c)** Cyst attachment points at the velum, deep draining veins, tela, and choroid must be carefully dissected to avoid vascular injury. (Adapted from Yahanda AT, Beaumont TL, Dacey RG Jr. Colloid cysts of the third ventricle. In: Winn HR, ed. Youmans & Winn's Neurological Surgery. 8th ed. Philadelphia: Elsevier; 2023.)

was based on relatively few cases.[11,19] In a recent, well-powered single-center study of 74 patients who underwent surgery via flexible endoscopy, there were no recurrence in patients with coagulated cyst wall remnants with a mean follow-up of 10.3 years.[9]

At Washington University, there was a transition in approach selection between 2008 and 2010, from exclusively MR to primarily ER. This was the result of a dramatic reduction in complications and improved patient satisfaction with the endoscopic approach. Prior to this transition, 95% (41/43 cases) of patients were treated microsurgically, while after the transition 89% (31/35 cases) were treated endoscopically (▶ Fig. 12.2). Aggregating the decades before and after the transition created three distinct epochs: microsurgical, transitional, and endoscopic. Although surgeon's experience, surgical strategy, and technology continued to evolve over the study period, this provided an excellent opportunity to compare the two surgical strategies within the institution. We performed a retrospective analysis of all patients with colloid cysts of the third ventricle who underwent surgery at Washington University between 1998 and 2018.[8] Patients underwent colloid cyst resection by either open microsurgery with standard IHTC or TCTV technique, or a single burr hole endoscopic technique. The primary endpoint was the rate of complications, although specific emphasis was placed on comparing procedure-related variables, the rate of residual cyst wall remnants and associated recurrence, as well as total inpatient costs.

## 12.2 Endoscopic Technique

The patient is positioned supine with the neck flexed and the head immobilized in Mayfield pins. A burr hole is planned approximately 4 cm lateral to midline and 5 cm anterior to coronal suture (approximately 8 cm posterior to the nasion) (▶ Fig. 12.3). The final location is optimized using image guidance to provide maximal access below the fornix while avoiding the caudate nucleus. A curvilinear, 3.5-cm coronally oriented incision is placed behind the hairline and a 14-mm burr hole is made with a high-speed drill and a perforator. Following this, a 19-French peel-away introducer (Aesculap) is passed into the ventricle under image guidance. A 30-degree ventriculoscope (LOTTA, Karl Storz, Tuttlingen, Germany) is then passed through the introducer into the lateral ventricle with gentle constant irrigation with warm normal saline. Net fluid egress is set at one drip every 1 to 2 seconds using the inflow and outflow stopcocks on the endoscope. The septal vein and choroid plexus are quickly identified, as are the thalamostriate and anterior caudate veins (see video in section Illustrated Cases). The cyst is then thoroughly inspected, and overlying choroid plexus is coagulated using a ball-tip monopolar electrode and/or bipolar electrode (Karl Storz). The cyst wall is also thoroughly coagulated and then opened sharply with endoscopic microscissors. Cysts containing viscous fluid are evacuated with suction using a suction-morcellation device (Myriad, Nico Corp, Indianapolis, IN, USA), while those with mineralized contents are evacuated with a combination of grasping forceps and morcellation. Care is taken to ensure large pieces of debris are not released into the third ventricle, as this can block the cerebral aqueduct and cause obstructive hydrocephalus. Following internal decompression, any cyst-associated vessels are carefully coagulated, and the cyst margins are developed with a combination of blunt and sharp dissection. The cyst wall can then be resected piecemeal using the Myriad. Bimanual technique is employed whenever possible, using the main working channel and flexible instruments introduced via one of the side ports.[12] However, the side ports often constrain the instruments due to the curvilinear path down the endoscope, or the small caliber side port instruments are too delicate to dissect the adherent tissues, particularly if coagulated. Any residual cyst wall that remains adherent to the fornix, tela choroidia, or internal cerebral veins that cannot be safely resected is carefully coagulated using the bipolar electrode. In rare instances, the cyst wall can be circumferentially freed and delivered into the lateral ventricle, allowing sharp dissection of the pedicle and en bloc removal. Great care should be taken to avoid overly aggressive traction on the cyst wall, as this can result in catastrophic injury of the internal cerebral veins. Septostomy is performed at the end of the

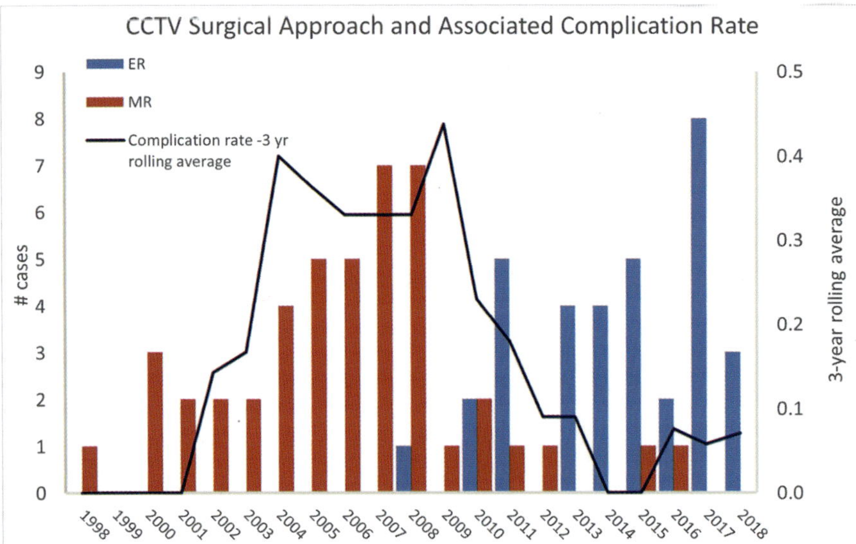


**Fig. 12.2** The evolution of approach selection for resection of colloid cysts of the third ventricle (CCTV). A distinct transition of approach selection occurred between 2008 and 2010, from exclusively microsurgical resection (MR, *red bars*) to primarily endoscopic resection (ER, *blue bars*). The 3-year rolling average complication rate is also shown. (Reproduced with permission from Beaumont TL, Limbrick DD, Patel B, Chicoine MR, Rich KM, Dacey RG. Surgical management of colloid cysts of the third ventricle: a single-institution comparison of endoscopic and microsurgical resection. J Neurosurg 2022:1–9. An Open Access or Creative Commons publishing model conveys no rights to use this material in any format without written permission from the JNS Publishing Group.)

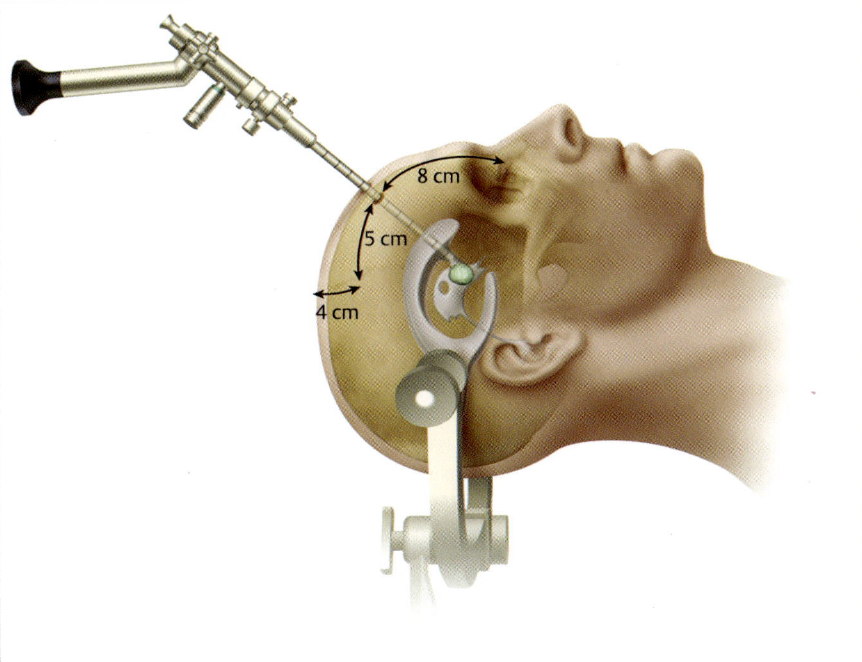


**Fig. 12.3** Head position and entry point for single burr hole endoscopic approach. The patient is positioned supine with the head in pin fixation. The burr hole is placed approximately 4 cm lateral to midline and 5 cm anterior to coronal suture. This is approximately 8 cm posterior to the nasion. The final location is optimized using image guidance to provide maximal access below the fornix while avoiding the caudate nucleus. (Adapted from Yahanda AT, Beaumont TL, Dacey RG Jr. Colloid cysts of the third ventricle. In: Winn HR, ed. Youmans & Winn's Neurological Surgery. 8th ed. Philadelphia: Elsevier; 2023.)

procedure unless the septum has spontaneously fenestrated. This is done by perforating the septum with the monopolar electrode while performing gentle cautery. Following this, balloon dilation to 6 mm is performed (NeuroBalloon, Integra Neurosciences, Princeton, NJ, USA). An external ventricular drain (EVD) is not routinely left in place at the end of the procedure unless there has been significant bleeding. The intraventricular compartment is then copiously irrigated. The endoscope is removed, a small piece of Gelfoam soaked in thrombin is placed into the corticotomy, and a burr hole cover is placed. The soft tissue is copiously irrigated and closed in layers with absorbable sutures in the galea and running 4–0 chromic in the skin. Following completion of the procedure the patient is observed in neurointensive care unit overnight and typically discharged home within 2 to 3 days.

## 12.3 Clinical Outcomes

During the study period, patients were subgrouped based on surgical approach: single burr hole ER ($n = 33$) and MR ($n = 45$). The microsurgical subgroup included either the TCTV approach ($n = 10$) or more commonly the IHTC approach ($n = 35$). More than 90% of the patients in both the groups had Colloid Cyst Risk Score (CCRS) of $\geq 4$ at the time of surgery.[2] The endoscopic subgroup ($n = 33$) was compared to the microsurgical subgroup ($n = 45$). The former procedures were performed by one of two primary endoscopic surgeons with the senior neuroendoscopist involved in 31/33 (94%) endoscopic cases, while the latter were performed by 12 different primary surgeons. ER of colloid cysts significantly optimized in nearly all procedure-related variables compared to microsurgery, with the single exception being the presence of residual cyst wall remnants noted at the conclusion of surgery (62.5% vs. 19.0%, $p = 0.002$, relative risk [RR] = 2.7). Operative time was significantly reduced in the endoscopic group compared to the microsurgical group (3.0 vs. 5.2 hours, $p < 0.001$). The use of temporary postoperative cerebrospinal fluid (CSF) drainage significantly decreased in the endoscopic group over time. If the endoscopic subgroup was evenly divided over the two decades interval, an EVD was left in place after surgery in 44% of the first half of the cases and only 13% of the second half ($p = 0.023$). Septostomy was performed more frequently in the endoscopic group (90.6% vs. 33.3%, $p < 0.001$) and has become a standard part of the procedure at Washington University. ER was associated with more than twofold reduction in LOS (4.1 ± 1.9 vs. 8.9 ± 7.5 days, $p < 0.001$) and all endoscopic patients were discharged home. In contrast, 24% of the patients who underwent microsurgery were discharged to a rehabilitation facility.

## 12.4 Complications

Nearly one-third of the microsurgical patients (31.1%) experienced a complication, and they tended to aggregate, with 46% of the patients who experienced complications having two or more events. These most commonly included venous thromboembolism (VTE) (11.1%) and persistent memory deficits (11.1%) at 1-year follow-up. Four patients (8.9%) developed postoperative wound infections, one occurred in a patient who had undergone urgent reoperation for venous infarction, while the remainder occurred after the initial surgery. Venous infarction, likely due to retraction injury, occurred in three patients in the microsurgical group (6.7%), all of whom had undergone an IHTC approach, while intraventricular hemorrhage (IVH) occurred in a single patient who had undergone a TCTV approach. All four patients with perioperative hemorrhage had at least one additional complication, most commonly seizures that occurred in three of four cases. The combination of infection and perioperative hemorrhage required return to the operating room in seven microsurgical patients (15.6%). Two additional patients who underwent MR required delayed return to the operating room for endoscopic septostomy due to unilateral trapped ventricle causing headache. Persistent memory deficits at 1-year postoperative follow-up were seen in two patients in the endoscopic group compared to five patients in the microsurgical group (6.3% vs. 12.2%, $p = 0.456$). There were no other immediate or delayed perioperative complications in the endoscopic group.

Analysis of variables potentially associated with the occurrence of complications was performed to identify independent predictors. Univariate analysis suggested a significant association of surgical approach ($p < 0.003$, RR 5.1). Surgeon's experience of < 3 colloid cyst cases also tended toward association with the occurrence of complications but did not achieve statistical significance ($p < 0.083$, RR 2.52). On multivariate analysis, only surgical approach remained an independent predictor of complications during surgery for colloid cysts ($p = 0.015$, odds ratio [OR] 7.35, $\beta = 2.9$). When the aforementioned two factors were further investigated with stepwise logistic regression, the effect size of surgical approach was reduced 7.2% by surgical experience suggesting a minimal confounding contribution.

## 12.5 Cyst Wall Remnants and Recurrence

All patients were followed with surveillance neuroimaging at 3 months, 6 months, and 1 year postoperatively. Following this, patients underwent annual imaging and clinic follow-up. Radiographic cyst recurrence was more frequent in the ER subgroup (22.6% vs. 7.1%, $p = 0.061$) although this was not associated with a significantly increased rate of reoperation (9.7% vs. 4.7%, $p = 0.347$) due to relatively few events. There were two microsurgical patients with recurrence, both of whom were symptomatic at the time of presentation due to obstructive hydrocephalus. One patient underwent endoscopic re-resection while the second underwent shunting only. Conversely, all three endoscopic patients with recurrence were asymptomatic and underwent elective endoscopic reoperation due to progressive growth on surveillance imagining. Mean time to recurrence was similar in both the endoscopic and microsurgical groups (2.7 ± 2.4 vs. 3.3 ± 3.2 years, $p = 0.758$).

## 12.6 Total Inpatient Cost

The United States consumer price index-adjusted total inpatient cost was reduced by 52.6% on average for the ER group compared to MR (22.5 ± 6.3 vs. 47.5 ± 34.7 K USD, $p < 0.001$). There was a notably large variance associated with the cost of microsurgery suggesting additional contributory factors. Further subgrouping demonstrated the significant impact of complications on procedure-related cost. When patients with complications were excluded, there was a 28% reduction in average inpatient cost for ER compared to MR (22.5 ± 6.3 vs. 31.3 ± 14.7 K USD, $p = 0.007$). However, the total inpatient cost for MR when complications occurred was fourfold (400%) greater compared to ER (22.5 ± 6.3 vs. 90.9 ± 33.0 K USD, $p < 0.001$). The reduction in inpatient cost associated with ER compared to MR remained during reoperation for recurrence (34.8 ± 4.4 vs. 71.2 ± 4.6 K USD).

## 12.7 Discussion and Current Strategy

Colloid cysts of the third ventricle can have dramatic clinical presentation and often represent a technical neurosurgical challenge. Although they have historically been approached microsurgically, more recently neuroendoscopy has demonstrated favorable outcomes with shorter hospital stay and markedly decreased complication rates, as further supported by the finding of the Washington University study.[7,10,11,20] For nearly all study endpoints ER was more favorable than MR. The endoscopic group had significantly reduced operative time, LOS, and need for discharge to inpatient rehabilitation. Importantly, ER eliminated major complications that were quite frequent in the microsurgical group, consistent with several prior reports.[1,7,13,14,21,22,23] Furthermore, the Washington University study demonstrated that this effect was not significantly confounded by surgeon's experience. Finally, not only did ER offer increased safety, shorter LOS, and improved outcomes, we also demonstrated for the first time that these benefits came with greater than 50% reduction in total inpatient cost. The latter cannot be overlooked given the increasing pressure on surgeons and health systems to contain the cost of surgical care.

The relatively high rate of complications associated with the MR of colloid cysts in the Washington University study was notable, yet unsurprising. Nearly one-third of patients in the microsurgical subgroup experienced a complication, consistent with several prior studies reporting complication rates from 3.5 to 33% (mean 19.1 ± 13.2%).[1,7,13,14,21,22] A recent analysis of an administrative claims database suggested similar complication profiles between the endoscopic and microsurgical approaches, although total admission costs and aggregated, 90-day postdischarge costs were significantly greater for microsurgical patients experiencing ≥ 1 complication, suggesting microsurgical patients had more severe complications.[24] Given the inherent selection bias of administrative database studies, particularly when only privately insured patients are captured as in the abovementioned study, it is challenging to appreciate the generalizability of these data. Nonetheless, these data appear consistent with the notion that ER of colloid cysts is more cost-effective, particularly in the setting of complications.

Interestingly, the Washington University microsurgical cohort included a comparatively large number of individual surgeons ($n = 12$) with a wide range of experience, while the endoscopic procedures were typically performed by two attending surgeons, at least one of whom was an expert neuroendoscopists and was present for nearly all cases. The adoption of this team approach may have contributed to the relatively low complication rate in the endoscopic group. Indeed, after accounting for other potential contributory factors, surgical approach was the only independent predictor of complications in the study. Nonetheless, it is noteworthy that when less experienced surgeons encountered a complication it was always during a microsurgical approach. This finding is consistent with the fact that over time, the endoscopic case volume became concentrated among only two surgeons, with the senior surgeon having participated in 94% of the endoscopic procedures at the institution. This represented threefold greater colloid cysts case volume than the highest volume surgeon in the microsurgical group.

In contrast to the abovementioned benefits, ER was associated with a threefold increase in frequency of coagulated residual cyst wall remnants. This is consistent with early case series reporting residual cyst wall remnants in 50 to 70% of patients who underwent ER.[13,14] The significance of residual cyst wall following ER remains unclear, and this is particularly the case when the remnant is small and thoroughly coagulated. In a recent well-powered single-center study of 74 patients who underwent surgery via flexible endoscopy, extent of resection (EOR) was categorized as en bloc removal (Grade I), complete removal of the cyst contents, and > 50% (Grade II) or < 50% (Grade III) resection or coagulation of the cyst wall.[9] There were no recurrences in Grade I or II patients with median follow-up of 10.3 years, strongly challenging the notion that coagulated cyst wall remnants lead to cyst recurrence. Although the mean time to cyst recurrence in our study was 2.2 years, other studies with extended follow-up have demonstrated mean time to recurrence of more than 7 years with late recurrences of up to 15 years.[11,19,25] Thus, determining the actual rate of cyst recurrence will require extended follow-up for at least 10 years.

It is possible that cyst wall remnants are more readily appreciated with the enhanced endoscopic visualization, as compared to the microscope, from "within the doorway" as opposed to "looking in from outside." This may further confound retrospective studies such as the present study. Whatever the actual frequency of cyst wall remnants and the associated recurrence rates may be, complete removal should be undertaken to avoid potential delayed recurrence, so long as it can be done safely. As reported by Hoffman et al, even with 6.9% overall rate of recurrence after ER, there was an increased frequency of recurrence in cases with coagulated cyst wall remnants (33%, 3/9 patients) compared to those with complete cyst resection (2%, 1/45 patients).[19] Nonetheless, the abovementioned report by Isaacs et al stands in stark contrast, as there were no recurrences in patients with > 50% cyst wall resection or coagulation.[9] Until the recurrence risk is better understood, any patient with coagulated residual cyst wall remnants must be followed with yearly surveillance imaging for at least a decade.

ER was found to be appreciably more cost-effective. The total inpatient cost associated with ER of colloid cysts was 53% less than MR, and this did not account for the additional costs associated with the rehabilitative services that were required for 24% of the patients in the latter group. This cost savings is further underscored by the fact that an open microsurgical procedure with a complication costs four times (400%) more on average than an endoscopic procedure without complications. Interestingly, the improved cost-effectiveness was maintained even for reoperations, where the microsurgical procedure remained more than twice as costly.

Whether the improved safety and cost-effectiveness of ER of colloid cysts justify the potentially increased rate of recurrence remains an open question, particularly since the EOR with the endoscopic technique has continued to improve, particularly as bimanual techniques become more common. Given the rarity of the lesion, this question can only be objectively addressed with a prospective, multicenter registry that includes preoperative grading, clearly defined indications for surgery, strict criteria for defining postoperative residual cyst wall remnants and EOR, neuropsychological testing, and patient satisfaction scores. Despite the statistics and ongoing debate, it is unlikely that one surgical approach will prove superior for *all* colloid cysts. Between single burr hole ER and traditional MR, there are hybrid port-based approaches that offer a minimally invasive approach with the benefit of true bimanual technique and dry-field dissection[26,27] (see Chapter 14). In cases where the cyst pedicle is posteriorly placed, the cyst contents are firm (hypointense on T2 MRI), or when the cyst wall is adherent to the fornix and/or internal cerebral veins, true bimanual technique along with dry-field dissection may allow for more complete resection with increased safety (▶ Fig. 12.4).

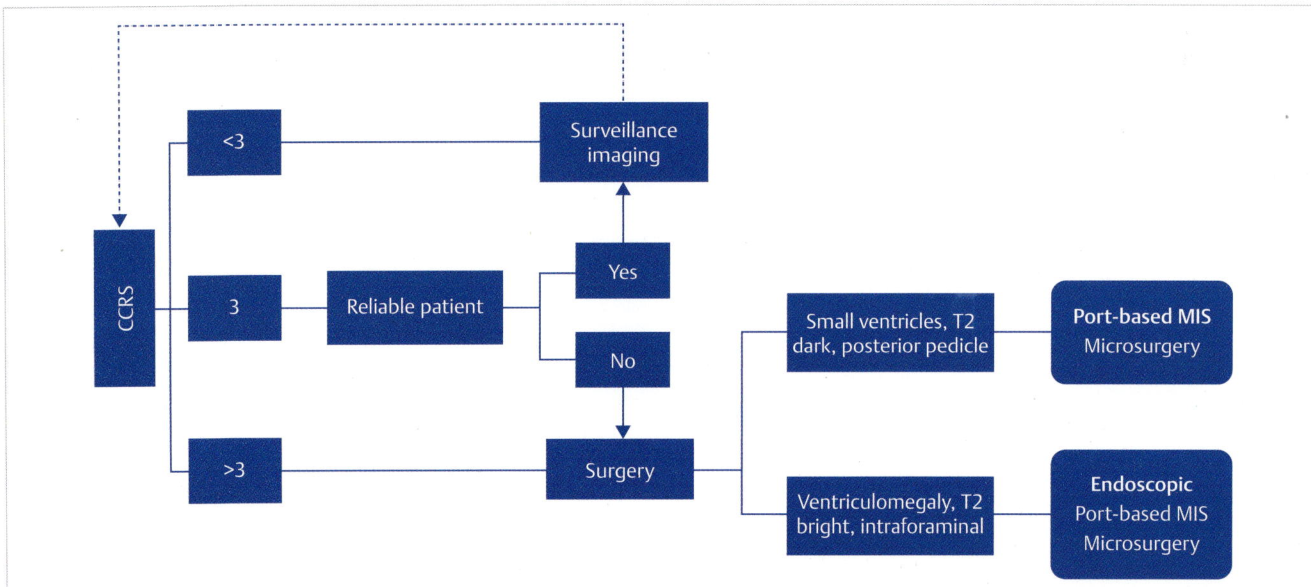


**Fig. 12.4** Clinical decision-making for colloid cysts of the third ventricle based on Colloid Cyst Risk Score (CCRS). Patients who have CCRS of ≤ 2 are considered low risk and can be observed with surveillance imaging, as they are not expected to present with obstructive hydrocephalus. Those with CCRS ≥ 4 are considered high risk, are commonly symptomatic, and have an increased risk of developing obstructive hydrocephalus (≥ 2% per year). CCRS 3 patients are intermediate risk and can be observed so long as the patient is reliable. T2 signal within the cyst suggests the character of cyst contents (T2 hypointense = firm, nonfluidic).[18]

# References


[1] Hernesniemi J, Romani R, Dashti R, et al. Microsurgical treatment of third ventricular colloid cysts by interhemispheric far lateral transcallosal approach—experience of 134 patients. Surg Neurol. 2008; 69(5):447–453, discussion 453–456

[2] Beaumont TL, Limbrick DD, Jr, Rich KM, Wippold FJ, II, Dacey RG, Jr. Natural history of colloid cysts of the third ventricle. J Neurosurg. 2016; 125(6):1420–1430

[3] Camacho A, Abernathey CD, Kelly PJ, Laws ER, Jr. Colloid cysts: experience with the management of 84 cases since the introduction of computed tomography. Neurosurgery. 1989; 24(5):693–700

[4] King WA, Ullman JS, Frazee JG, Post KD, Bergsneider M. Endoscopic resection of colloid cysts: surgical considerations using the rigid endoscope. Neurosurgery. 1999; 44(5):1103–1109, discussion 1109–1111

[5] Grondin RT, Hader W, MacRae ME, Hamilton MG. Endoscopic versus microsurgical resection of third ventricle colloid cysts. Can J Neurol Sci. 2007; 34(2):197–207

[6] Lewis AI, Crone KR, Taha J, van Loveren HR, Yeh HS, Tew JM, Jr. Surgical resection of third ventricle colloid cysts. Preliminary results comparing transcallosal microsurgery with endoscopy. J Neurosurg. 1994; 81(2):174–178

[7] Sampath R, Vannemreddy P, Nanda A. Microsurgical excision of colloid cyst with favorable cognitive outcomes and short operative time and hospital stay: operative techniques and analyses of outcomes with review of previous studies. Neurosurgery. 2010; 66(2):368–374, discussion 374–375

[8] Beaumont TL, Limbrick DD, Patel B, Chicoine MR, Rich KM, Dacey RG. Surgical management of colloid cysts of the third ventricle: a single-institution comparison of endoscopic and microsurgical resection. J Neurosurg. 2022:1–9. Online ahead of print

[9] Isaacs AM, Bezchlibnyk YB, Dronyk J, Urbaneja G, Yong H, Hamilton MG. Long-term outcomes of endoscopic third ventricle colloid cyst resection: case series with a proposed grading system. Oper Neurosurg (Hagerstown). 2020; 19(2):134–142

[10] Margetis K, Christos PJ, Souweidane M. Endoscopic resection of incidental colloid cysts. J Neurosurg. 2014; 120(6):1259–1267

[11] Vorbau C, Baldauf J, Oertel J, Gaab MR, Schroeder HWS. Long-term results after endoscopic resection of colloid cysts. World Neurosurg. 2019; 122:e176–e185

[12] Wilson DA, Fusco DJ, Wait SD, Nakaji P. Endoscopic resection of colloid cysts: use of a dual-instrument technique and an anterolateral approach. World Neurosurg. 2013; 80(5):576–583

[13] Horn EM, Feiz-Erfan I, Bristol RE, et al. Treatment options for third ventricular colloid cysts: comparison of open microsurgical versus endoscopic resection. Neurosurgery. 2007; 60(4):613–618, discussion 618–620

[14] Kehler U, Brunori A, Gliemroth J, et al. Twenty colloid cysts—comparison of endoscopic and microsurgical management. Minim Invasive Neurosurg. 2001; 44(3):121–127

[15] Boogaarts H, El-Kheshin S, Grotenhuis J. Endoscopic colloid cyst resection: technical note. Minim Invasive Neurosurg. 2011; 54(2):95–97

[16] Hellwig D, Bauer BL, Schulte M, Gatscher S, Riegel T, Bertalanffy H. Neuroendoscopic treatment for colloid cysts of the third ventricle: the experience of a decade. Neurosurgery. 2003; 52(3):525–533, discussion 532–533

[17] Longatti P, Godano U, Gangemi M, et al. Italian neuroendoscopy group. Cooperative study by the Italian neuroendoscopy group on the treatment of 61 colloid cysts. Childs Nerv Syst. 2006; 22(10):1263–1267

[18] Samadian M, Ebrahimzadeh K, Maloumeh EN, et al. Colloid cyst of the third ventricle: long-term results of endoscopic management in a series of 112 cases. World Neurosurg. 2018; 111:e440–e448

[19] Hoffman CE, Savage NJ, Souweidane MM. The significance of cyst remnants after endoscopic colloid cyst resection: a retrospective clinical case series. Neurosurgery. 2013; 73(2):233–237, discussion 237–239

[20] Sribnick EA, Dadashev VY, Miller BA, Hawkins S, Hadjipanayis CG. Neuroendoscopic colloid cyst resection: a case cohort with follow-up and patient satisfaction. World Neurosurg. 2014; 81(3–4):584–593

[21] Desai KI, Nadkarni TD, Muzumdar DP, Goel AH. Surgical management of colloid cyst of the third ventricle—a study of 105 cases. Surg Neurol. 2002; 57(5):295–302, discussion 302–304

[22] Shapiro S, Rodgers R, Shah M, Fulkerson D, Campbell RL. Interhemispheric transcallosal subchoroidal fornix-sparing craniotomy for total resection of colloid cysts of the third ventricle. J Neurosurg. 2009; 110(1):112–115

[23] Sheikh AB, Mendelson ZS, Liu JK. Endoscopic versus microsurgical resection of colloid cysts: a systematic review and meta-analysis of 1,278 patients. World Neurosurg. 2014; 82(6):1187–1197

[24] Connolly ID, Johnson E, Lamsam L, Veeravagu A, Ratliff J, Li G. Microsurgical vs. endoscopic excision of colloid cysts: an analysis of complications and costs using a longitudinal administrative database. Front Neurol. 2017; 8:259

[25] Greenlee JD, Teo C, Ghahreman A, Kwok B. Purely endoscopic resection of colloid cysts. Neurosurgery. 2008; 62(3) Suppl 1:51–55, discussion 55–56

[26] Eichberg DG, Buttrick SS, Sharaf JM, et al. Use of tubular retractor for resection of colloid cysts: single surgeon experience and review of the literature. Oper Neurosurg (Hagerstown). 2019; 16(5):571–579

[27] Engh JA, Lunsford LD, Amin DV, et al. Stereotactically guided endoscopic port surgery for intraventricular tumor and colloid cyst resection. Neurosurgery. 2010; 67(3) Suppl Operative:ons198–ons204, discussion ons204–ons205

# Part V

## Atlas of Illustrated Clinical Cases



V

# 13 Case Vignette: The Interhemispheric Transcallosal Approach for Resection of Colloid Cysts

*Sean D. McEvoy*

**Abstract**

Large colloid cysts present a particular challenge for surgical approach. This chapter describes the management of a large (3 cm) colloid cyst positioned predominately in the region of the velum interpositum and septum pellucidum. This chapter also describes a transcallosal approach to resection and accompanying figures help to delineate relevant anatomy. Intraoperative video further demonstrates the surgical technique.

*Keywords:* giant colloid cyst, transcallosal, interhemispheric, video, velum interpositum, internal cerebral veins

## 13.1 Clinical Course

A 13-year-old young woman presented after 4 months of progressive headaches. She had no complaints of visual change, altered mental status, nausea, or vomiting. After failure of medical headache management, she had been referred for a magnetic resonance imaging (MRI) which showed a 3.5 × 3.5 × 3.0 cm mass centered within the septum pellucidum (▶ Fig. 13.1).

The mass extended from the corpus callosum to the internal cerebral veins and inferiorly displaced the velum interpositum. It did not appear to enter the third ventricle. Its mass effect shifted the bilateral thalami inferolaterally. The lesion was isointense to the gray matter on T1, T2, and fluid-attenuated inversion recovery (FLAIR) sequences and did not show restricted diffusion. It showed rim enhancement with an enhancing nodule in the anterior left-lateral ventricle.

The initial differential diagnosis included colloid cyst. However, because of its atypically large size and relative lack of involvement of the third ventricle, we maintained a broad differential diagnosis of a supratentorial intraventricular mass with limited/mixed enhancement. This included ependymoma, subependymoma, choroid plexus tumor, craniopharyngioma, central neurocytoma, astrocytoma/glioma, primitive neuroectodermal tumor, neurocysticercosis, neurosarcoid, and teratoma.

An endoscopic approach was considered but rejected because debris from such a large mass would likely obscure the view through the cerebrospinal fluid (CSF). Transcortical and transcallosal open approaches were both considered. Given the preoperative uncertainty of the pathology and its proximity to the corpus callosum, the transcallosal approach was chosen to optimize access to the lesion in the bilateral ventricles.

## 13.2 Surgical Technique (▶ Video 13.1)

The patient was positioned supine on the operating table. The head was held in an anterolateral (AP) position with mild neck flexion in Mayfield pins. Mannitol, levetiracetam, and dexamethasone were given perioperatively. A zig-zag three-fourth coronal incision was used to allow for optimal cosmesis of her scar (▶ Fig. 13.2, *left*). Alternatively, the galea may be opened using a trap door incision hinged medially. The bone flap was planned to incorporate the coronal suture and crossed the sagittal sinus (▶ Fig. 13.2, *right*) to allow for retraction of the sinus to better visualize the anterior corpus callosum in the interhemispheric fissure.

The dura was flapped medially, and great care was exercised to avoid cortical vessels which may enter the dura lateral to the sinus (▶ Fig. 13.3). The dura was trimmed to the lateral margin of the sagittal sinus for visualization of the interhemispheric fissure. The sagittal sinus may create venous lakes which extend laterally between the periosteal and meningeal layers of the dura (▶ Fig. 13.3). The surgeon must maintain suspicion for their presence to allow early detection and prevention of significant

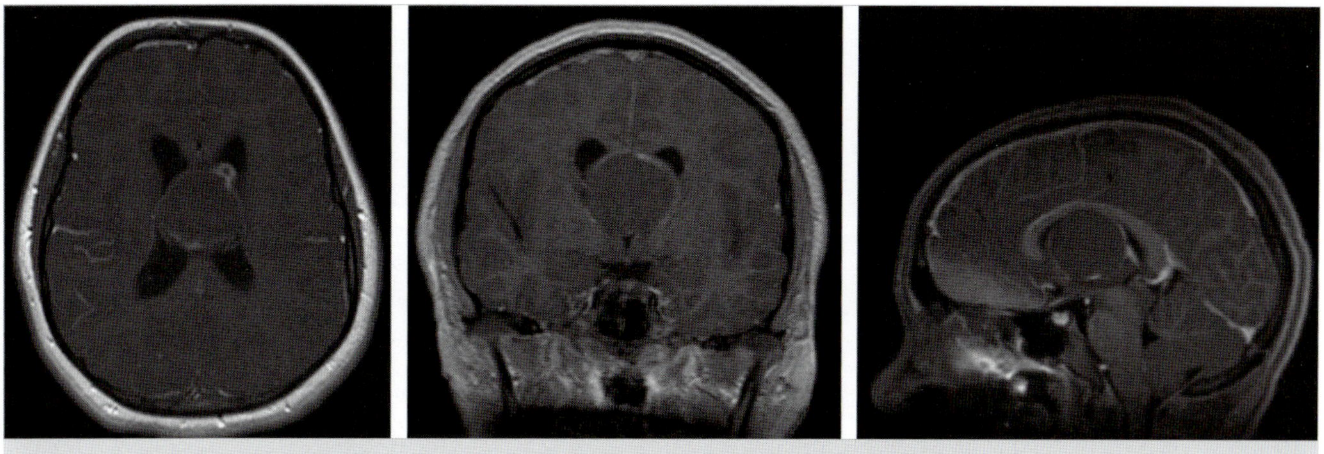

**Fig. 13.1** Preoperative axial, coronal, and sagittal postcontrast magnetic resonance imaging (MRI) views of the mass extending from the corpus callosum to the velum interpositum with lateral displacement of the thalami and obstructive hydrocephalous.

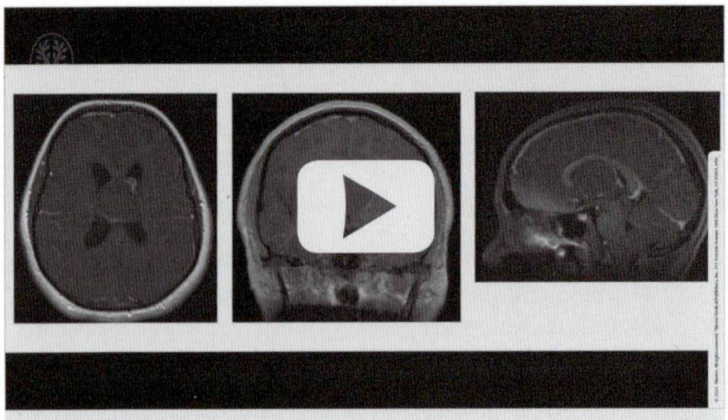

**Video 13.1** Operative video of interhemispheric transcallosal approach to giant colloid cyst.

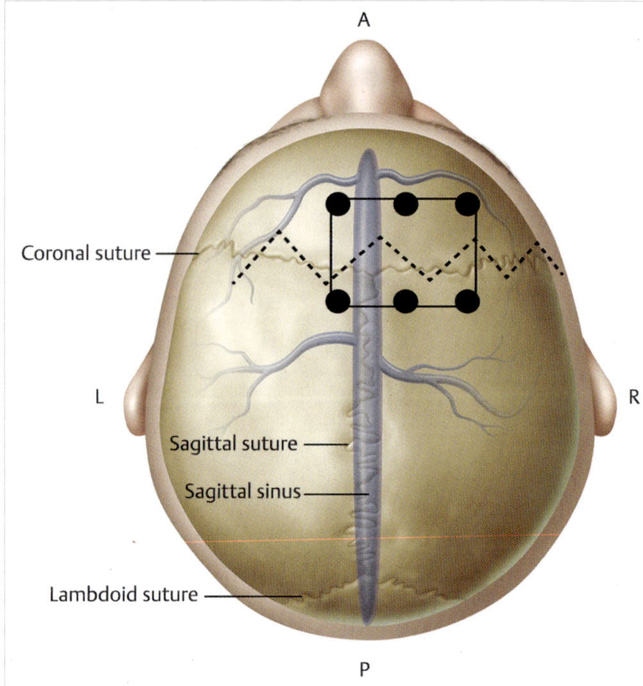


**Fig. 13.2** *Left*: The galea was opened with a zig-zag three-fourth coronal incision to allow obscuring of the scar in her hair for cosmesis. *Right*: The bone flap crossed the midline to allow for exposure and eventual retraction of the sagittal sinus. The flap incorporated the coronal suture to position the approach over the anterior corpus callosum.

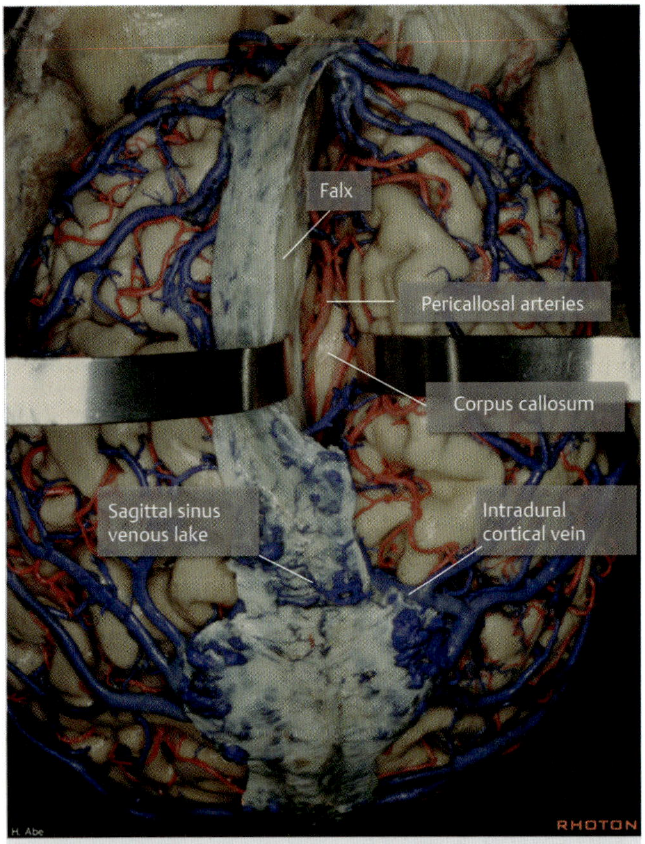


**Fig. 13.3** Superior view of interhemispheric fissure as encountered in the transcallosal approach. Venous lakes of the sagittal sinus as well as bridging cortical veins in the dura present hazards for significant hemorrhage. The corpus callosum may be seen deep to the pericallosal arteries. (Used with permission from the Rhoton Collection, American Association of Neurological Surgeons [(AANS]/Neurosurgical Research and Education Foundation [NREF].)

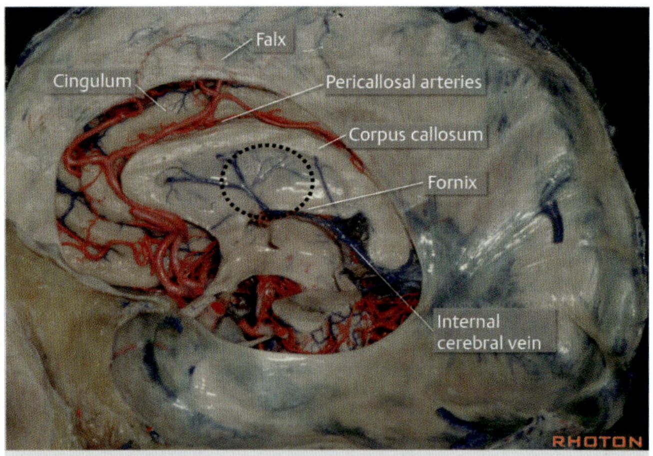


**Fig. 13.4** Lateral view of interhemispheric fissure. The inferior border of the falx terminates near the level of the cingulate sulcus. This is often an area of strong pial adhesions. The colloid cyst described here (*dashed circle*) abuts the corpus callosum superiorly and the fornices and internal cerebral veins inferiorly. (Used with permission from the Rhoton Collection, American Association of Neurological Surgeons [(AANS]/ Neurosurgical Research and Education Foundation [NREF].)

bleeding. The dural flap was used to retract the sinus toward the contralateral hemisphere. Over-retraction may inadvertently occlude the sagittal sinus. This may be assessed intraoperatively with a vascular Doppler. An external ventricular drain was passed through the lateral aspect of the incision to drain CSF and reduce the force required for retraction.

The initial dissection follows the firm border of the falx medially (► Fig. 13.3, ► Fig. 13.4).

Retraction against the medial portion of the precentral gyrus should be avoided to prevent injury to the leg motor area. Just below the inferior margin of the falx, the cingulate sulcus and gyrus are encountered (▶ Fig. 13.4). Because the falx no longer separates the pial surfaces of the bilateral cingulum here, this is often an area of particularly strong adhesions. After dividing the adhesions, the pericallosal branches of the anterior cerebral arteries (ACA) become visible (▶ Fig. 13.3, ▶ Fig. 13.4). The corpus callosum appears noticeably white in contrast to the surrounding cerebral cortex.

A plane may be dissected between the left and right pericallosal arteries to cross the corpus callosum and enter between leaflets of the septum pellucidum. On rare occasions, as in this case, firm adhesions between the arteries may require a paramedian dissection of the corpus callosum. Our dissection led into the right lateral ventricle. We immediately encountered the septum pellucidum and cyst wall bulging laterally into the ventricle. In order to improve visualization, we fenestrated the cyst, which released thick mucinous fluid.

We then began to remove the cyst wall in a piecemeal fashion using sharp and blunt dissection as well as cavitational aspiration. We carefully dissected it away from the surrounding corpus callosum and ependymal lining of the ventricle and rolled the cyst wall into itself. Branches of the internal cerebral vein could be seen running through the inferior portion of the cyst. The most inferior and posterior portion of the cyst was particularly adherent to the surrounding tissue. This placed the bilateral fornices and internal cerebral veins at risk of injury from further aggressive dissection (▶ Fig. 13.4). We therefore chose to allow a remnant of the cyst to remain. Postoperative MRI showed extensive debulking of the colloid cyst with the expected small posterior–inferior remnant adherent to the velum interpositum (▶ Fig. 13.5). The patient had complete resolution of her hydrocephalous and no postoperative memory deficit or disconnection syndrome.

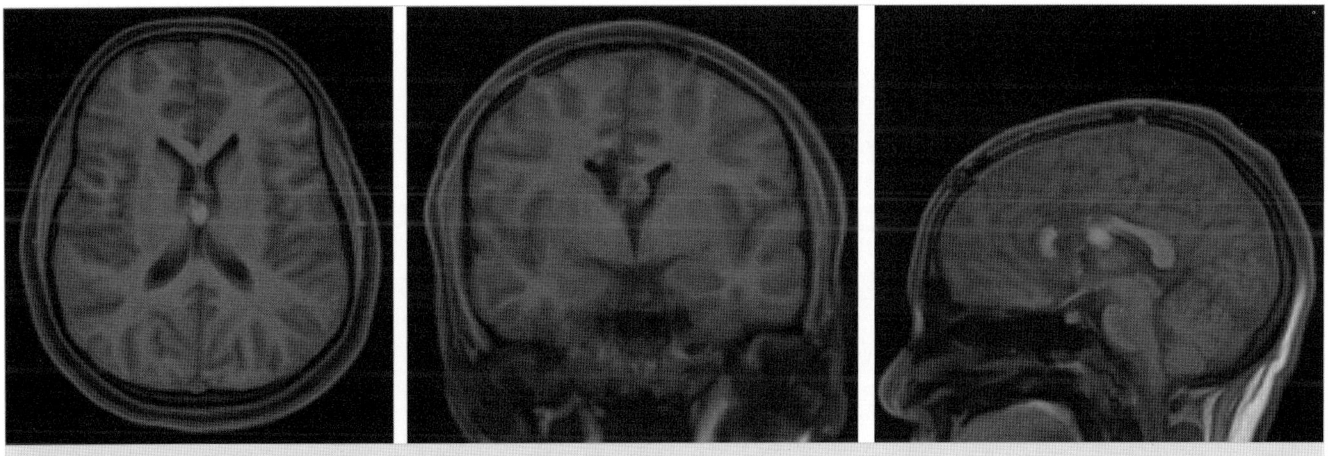

**Fig. 13.5** Postoperative axial, coronal, and sagittal T1 magnetic resonance imaging (MRI) scan showing the callosotomy and debulking of the colloid cyst. A small remnant of the posterior inferior cyst wall remains attached to the velum interpositum.

# 14 Principles of Surgical Management: Transcortical Approaches

*Hussein A. Zeineddine, David M. Panczykowski, and Arthur Day*

**Abstract**
Colloid cyst can lead to significant life-threatening consequences including hydrocephalus and sudden death. Surgical resection of these lesions should be in the arsenal of all neurosurgeons. This case illustration and associated video describe the surgical steps involved in the transcortical approach.

*Keywords:* colloid cyst, transcortical approach, lateral ventricle, fornix, open surgery

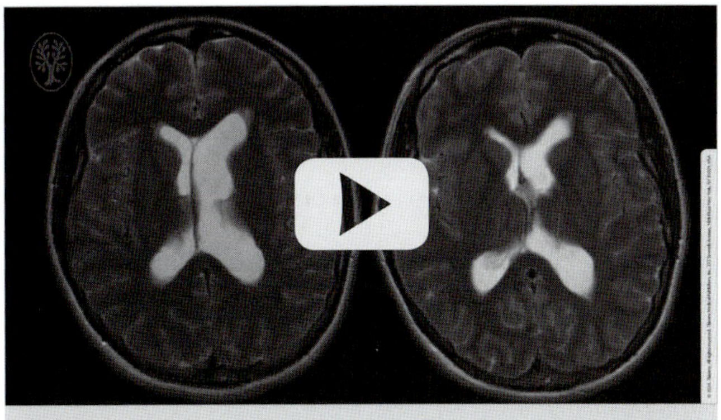

**Video 14.1** Surgical resection of a colloid cyst using a transcortical approach.

## 14.1 History and Physical Examination

A 24-year-old female presented to our clinic for consultation regarding management of her recently discovered colloid cyst. Her history began many years ago, with long-standing headaches that started in adolescence. Her typical headache would be nonspecific in location and would last approximately 24 hours, and then resolve. Recently, she had a severe headache, associated with vague anxiety, which persisted for over a week. She denied any visual obscurations or alterations of consciousness during this period. Over the last few days, her symptoms have largely resolved. Her neurological examination was normal.

## 14.2 Imaging

A cranial computed tomography (CT) followed by a magnetic resonance imaging (MRI) demonstrated a 1-cm, anterior, third ventricular lesion consistent with a colloid cyst. The left lateral ventricle was markedly dilated compared to the right side, with a left-to-right midline shift. A diagnosis of unilateral obstructive hydrocephalus at the level of the left foramen of Monro was made, and the decision was made to proceed with a left-sided, transcortical transventricular approach.

## 14.3 Operative Procedure

The patient was placed on the operating room table in the supine position with the neck slightly flexed and looking straight ahead (▶ Video 14.1; see ▶ Fig. 8.1, ▶ Fig. 8.2, ▶ Fig. 8.3, ▶ Fig. 8.4, ▶ Fig. 8.5). A linear midline incision was made starting from the hairline and going posteriorly to 3 cm behind the coronal suture, and then arched laterally toward the left ear. The scalp was reflected anteriorly and laterally with fishhook retractors. A free bone flap was turned in the left frontal region, partly in front of and partly behind the coronal suture in the parasagittal region, using stereotactic guidance to identify the midline and to avoid entry into the frontal sinus. The dura was opened and reflected toward the midline. A 1.5-cm superficial corticectomy was made in the left middle frontal gyrus, roughly paralleling the midline. Great care was taken to coagulate the pia carefully, so as to avoid any significant subarachnoid hemorrhage outside the confines of the operative plane. A ventricular catheter was inserted into the frontal horn aided by stereotactic guidance. Once cerebrospinal fluid (CSF) was encountered, the catheter tract was followed through the white matter in the same plane as the corticectomy, down to the frontal horn of left lateral ventricle.

The choroid plexus was identified and followed to the point where it entered into the foramen of Monro. A single medially directed self-retaining retractor was then added to create a semi-elliptical-shaped aperture for visualization and bimanual dissection.

Cotton balls were inserted in the lateral ventricle both anterior and posterior to the foramen of Monro so as to displace the lateral ventricular walls wider, greatly enhancing our operative working space and view. The choroid fissure was clarified by coagulating portions of the choroid plexus, carefully avoiding injury to any adjacent veins. The base of the choroid plexus where it inserted along the fornix (the taenia fornix) was then sectioned sharply to widen the foraminal aperture and obtain easier access to the entire cyst and its adherent structures. The attachments of the cyst to the third ventricle roof structures (the internal cerebral veins, medial posterior choroidal arteries, and choroid plexus) were separated from the lesion using the turgor of the intact cyst to guide the proper plane of dissection. Once the posterior aspect of the cyst was conceptually defined, the cyst was punctured and aspirated. The collapsed cyst wall was then peeled away from the fornix and adjacent veins, coagulating tiny arterial feeders coming from the posterior medial choroidal arteries and the choroid plexus until the entire mass was delivered.

The cotton balls were removed from the ventricle, and the corticectomy was carefully examined for any bleeding as the single retractor was removed, and several longitudinal strips of

Surgicel were placed to ensure perfect hemostasis. The dura was then closed with running 3–0 silk suture. A subdural drain was left in place, brought out through a separate stab wound to the posterior aspect of the incision, and connected to straight drainage without suction. The bone flap was repositioned and held in place with titanium plates and screws. Methyl methacrylate was added for cosmesis. The skin was closed in two layers using Vicryl on the galea and simple interlocking nylon suture on the skin.

## 14.4 Postoperative Course

The patient was admitted to the intensive care unit overnight and transferred to the floor the following day. The subdural drain was removed once blood has cleared and drain output is low. She was discharged home on day 2. She was seen at 2 weeks and at 2 months postoperatively, with complete resolution of her symptoms. A 6-month follow-up visit is planned, with a repeat MRI with or without contrast planned at that time.

# 15 Colloid Cysts of the Third Ventricle: The Tubular Retractor Approach

*Thiago Albonette-Felicio, Douglas A. Hardesty, Johnathan Engh, and Daniel M. Prevedello*

**Abstract**
Colloid cysts, rare benign intraventricular tumors primarily located near the foramen of Monro, pose significant surgical challenges due to their deep location within the ventricular system surrounded by critical neurovascular structures. Despite the existence of various surgical techniques, there is no consensus among neurosurgeons on a standardized approach. The tubular retractor approach, first introduced in 1980, has gained favor for its ability to minimize tissue damage compared to traditional methods. This technique involves the use of a cylindrical tube to displace brain tissue gently, allowing for bimanual microsurgery under air, enhancing the surgeon's ability to control bleeding and achieve hemostasis. Although complete resection remains the goal due to the high recurrence rate associated with simpler decompression methods, the tubular retractor has shown promising results in reducing surgical trauma and improving outcomes. An illustrative case is presented.

*Keywords:* colloid cyst, endoscopy, ventricular tumors, tubular retractor, third ventricle tumors

## 15.1 Introduction

Colloid cysts represent a formidable surgical challenge due to their location deep within the ventricular system surrounded by critical neurovascular structures. Although there have been many surgical approaches described to reach these lesions, a unified consensus among neurosurgeons remains lacking. Colloid cysts are rare benign intraventricular lesions, primarily arising from the anterior aspect of the *velum interpositum* around the foramen of Monro. They represent about 2% of all intracranial tumors. Because of their critical location, patient symptomology is often attributable to obstructive hydrocephalus, which sometimes may be acute in onset, requiring prompt intervention.[1] Simple decompression of the cyst, through stereotactic drainage or endoscopic marsupialization, is associated with a high rate of recurrence.[2,3] Therefore, complete resection of the colloid cyst is usually the surgical goal, and authors have shown promising results utilizing the tubular retractor approach.[4,5,6,7,8,9,10]

The tubular retractor approach was first reported by Kelly and Alker Jr.[11] in 1980, using a stereotactic arc to deploy a cylindrical access tube to visualize deep subcortical lesions for resection, as an alternative to the traditional brain spatula retractors. Since then, the interest in such approaches has grown. Many neurosurgeons advocated for the safe use and less traumatic profile of the tubular retractor compared to the spatula retractor because of the pressure the latter exerted on adjacent brain tissue.[12,13] The reason for this could be explained by the variance in dispersion of retraction forces with each technique. The flat spatula retractor features abrupt edges with a very small surface area of tissue contact, resulting in extremely high-pressure points, which may lead to laceration of surrounding tissue. In contrast, the tubular retractor system circumferentially disperses tissue forces, leading to reduced focal pressure points. In comparison to traditional neuroendoscopy that is performed within a liquid medium, the tubular retractor allows ventricular microsurgery to be carried out bimanually and under an air medium, which significantly increases the surgeon's ability to dissect, visualize and control bleeding, and achieve hemostasis.[4,14,15]

The tubular retractor consists of an inner dilator and an outer tube, which are introduced into the brain parenchyma, after a proper craniotomy and durotomy, through a trans-sulcal or transcortical route. This device is introduced into the brain and gently parts the subcortical white matter tracts rather than cutting them, theoretically resulting in less collateral damage. Mechanistically this has been studied and may be supported by postoperative imaging studies.[16,17,18] When the target location is reached, the inner dilator is removed, and the surgery is performed within the tube, with any preferred optical device aid. Currently, there are two commercial tubular retractor systems approved by the FDA: the ViewSite Brain Access System (Vycor Medical Inc., Boca Raton, FL)[19] and the BrainPath (Nico Corp., Indianapolis, IN).[20] Both can be used with frameless stereotactic navigation system and have a variety of lengths and widths available (▶ Fig. 15.1). More recently, newer visualization devices, such as exoscopes, as well as recent advances in traditional microscope technology and endoscopes have allowed for better utilization of the tubular retractor approach for deep subcortical lesions.[6,18,21,22]

Among the subcortical lesions in which the tubular approach is indicated, colloid cysts are an ideal lesion for this approach, being both subcortical and intraventricular.

The ideal method for visualization remains a matter of controversy, and in our institution, we use the operative microscope for visualization since it provides increased freedom of movements inside the tubular retractor. Furthermore, the operative microscope provides a three-dimensional view and fast repositioning when the tubular retractor is adjusted into a different angle. These characteristics allow us to perform more complete resections when utilizing the microscope particularly for intraparenchymal lesions.[23]

## 15.2 Illustrative Case

A 36-year-old woman, with no past medical history, presented to the emergency department with approximately 1 week of a progressive headache. The headaches were associated with blurry vision and nausea, but no loss of consciousness. Her neurological examination was unremarkable. Subsequently, she had a head computed tomography (CT) scan which demonstrated a hyperdense lesion in the third ventricle obstructing the foramen of Monro and causing moderate hydrocephalus. Her brain magnetic resonance imaging (MRI) showed moderate

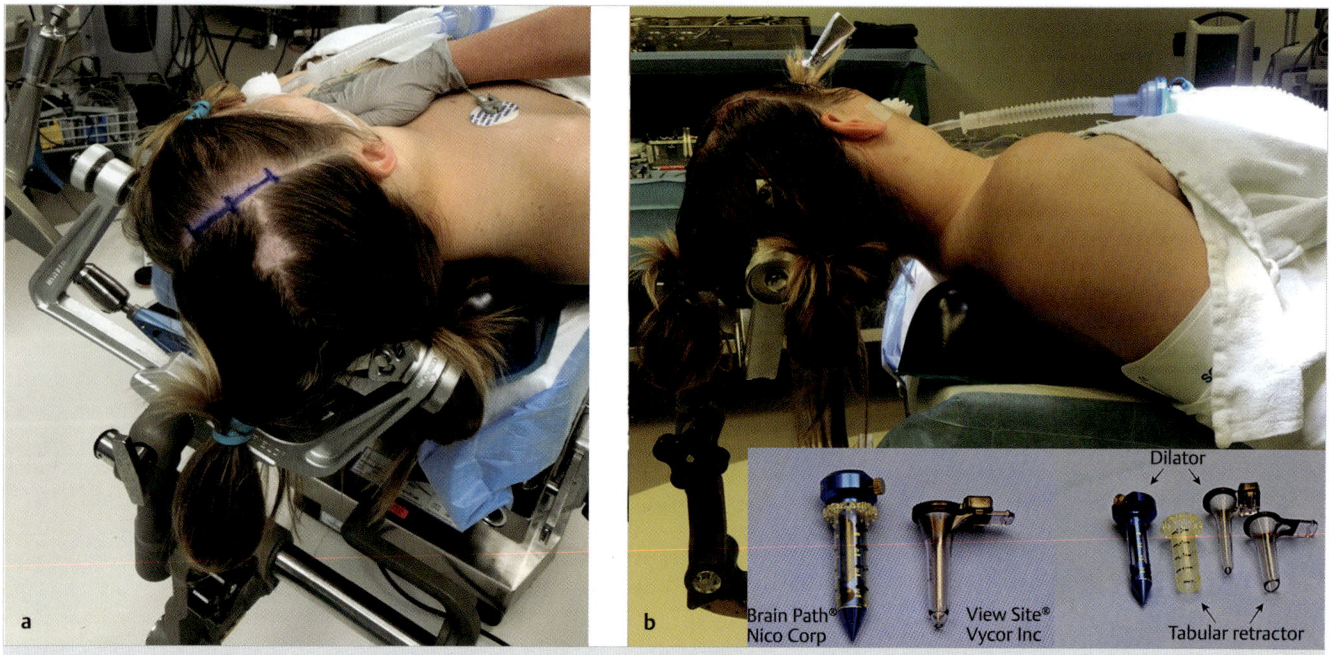


**Fig. 15.1** Patient positioning. The patient is positioned supine with a small shoulder bump to turn the head without disrupting venous return in the neck. The patient's head is immobilized in Mayfield pins and stereotactic neuronavigation is used to map out the patient's incision and trajectory to the lesion via a right frontal approach. **(a)** The patient's head should be turned such that the long axis of the foramen of Monro is orthogonal to the surgeon to give the surgeon bimanual access along the long access of the foramen. **(b)** The head should be positioned with the vertex up about 30 degrees for optimized trajectory toward the third ventricle. The two commercially available, FDA-approved tubular retractors are shown in the *right lower panel.*

hydrocephalus with transependymal flow and a 7- to 8-mm lesion in the bilateral foramina of Monro, consistent with a colloid cyst of the third ventricle. There were no other significant findings other than the hydrocephalus and cyst. Given her progressive symptomatology, age, hydrocephalus on imaging, and the diagnosis of a colloid cyst, surgical removal of the cyst was recommended in order to prevent clinical deterioration.

A transcortical tubular, right-sided (nondominant) approach, using the operative microscope, was selected for this lesion.

## 15.3 Operative Technique

Once the patient was induced under general anesthesia, the patient's head was immobilized in Mayfield pins and stereotactic neuronavigation was registered. Then, a trajectory from the surface to the cyst, via the right foramen of Monro, was selected and extrapolated to the entry position on the right frontal convexity around the coronal suture. The trajectory should be as parallel as possible to the important white matter tracts, and the entry point should be in a noneloquent cortical surface. Roughly, this means a location 1 to 3 cm anterior to the coronal suture and slightly more lateral than the midpupillary line (3–6 cm from midline) to allow for a more caudal to cranial visualization. It is very important to make sure the trajectory is not crossing the position of the head of the caudate. The trajectory is analyzed on the image guidance system. The patient's positioning is illustrated in ▶ Fig. 15.1.

A linear incision is made over the right frontal region and the craniotomy is performed accordingly. The dura is opened and retracted. The size of the craniotomy is important in considering the movements that will be made by the retractor. The size of the craniotomy should be big enough to allow the tubular retractor to be tilted in various angles during the surgery without being limited by the craniotomy edges. Similarly, the dural opening should be adequate to accommodate the tubular retractor as well in order to prevent displacement of the retractor and constriction of movements. A small 1-cm corticectomy is made, and hemostasis is achieved prior to cannulating the brain with a peel-away trochar that is used to access the ventricle under direct neuronavigation. Once the trochar is removed and an established trajectory is made, the tubular retractor system (Vycor) is placed and fixed to a Greenberg retractor system for optimized positioning during surgery. Once the retractor is placed, the operative microscope is brought in. The above-described procedure is illustrated in ▶ Fig. 15.2.

To enter and visualize the ventricle, if there is ependyma obstructing ventricular visualization, a small amount of white matter can be coagulated and suctioned to penetrate the ventricular system with the tubular retractor (▶ Fig. 15.3). Care must be taken not to cannulate too deep, as the port must be docked in the frontal horn superficial to the cyst and surrounding neurovascular structures. The port is angled toward the midline to identify the septum pellucidum, and an initial septostomy may be performed with a bipolar cautery, well above the fornix, in order to achieve communication with the contralateral side of the lateral ventricle. This maneuver also helps to decompress the septum, widening access to the cyst. In sequence, a 12-mm Vycor port is exchanged for a 17-mm diameter port, which is angled toward the foramen of Monro.

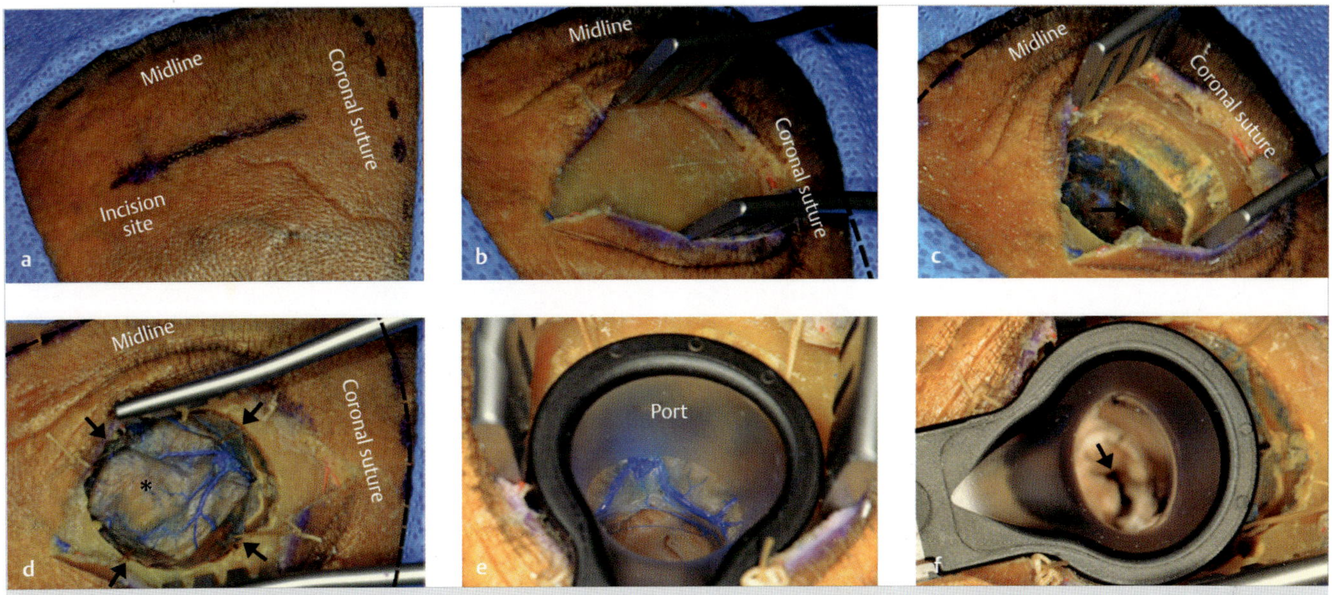


**Fig. 15.2** Cadaveric dissection of the left frontal region showing the tubular approach to the lateral/third ventricle. **(a–f)** Sequential steps of dissection. **(a)** Site of skin incision. **(b)** After skin incision showing the bone surface. **(c)** After craniotomy showing the dura mater (*arrow*). **(d)** After dural opening, showing the brain surface (*); dura is retracted with sutures (*arrows*). **(e)** Port inside the brain. **(f)** Port inside the brain with partial visualized lateral ventricle (*arrow*).

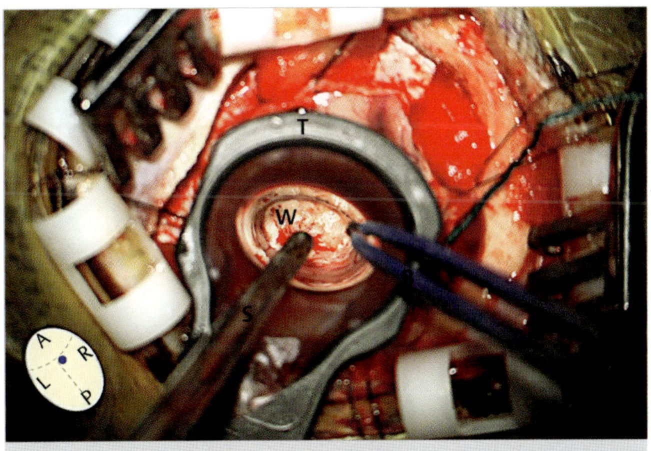


**Fig. 15.3** Intraoperative microscopic view showing the tubular retractor (T) inside the brain. It is possible to see white matter (W) surrounding the outside of the port; bipolar (B) and suction tip (S) are shown. Orientation of the patient's head is indicated in the left inferior corner of the image.

The foramen may be challenging to visualize, especially if it is obstructed by the colloid cyst. However, it can be localized by following the choroid plexus anteriorly until it reaches the anterior septal vein. Then, the choroid plexus is identified and coagulated around the foramen of Monro to allow for better visualization and working space to resect the cyst (▶ Fig. 15.4). Better visualization will allow the identification of the fornix, the thalamostriate vein, and the anterior septal veins, which should be preserved (▶ Fig. 15.5). Alternatively, a small amount of the choroidal fissure can be opened in order to develop some working space to reach down in the third ventricle for larger cysts. Subsequently, once the colloid cyst is visualized (▶ Fig. 15.5), it can be incised with microscissors or an arachnoid knife, taking care to not allow its contents to spill into the intraventricular space. This maneuver debulks the cyst and makes it easier to dissect the cyst from the surrounding structures. This allows the surgeon to grasp the cyst wall with toothed micro-forceps and precisely dissect the wall from the choroid plexus and surrounding structures. The remaining attachments of the cyst are coagulated, allowing for en bloc resection of the cyst wall (▶ Fig. 15.6). Next, hemostasis is achieved, and the ventricle is inspected and irrigated carefully (▶ Fig. 15.6). A vast majority of small choroidal and ependymal bleeders will stop with gentle irrigation. Then, an antibiotic-coated external ventricular drain (EVD) is placed in the third ventricle, under direct visualization. We routinely use EVDs and keep them clamped postoperatively for 24 hours in the event they are needed for acute events in the postoperative window. Frequently ICP is monitored during this period until EVD is removed. The Vycor port is slowly removed and, at the same time, the surrounding white matter is inspected for any bleeding. Hemostatic collagen matrix is placed over the cortex, and the EVD is tunneled out through the scalp. Copious irrigation with saline is used to wash the superficial surgical field, and the dura, craniotomy, and soft tissues are closed in a standard multilayer fashion. The patient in this case was extubated and observed for 24 hours in the intensive care unit with the EVD clamped. She remained neurologically intact, and a postoperative CT demonstrated resolution of the hydrocephalous with expected postsurgical changes and minimal blood products in the ventricular system (▶ Fig. 15.7). The EVD was therefore removed after 24 hours, and the patient was discharged on postoperative day 2. On her last follow-up visit, she had no headaches or neurologic complaints, and she had returned to work with normal memory function.

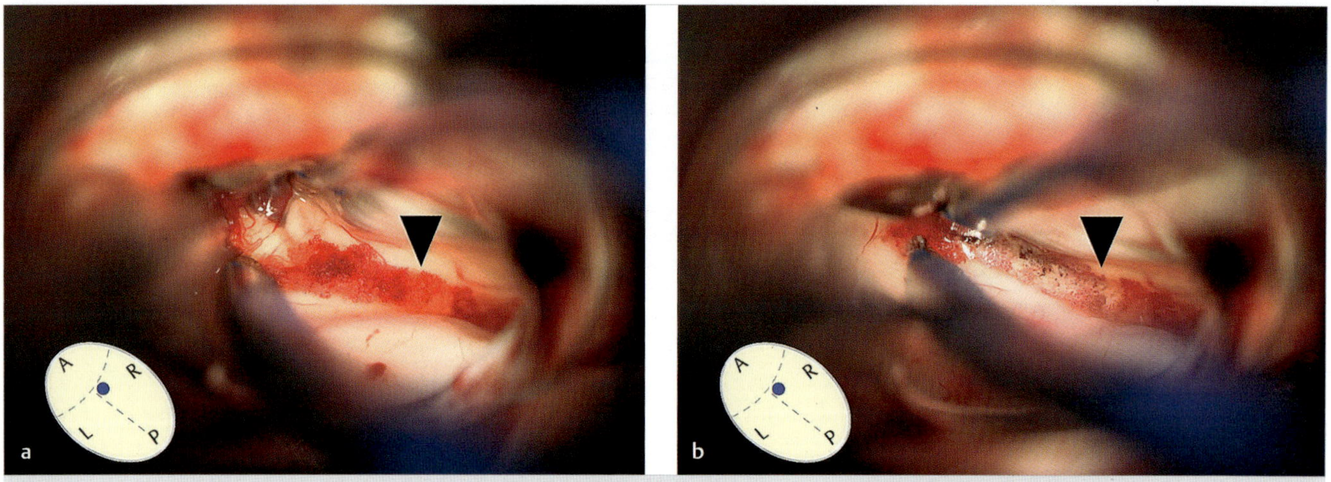


Fig. 15.4 Intraoperative microscopic view inside the body of the right lateral ventricle. Choroid plexus (*arrowhead*) before **(a)** and after **(b)** bipolar coagulation. Orientation of the patient's head is indicated in the left inferior corner of the image.

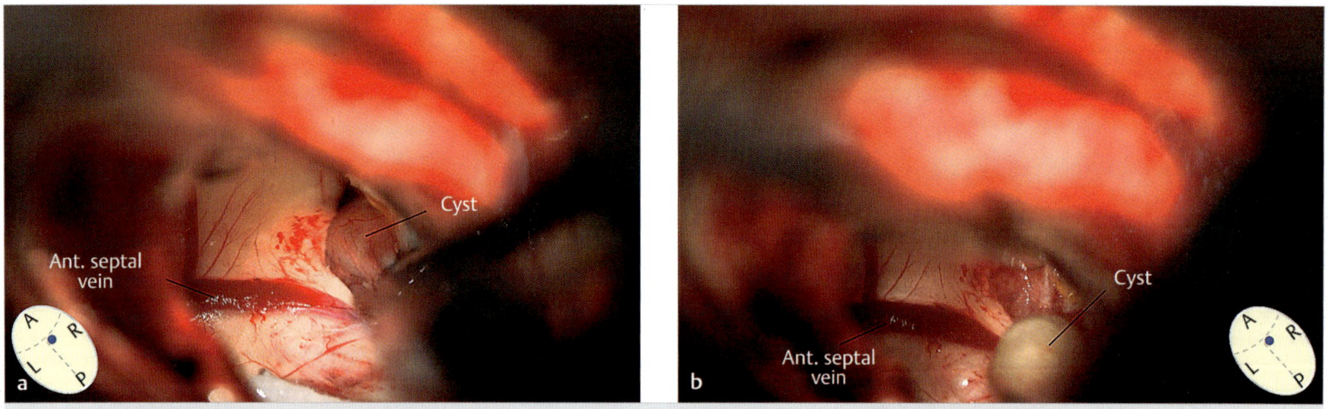


Fig. 15.5 Intraoperative microscopic view inside the body of the right lateral ventricle, same position as in ▶ Fig. 15.4, showing sequential dissection of the colloid cyst from the third ventricle/foramen of Monro **(a,b)**. Anterior septal vein can also be seen. Orientation of the patient's head is indicated in the left inferior corner of the image.

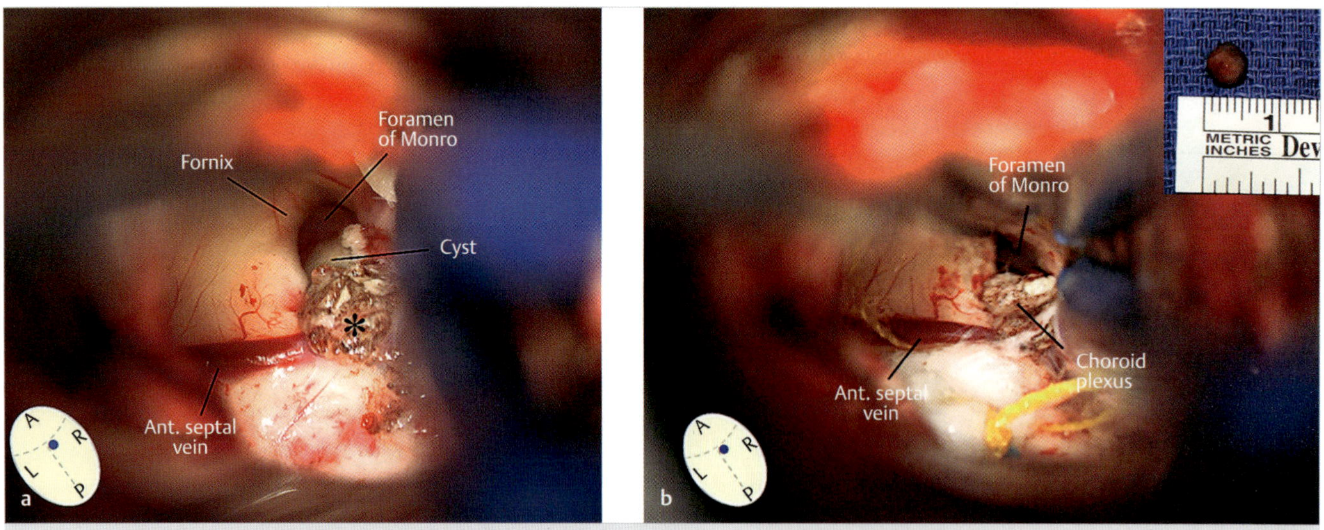


Fig. 15.6 Intraoperative microscopic view inside the body of the right lateral ventricle, same position as in ▶ Fig. 15.5, showing the comparison pre **(a)** and post **(b)** complete cyst removal. Anterior septal vein, foramen of Monro, and choroid plexus (*) can also be seen. Superior right inset depicts the intraoperative specimen. Orientation of the patient's head is indicated in the left inferior corner.

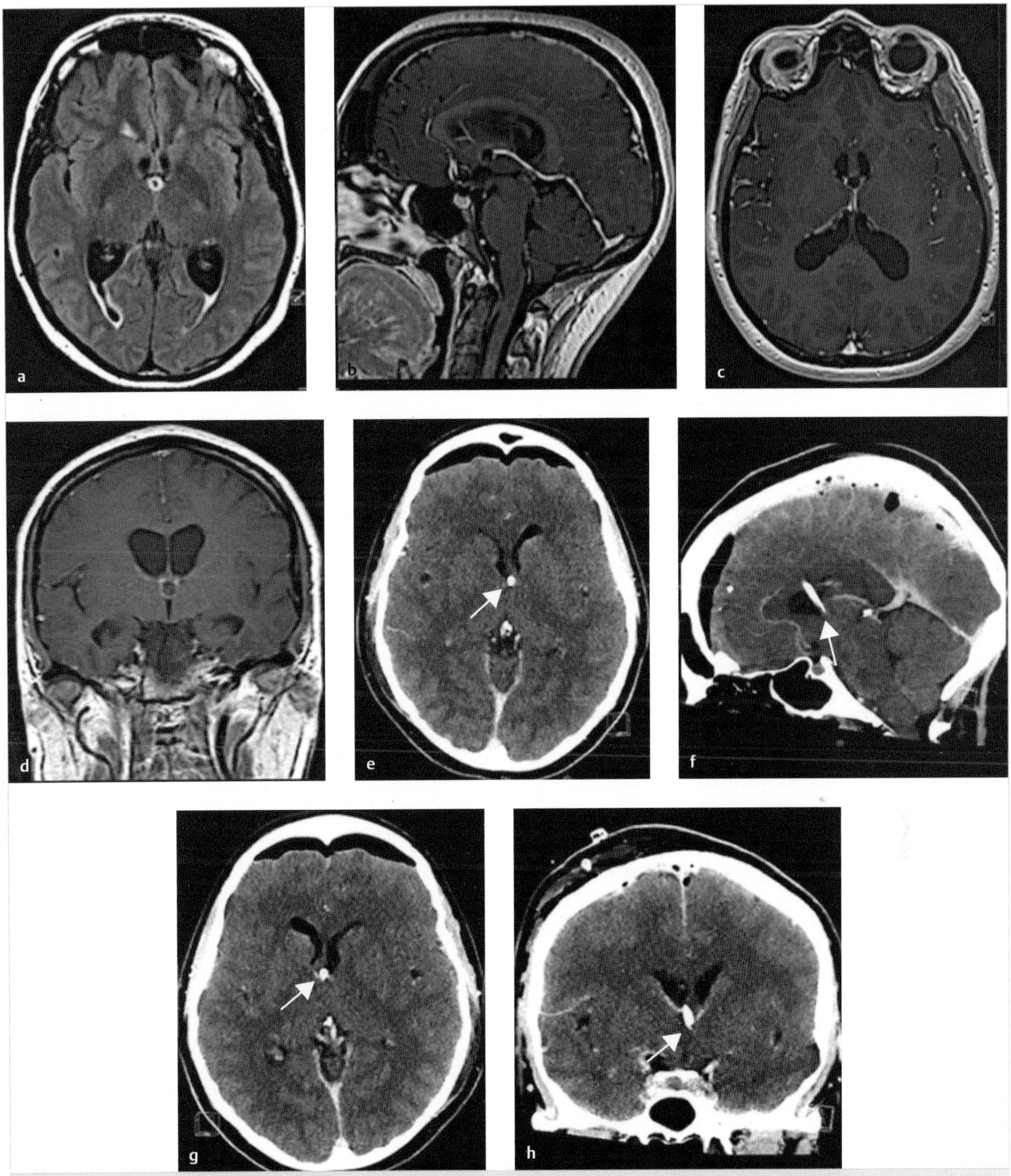


**Fig. 15.7** Neuroimaging. Upper panels showing preoperative brain magnetic resonance imaging (MRI). **(a)** Axial fluid-attenuated inversion recovery (FLAIR), **(b)** sagittal, **(c)** axial, and **(d)** coronal, T1-weighted postcontrast sequences showing a colloid cyst in the third ventricle, obstructing the foramen of Monro. Moderate ventriculomegaly can also be appreciated. Lower half showing postoperative head computed tomography (CT) scan. **(e)** Axial, **(f)** sagittal, **(g)** axial, and **(h)** coronal postcontrast showing removal of the lesion. A decrease in size of the ventricles can be observed, as well as an external ventricular drain (EVD) catheter (*arrow*) within the right lateral and third ventricle.

## 15.4 Conclusion

Colloid cysts are rare benign intraventricular lesions that can present with hydrocephalus. If untreated, this may lead to death. Most of the symptoms are usually attributable to hydrocephalus, which sometimes may present as an acute-onset neurological event, requiring prompt intervention.[1] Simple decompression of the cyst is associated with a high rate of recurrence and should be avoided.[2,3] Most colloid cysts are cured with proper surgical removal.

Hemiparesis, aseptic meningitis, postoperative seizures, continued hydrocephalus, venous infarctions, and even death have all been documented complications of colloid cyst removal.[24] All surgical approaches to these lesions have been associated with some type of morbidity or possibility of recurrence. A decision on which approach to take is guided by the size and location of the lesion, the patient's anatomy and medical condition, and the experience and degree of comfort of the surgeon with each approach. Tubular approaches are a minimally invasive option to treat these lesions. This approach has shown promising results regarding gross total resection and functional outcomes.[25,26] When using these techniques, detailed image-based preoperative planning and navigation are paramount, along with a profound understanding of the subcortical and intraventricular anatomy. The operative microscope provides three-dimensional visualization of the anatomy, which may contribute to a complete and more effective resection, although other visualization devices have been shown to be effective. The tubular approach to the ventricle provides an air-medium environment and bimanual surgical manipulation, which allow for microsurgical technique and better hemostasis. Although more invasive than working channel endoscopic approaches for cyst resection, the tubular retractor approach allows the opportunity for complete cyst wall removal using microsurgical technique. However, the tubular retractor approach remains less invasive than traditional transcortical microsurgical approaches and avoids many of the concerns of transcallosal approaches for cyst removal such as manipulating of the cingular gyrus and the anterior cerebral arteries. In summary, the tubular approach for the colloid cyst represents an excellent treatment option in the neurosurgical armamentarium.

## References


[1] Beaumont TL, Limbrick DD, Jr, Rich KM, Wippold FJ, II, Dacey RG, Jr. Natural history of colloid cysts of the third ventricle. J Neurosurg. 2016; 125(6):1420–1430

[2] Mathiesen T, Grane P, Lindquist C, von Holst H. High recurrence rate following aspiration of colloid cysts in the third ventricle. J Neurosurg. 1993; 78 (5):748–752

[3] Mathiesen T, Grane P, Lindgren L, Lindquist C. Third ventricle colloid cysts: a consecutive 12-year series. J Neurosurg. 1997; 86(1):5–12

[4] Barlas O, Karadereler S. Stereotactically guided microsurgical removal of colloid cysts. Acta Neurochir (Wien). 2004; 146(11):1199–1204

[5] Engh JA, Lunsford LD, Amin DV, et al. Stereotactically guided endoscopic port surgery for intraventricular tumor and colloid cyst resection. Neurosurgery. 2010; 67(3) Suppl Operative:ons198–ons204, discussion ons204–ons205

[6] McLaughlin N, Prevedello DM, Engh J, Kelly DF, Kassam AB. Endoneurosurgical resection of intraventricular and intraparenchymal lesions using the port technique. World Neurosurg. 2013; 79(2) Suppl:18.e1–18.e8

[7] Harris AE, Hadjipanayis CG, Lunsford LD, Lunsford AK, Kassam AB. Microsurgical removal of intraventricular lesions using endoscopic visualization and stereotactic guidance. Neurosurgery. 2005; 56(1) Suppl:125–132, discussion 125–132

[8] Cabbell KL, Ross DA. Stereotactic microsurgical craniotomy for the treatment of third ventricular colloid cysts. Neurosurgery. 1996; 38(2):301–307

[9] Eichberg DG, Buttrick S, Brusko GD, Ivan M, Starke RM, Komotar RJ. Use of tubular retractor for resection of deep-seated cerebral tumors and colloid cysts: single surgeon experience and review of the literature. World Neurosurg. 2018; 112:e50–e60

[10] Eichberg DG, Buttrick SS, Sharaf JM, et al. Use of tubular retractor for resection of colloid cysts: single surgeon experience and review of the literature. Oper Neurosurg (Hagerstown). 2019; 16(5):571–579

[11] Kelly PJ, Alker GJ, Jr. A method for stereotactic laser microsurgery in the treatment of deep-seated CNS neoplasms. Appl Neurophysiol. 1980; 43(3–5):210–215

[12] Ogura K, Tachibana E, Aoshima C, Sumitomo M. New microsurgical technique for intraparenchymal lesions of the brain: transcylinder approach. Acta Neurochir (Wien). 2006; 148(7):779–785, discussion 785

[13] Waran V, Vairavan N, Sia SF, Abdullah B. A new expandable cannula system for endoscopic evacuation of intraparenchymal hemorrhages. J Neurosurg. 2009; 111(6):1127–1130

[14] Engh JA, Lunsford LD, Amin DV, et al. Stereotactically guided endoscopic port surgery for intraventricular tumor and colloid cyst resection. Neurosurgery. 2010; 67(3) Suppl Operative:ons198–ons204, discussion ons204–ons205

[15] Jho H-D, Alfieri A. Endoscopic removal of third ventricular tumors: a technical note. Minim Invasive Neurosurg. 2002; 45(2):114–119

[16] Raza SM, Recinos PF, Avendano J, Adams H, Jallo GI, Quinones-Hinojosa A. Minimally invasive trans-portal resection of deep intracranial lesions. Minim Invasive Neurosurg. 2011; 54(1):5–11

[17] Recinos PF, Raza SM, Jallo GI, Recinos VR. Use of a minimally invasive tubular retraction system for deep-seated tumors in pediatric patients. J Neurosurg Pediatr. 2011; 7(5):516–521

[18] Bauer AM, Rasmussen PA, Bain MD. Initial single-center technical experience with the BrainPath system for acute intracerebral hemorrhage evacuation. Oper Neurosurg (Hagerstown). 2017; 13(1):69–76

[19] Vycor Medical. ViewSite Brain Access System (VBAS). Accessed April 12, 2018 at: http://www.vycorvbas.com

[20] NICO Corporation. BrainPath. Accessed April 12, 2018 at: http://www.nico-neuro.com/nico-product-line/

[21] Day JD. Path for Subcortical Lesions. 2017; 64(1):151–156

[22] Labib MA, Shah M, Kassam AB, et al. The safety and feasibility of image-guided BrainPath-mediated transsulcul hematoma evacuation: a multicenter study. Neurosurgery. 2017; 80(4):515–524

[23] Hong CS, Prevedello DM, Elder JB. Comparison of endoscope- versus microscope-assisted resection of deep-seated intracranial lesions using a minimally invasive port retractor system. J Neurosurg. 2016; 124(3):799–810

[24] Symss NP, Ramamurthi R, Kapu R, et al. Complication avoidance in transcallosal transforaminal approach to colloid cysts of the anterior third ventriclen: an analysis of 80 cases. Asian J Neurosurg. 2014; 9(2):51–57

[25] Eichberg DG, Sedighim S, Buttrick S, Komotar RJ. Postoperative seizure rate after transcortical resection of subcortical brain tumors and colloid cysts: a single surgeon's experience. Cureus. 2018; 10(1):e2115

[26] Milligan BD, Meyer FB. Morbidity of transcallosal and transcortical approaches to lesions in and around the lateral and third ventricles: a single-institution experience. Neurosurgery. 2010; 67(6):1483–1496, discussion 1496

# 16 Endoscopic Resection of Colloid Cyst of the Third Ventricle Using a Suction-Morcellation Device

*Thomas L. Beaumont*

**Abstract**

Colloid cysts of the third ventricle have historically been removed by open microsurgical approaches, most commonly the interhemispheric transcallosal approach. More recently minimally invasive endoscopic and port-based techniques have offered decreased complications and length of stay, with improved patient satisfaction. Here we describe the case of a colloid cyst causing obstructive hydrocephalus that was managed by a single burr hole endoscopic approach using a suction-morcellation device. Complete resection of the lesion was achieved with a small, coagulated cyst wall remnant left on the tela choroidea. The patient had an uneventful postoperative course and was headache-free at 1-month postoperative follow-up. The patient remained symptom-free and without evidence of radiographic recurrence at 4-year postoperative follow-up. Single burr hole endoscopic resection using a suction-morcellation device is an effective minimally invasive approach for appropriately selected patients with colloid cysts.

*Keywords:* colloid cyst, endoscopic, neuroendoscopy, third ventricle

## 16.1 Introduction

Colloid cysts can represent a formidable neurosurgical challenge due to their location deep within the brain, intimate association with the fornix, and critical deep draining veins to which they are commonly adherent. Historically, they have been removed with transcranial microsurgery by an interhemispheric transcallosal (IHTC) or transcortical transventricular (TCTV) approach. The former has been favored due to concern for an increased likelihood of seizures following transcortical approaches, although reported data are somewhat anecdotal.[1,2,3] Open microsurgical approaches have a relatively high rate of complications in reported series, ranging from 3.5 to 33%, with an average rate of at least 20%.[4,5,6] Over the past two decades, neuroendoscopic techniques have offered increasingly favorable results with significantly decreased complication rates ranging from 3 to 10%, along with optimal procedure-related variables and improved patient satisfaction.[6,7,8,9]

Early case series comparing endoscopic resection (ER) to microsurgical resection (MR) consistently demonstrated decreased operative time and decreased perioperative complications, including the elimination of perioperative death, and reduced length of stay (LOS).[4,5,10,11] However, these studies also demonstrated an increased rate of residual cyst wall remnants and cyst recurrence following ER, which was confirmed in several subsequent case series.[11,12,13,14] As the endoscopic technique has continued to evolve, more recent series describe rates of gross total resection (GTR) and recurrence similar to that achieved by microsurgical techniques.[9,15] Nonetheless, it remains unclear how the presence of coagulated cyst wall remnants after ER is associated with radiographic recurrence and the need for reoperation, as the data have been somewhat inconsistent.[16,17,18]

## 16.2 Case Description and Surgical Decision-Making

We present the case of a 42-year-old right-handed female with a long history of chronic migraine-type headaches with retro-orbital onset and a constellation of symptoms including colorful scotoma, photophobia, phonophobia, and nausea. These headaches were sometimes severe and occurred sporadically every 1 to 3 months. Over the year prior to presentation, the patient noted a distinct change in the frequency and character of her headaches which she described as daily, bifrontal, "sharp," 10/10 in severity, and associated with dizziness and blurred vision. At the time of presentation, the patient was neurologically intact on examination with stable vital signs. Neuroimaging demonstrated marked ventriculomegaly with a 1-cm hyperdense lesion at the foramen of Monro (▶ Fig. 16.1). Subsequent magnetic resonance imaging (MRI) demonstrated an 8 × 11 × 9 mm, T1 hyperintense, T2 hypointense, fluid-attenuated inversion recovery (FLAIR) hypointense lesion of the third ventricle consistent with a colloid cyst (▶ Fig. 16.2). This was associated with symmetric ventriculomegaly of the lateral ventricles without transependymal flow as well as thinning of the corpus callosum, suggesting chronic obstructive hydrocephalus. Colloid Cyst Risk Score (CCRS) at that time was 4.

Given the new progressive symptoms of obstructive hydrocephalus in the setting of a colloid cyst of the third ventricle, urgent neurosurgical intervention was indicated. Both craniotomy with port-based transventricular approach and a single burr hole endoscopic approach were discussed with the patient. Although the ventriculomegaly and cyst location were favorable for the latter, the T2 hypointensity suggested the cyst contents would be

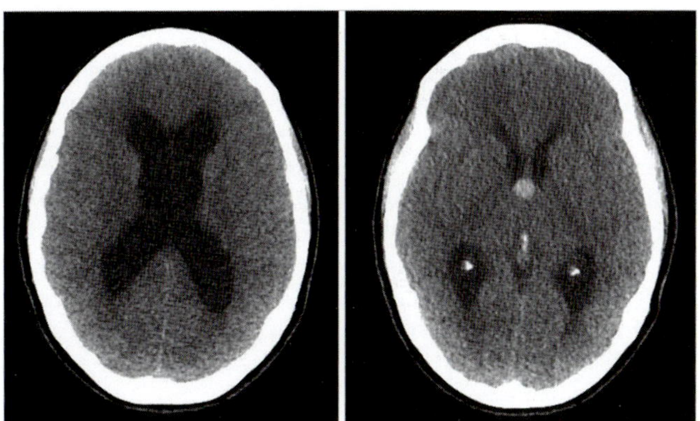

**Fig. 16.1** Preoperative computed tomography (CT) scan demonstrating marked ventriculomegaly with a 1-cm hyperdense lesion at the foramen of Monro, consistent with a colloid cyst of the third ventricle.

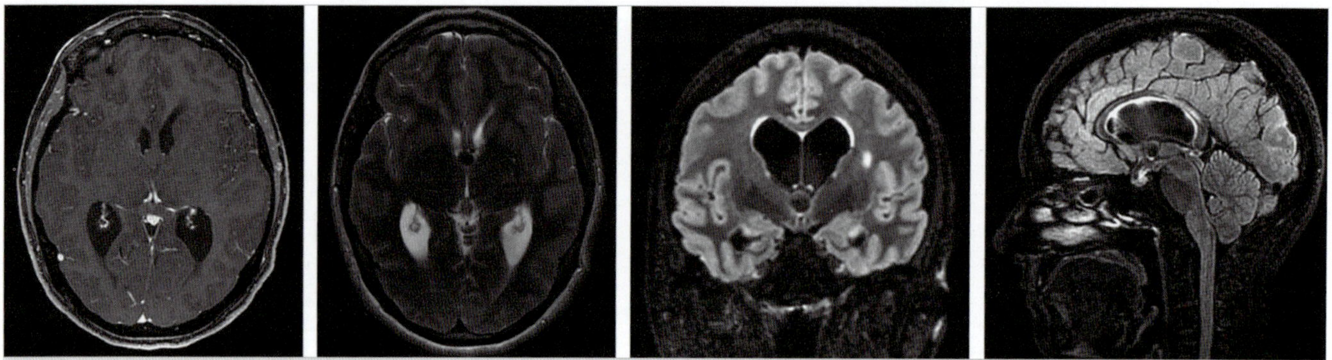

**Fig. 16.2** Preoperative postcontrast magnetic resonance imaging (MRI) demonstrating an 8 × 11 × 9 mm, nonenhancing, T2 hypointense, fluid-attenuated inversion recovery (FLAIR) hypointense lesion of the third ventricle consistent with a colloid cyst. There is obstruction of the foramen of Monro with marked ventriculomegaly and mild transependymal flow.

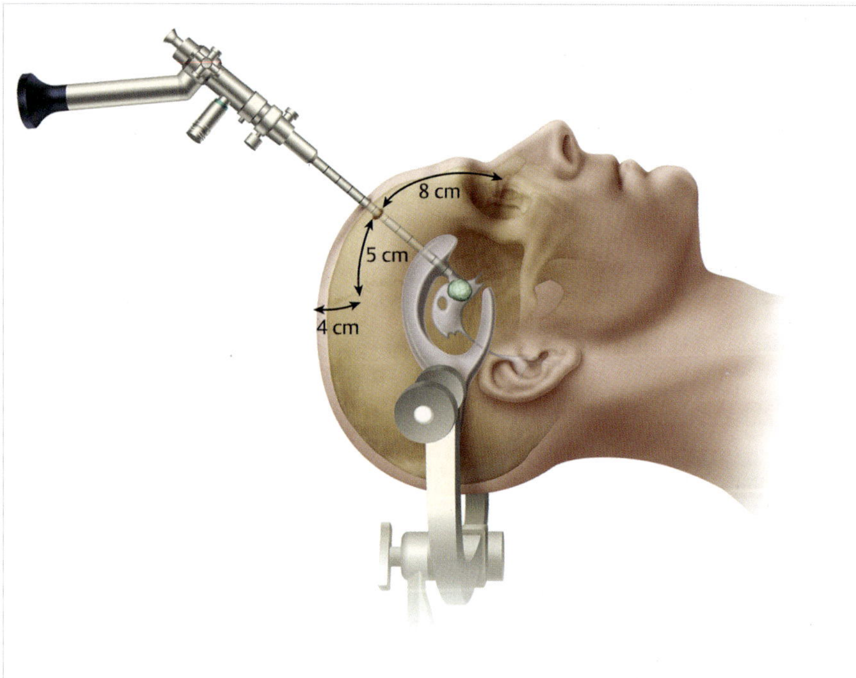


**Fig. 16.3** Head position and entry point for single burr hole endoscopic approach. The patient is positioned supine with the head in pin fixation. The burr hole is placed approximately 4 cm lateral to midline and 5 cm anterior to coronal suture. This is approximately 8 cm posterior to the nasion. The final location is optimized using image guidance to provide maximal access below the fornix while avoiding the caudate nucleus. (Reproduced with permission from Yahanda AT, Beaumont TL, Dacey RG Jr. Colloid cysts of the third ventricle. In: Winn HR, ed. Youmans & Winn's Neurological Surgery. 8th ed. Philadelphia: Elsevier; 2023.)

solid and non-suckable.[15] Also, the cyst appeared to have some posterior attachments to the tela choroidea and velum interpositum that could be more effectively dissected with true bimanual dissection. As a compromise between the desire for a minimally invasive approach and the need for sharp dissection and an effective means to address firm cyst contents, a single burr hole endoscopic approach with a multi-port endoscope (Karl Storz, Tutlingen, Germany) along with a suction-morcellation device (Nico Corp, Indianapolis, IN, USA) was planned. Admission to the hospital from clinic for surgery the following day was recommended but the patient declined. She was therefore given detailed instructions regarding warning signs that should prompt immediate presentation to the emergency department, and surgery was scheduled the following week (6 days later).

## 16.3 Surgical Technique

The patient was positioned supine with her neck flexed and her head immobilized in Mayfield pins. A burr hole was planned approximately 4 cm lateral to midline and 5 cm anterior to coronal suture (approximately 8 cm posterior to the nasion) using image guidance (▶ Fig. 16.3). The final location was optimized to provide maximal access below the fornix while avoiding the caudate nucleus. A curvilinear, 2.5-cm, coronally oriented incision was placed behind the hairline and a 14-mm burr hole was made with a high-speed drill and a perforator. Following this, a 19-French peel-away introducer (Aesculap) was passed into the ventricle under image guidance. A 30-degree ventriculoscope (LOTTA, Karl Storz) was then passed through the introducer into the lateral ventricle with gentle constant irrigation with warm normal saline. Net fluid egress was set at 1 drip every 1 to 2 seconds using the inflow and outflow stopcocks. The right septal veins were quickly identified, as was the choroid plexus, thalamostriate, and anterior caudate veins (▶ Video 16.1). The colloid cyst could be seen below the columns of the fornix anteriorly, partially obscured by overlying choroid plexus. Upon inspection of the septum pellucidum, a large fenestration was noted posterior to the septal veins; thus, septostomy was not necessary.

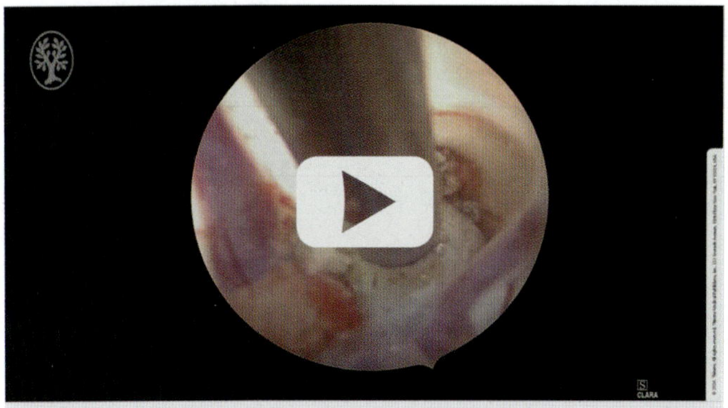

Video 16.1 Single burr hole endoscopic resection of a colloid cyst using a suction morcellation device.

Cyst resection began with coagulation of the overlying choroid plexus using a ball-tip monopolar electrode (Karl Storz). Care was taken to coagulate all the small penetrating arterioles on the colloid cyst wall. Following this, the cyst was opened sharply with endoscopic scissors and the mineralized contents were evacuated with a combination of grasping forceps and a suction-morcellation device (Myriad, Nico Corp, Indianapolis, IN, USA). Following internal decompression, we gained transforaminal access to the anterior interval between the cyst and the fornix. Any cyst-associated vessels were coagulated, the cyst margins were developed with blunt and sharp dissection, and the cyst wall was resected using the Myriad. Multiple cycles of resection followed by bipolar cautery were performed to reduce the cyst mass in piecemeal fashion. During resection of the posterolateral cyst wall just anterior to the thalamostriate vein, mild bleeding was encountered from a penetrating arteriole. This was initially controlled with tamponade and irrigation, with bipolar cautery subsequently. A small vascular complex emanating from the contralateral body of the fornix was adherent to the superior wall of the colloid cyst. This was coagulated and divided sharply using endoscopic scissors. Pulsatile irrigation and inspection of the ipsilateral and contralateral foramen of Monro were performed. The residual cyst wall that remained adherent to the fornix, tela choroidea, and internal cerebral veins was carefully coagulated (▶ Fig. 16.4). An external ventricular drain (EVD) was left in the lateral ventricle at the end of the case and a burr hole cover was placed. The operative site was irrigated, and the soft tissue was closed in layers with absorbable sutures in the galea and running 4–0 chromic in the skin. Following completion of the procedure the patient was extubated and transported to the neurointensive care unit for overnight observation.

## 16.4 Surgical Outcome

The patient had an uneventful postoperative course with complete resolution of headache, dizziness, and nausea. The EVD remained clamped and was only used to transduce intracranial pressure (ICP) for 24 hours postoperatively. ICP remained within normal limits, ranging between 7 to 16 cm $H_2O$. A computed tomography (CT) scan of the head on postoperative day 1 demonstrated GTR of colloid cyst (▶ Fig. 16.5). The patient was seen in clinic at 1 month postoperatively; she was headache-free, neurologically intact, and without complaints. New baseline neuroimaging was planned at 3 months postoperatively but was delayed until 6 months due to the COVID-19 pandemic. At 6-month follow-up she remained headache-free, physically active and well, stating she had returned to her baseline from 5 years prior. Neuroimaging demonstrated decreased maximum frontal horn diameter and decreased caliber of temporal horns with resolution of transependymal flow (▶ Fig. 16.6). At 4 years postoperatively, she remains symptom-free and without radiographic evidence of recurrence.

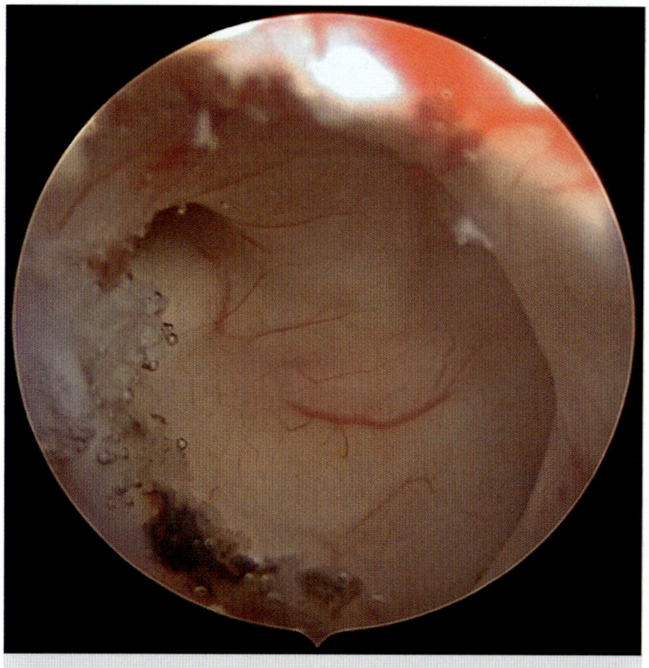

Fig. 16.4 Coagulated cyst wall remnant on the internal cerebral vein following endoscopic resection of colloid cyst. The fornix is seen on the right, contralateral foramen of Monro is seen in the background at 9 o'clock.

## 16.5 Discussion

Colloid cysts remain a technical neurosurgical challenge. Although they have historically been approached microsurgically, neuroendoscopy offers favorable outcomes with reduced operative time and reduced LOS with markedly decreased complication rates.[6,7,8,9] Importantly, endoscopy essentially eliminates major complications that were quite frequent with MR.[1,3,6,10,11,19,20,21] In contrast to the abovementioned benefits, ER is associated with a significantly increased frequency of coagulated residual cyst wall remnants, the significance of which remains unclear. Reported colloid cyst recurrence rates in the setting of coagulated cyst wall remnants range widely from 11.1 to 33.3%, although the latter was based on relatively few cases.[9,17] In a recent, well-powered single-center study of patients who underwent surgery via flexible endoscopy, the extent of resection (EOR) was categorized as en bloc removal (Grade I), complete removal of the cyst contents and > 50% (Grade II) or < 50% (Grade III) resection, or coagulation of the cyst wall.[18] There were no recurrences in Grade I or II patients

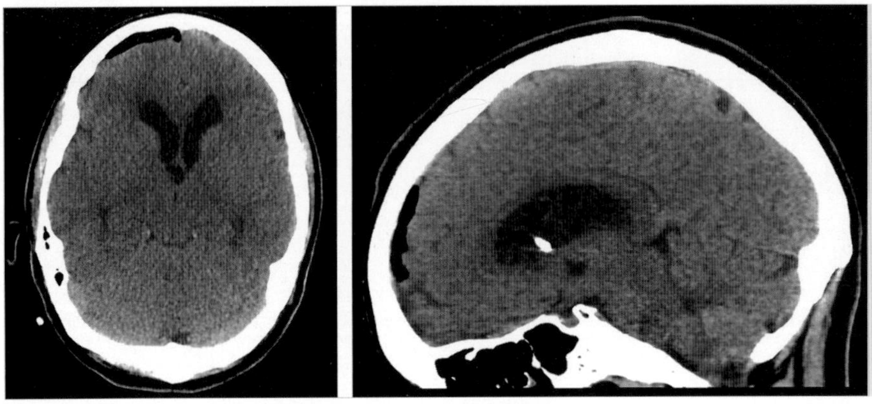

**Fig. 16.5** Postoperative computed tomography (CT) scan demonstrating complete resection of the colloid cyst with mild pneumocephalus. A clamped right frontal external ventricular drain remains in place.

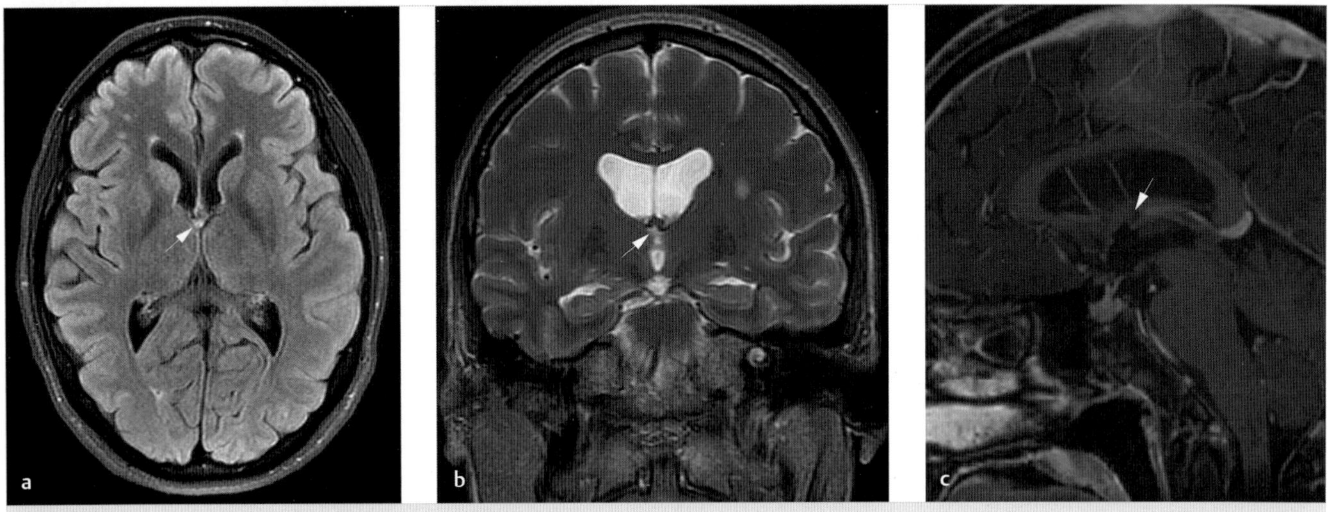

**Fig. 16.6** Postcontrast magnetic resolution imaging (MRI) at 2 years postoperatively. Axial fluid-attenuated inversion recovery (FLAIR) **(a)** demonstrating resolution of ventriculomegaly with a small focus of hyperintensity representing coagulated cyst wall remnant (arrow). Coronal T2-weighted sequence **(b)** and sagittal, postcontrast T1-weighted sequences **(c)** through the region of hyperintensity seen on FLAIR (*arrows*). There is resolution of ventriculomegaly and transependymal flow and no residual enhancement.

with median follow-up of 10.3 years, directly challenging the notion that coagulated cyst wall remnants lead to cyst recurrence. Nonetheless, studies reporting extended follow up have demonstrated mean time to recurrence of more than 7 years with late recurrences as long as 15 years postoperatively.[9,17,22] Thus, all patients should have annual surveillance imaging for at least 10 years, particularly in the setting of coagulated cyst wall remnants.

Whether the improved safety and cost-effectiveness of ER of colloid cysts justifies the potentially increased rate of recurrence remains an open question, particularly since endoscopic EOR has continued to improve as bimanual endoscopic techniques evolve.[23] Given the rarity of the lesion, this question will need to be addressed with a prospective, multicenter registry that includes preoperative grading, clearly defined indications for surgery, strict criteria for defining postoperative residual cyst wall remnants and EOR, neuropsychological testing, and patient satisfaction scores. Despite the ongoing debate, it seems unlikely that one surgical approach will prove superior for *all* colloid cysts. Although beyond the scope of the present study, between single burr hole ER and traditional MR, hybrid port-based approaches offer a minimally invasive approach with the benefit of true bimanual technique and dry-field dissection.[24,25] In cases where the cyst pedicle is posteriorly placed, the cyst contents are firm (hypointense on T2 MRI), or when the cyst wall is adherent to the fornix and/or internal cerebral veins, true bimanual technique along with dry-field dissection may offer increased EOR with increased safety.

Finally, there are presently no defined indications for the various approaches for colloid cysts of the third ventricle, and approach selection typically relies on how a particular surgeon was trained and what has been the institutional preference.[19] There is a steep learning curve associated with intraventricular endoscopy and a significant initial capital investment for institutions implementing neuroendoscopy. Furthermore, colloid cysts occur in intimate association with critical neurovascular anatomy where complications are poorly to tolerated and can be catastrophic. Surgeons with limited experience with neuroendoscopy should therefore select cases that are most favorable for success. These include patients with mild ventriculomegaly and anteriorly positioned cysts that are T2 hyperintense.

## References


[1] Desai KI, Nadkarni TD, Muzumdar DP, Goel AH. Surgical management of colloid cyst of the third ventricle—a study of 105 cases. Surg Neurol. 2002; 57(5): 295–302, discussion 302–304

[2] Milligan BD, Meyer FB. Morbidity of transcallosal and transcortical approaches to lesions in and around the lateral and third ventricles: a single-institution experience. Neurosurgery. 2010; 67(6):1483–1496, discussion 1496

[3] Sheikh AB, Mendelson ZS, Liu JK. Endoscopic versus microsurgical resection of colloid cysts: a systematic review and meta-analysis of 1,278 patients. World Neurosurg. 2014; 82(6):1187–1197

[4] Grondin RT, Hader W, MacRae ME, Hamilton MG. Endoscopic versus microsurgical resection of third ventricle colloid cysts. Can J Neurol Sci. 2007; 34 (2):197–207

[5] Lewis AI, Crone KR, Taha J, van Loveren HR, Yeh HS, Tew JM, Jr. Surgical resection of third ventricle colloid cysts. Preliminary results comparing transcallosal microsurgery with endoscopy. J Neurosurg. 1994; 81(2):174–178

[6] Sampath R, Vannemreddy P, Nanda A. Microsurgical excision of colloid cyst with favorable cognitive outcomes and short operative time and hospital stay: operative techniques and analyses of outcomes with review of previous studies. Neurosurgery. 2010; 66(2):368–374, discussion 374–375

[7] Margetis K, Christos PJ, Souweidane M. Endoscopic resection of incidental colloid cysts. J Neurosurg. 2014; 120(6):1259–1267

[8] Sribnick EA, Dadashev VY, Miller BA, Hawkins S, Hadjipanayis CG. Neuroendoscopic colloid cyst resection: a case cohort with follow-up and patient satisfaction. World Neurosurg. 2014; 81(3–4):584–593

[9] Vorbau C, Baldauf J, Oertel J, Gaab MR, Schroeder HWS. Long-term results after endoscopic resection of colloid cysts. World Neurosurg. 2019; 122:e176–e185

[10] Horn EM, Feiz-Erfan I, Bristol RE, et al. Treatment options for third ventricular colloid cysts: comparison of open microsurgical versus endoscopic resection. Neurosurgery. 2007; 60(4):613–618, discussion 618–620

[11] Kehler U, Brunori A, Gliemroth J, et al. Twenty colloid cysts—comparison of endoscopic and microsurgical management. Minim Invasive Neurosurg. 2001; 44(3):121–127

[12] Boogaarts H, El-Kheshin S, Grotenhuis J. Endoscopic colloid cyst resection: technical note. Minim Invasive Neurosurg. 2011; 54(2):95–97

[13] Hellwig D, Bauer BL, Schulte M, Gatscher S, Riegel T, Bertalanffy H. Neuroendoscopic treatment for colloid cysts of the third ventricle: the experience of a decade. Neurosurgery. 2003; 52(3):525–533, discussion 532–533

[14] Longatti P, Godano U, Gangemi M, et al. Italian neuroendoscopy group. Cooperative study by the Italian neuroendoscopy group on the treatment of 61 colloid cysts. Childs Nerv Syst. 2006; 22(10):1263–1267

[15] Samadian M, Ebrahimzadeh K, Maloumeh EN, et al. Colloid cyst of the third ventricle: long-term results of endoscopic management in a series of 112 cases. World Neurosurg. 2018; 111:e440–e448

[16] Boogaarts HD, Decq P, Grotenhuis JA, et al. Long-term results of the neuroendoscopic management of colloid cysts of the third ventricle: a series of 90 cases. Neurosurgery. 2011; 68(1):179–187

[17] Hoffman CE, Savage NJ, Souweidane MM. The significance of cyst remnants after endoscopic colloid cyst resection: a retrospective clinical case series. Neurosurgery. 2013; 73(2):233–237, discussion 237–239

[18] Isaacs AM, Bezchlibnyk YB, Dronyk J, Urbaneja G, Yong H, Hamilton MG. Long-term outcomes of endoscopic third ventricle colloid cyst resection: case series with a proposed grading system. Oper Neurosurg (Hagerstown). 2020; 19(2): 134–142

[19] Beaumont TL, Limbrick DD, Patel B, Chicoine MR, Rich KM, Dacey RG. Surgical management of colloid cysts of the third ventricle: a single-institution comparison of endoscopic and microsurgical resection. J Neurosurg. 2022: 1–9.-Online ahead of print

[20] Hernesniemi J, Romani R, Dashti R, et al. Microsurgical treatment of third ventricular colloid cysts by interhemispheric far lateral transcallosal approach—experience of 134 patients. Surg Neurol. 2008; 69(5):447–453, discussion 453–456

[21] Shapiro S, Rodgers R, Shah M, Fulkerson D, Campbell RL. Interhemispheric transcallosal subchoroidal fornix-sparing craniotomy for total resection of colloid cysts of the third ventricle. J Neurosurg. 2009; 110(1):112–115

[22] Greenlee JD, Teo C, Ghahreman A, Kwok B. Purely endoscopic resection of colloid cysts. Neurosurgery. 2008; 62(3) Suppl 1:51–55, discussion 55–56

[23] Wilson DA, Fusco DJ, Wait SD, Nakaji P. Endoscopic resection of colloid cysts: use of a dual-instrument technique and an anterolateral approach. World Neurosurg. 2013; 80(5):576–583

[24] Eichberg DG, Buttrick SS, Sharaf JM, et al. Use of tubular retractor for resection of colloid cysts: single surgeon experience and review of the literature. Oper Neurosurg (Hagerstown). 2019; 16(5):571–579

[25] Engh JA, Lunsford LD, Amin DV, et al. Stereotactically guided endoscopic port surgery for intraventricular tumor and colloid cyst resection. Neurosurgery. 2010; 67(3) Suppl Operative:ons198–ons204, discussion ons204–ons205

# 17 Bimanual Endoscopic Technique Using an Anterolateral Approach for the Resection of Colloid Cysts

*Roland Jabre and Peter Nakaji*

**Abstract**

Endoscopic resection of colloid cysts is a minimally invasive technique that can successfully completely remove colloid cyst contents and membrane, manage hydrocephalus, treat hydrocephalus, and preserve forniceal function. Keys to achieving success are avoidance of swinging the endoscope from side to side and up and down, using two instruments through two working channels, and approaching from as anterolateral a trajectory as the patient's anatomy permits, which allows the surgeon an improved view of the attachment point of the cyst on the roof of the third ventricle. Meticulous technique must be employed, which optimally involves holding the cyst under tension with a small grasping forceps through a side channel while coagulating, draining, or cutting the cyst with instruments introduced through a primary channel. Excellent results can be obtained through a small burr hole and incision with high efficacy and low complications.

*Keywords:* endoscopic resection, fornices, bimanual technique, anterolateral trajectory, working channels

## 17.1 Introduction

As has been seen with the treatment of many other neurosurgical pathologies, there is a trend toward minimally invasive approaches using endoscopy for the treatment of many colloid cysts. The advantage of this technique is its lower morbidity rates compared to open transcranial approaches.[1] However, this advantage is usually counterbalanced by a higher risk of postoperative residue and recurrence.[1] The "one-handedness" of the endoscopic removal technique and inadequate visualization of the attachment site of the colloid cyst could explain this lower rate of complete resection. Here, we describe an improved technique that has been developed to partially overcome these issues which uses two instruments simultaneously through two channels to achieve bimanuality and an anterolateral approach to improve visualization.[2] Given that the more general aspects of the endoscopic technique are discussed by multiple authors in this volume, we will focus on the details and nuances of our specific technique rather than an exhaustive general review of the subject.

## 17.2 Preoperative Planning

The first step in endoscopic removal consists in studying the imaging and the anatomy of each specific case before undertaking surgery. The size of the colloid cyst, its relationship to the fornices, its point of attachment, and the presence of enlarged ventricles are important characteristics to take into consideration in order to choose the best approach.

A colloid cyst of larger size (> 1.2–1.5 cm) makes endoscopic resection substantially longer and more complex in many cases both because of the larger volume and because the fornices may become thinner and more adherent. Larger cysts can be removed if the cyst is both pedunculated and soft, as its contents can be evacuated with a cannula or an endoscopic shaver and then the cyst wall gathered and detached. However, it can be challenging to determine reliably in advance if this is the case or not; this may lead some surgeons to limit the size of cysts that are removed endoscopically or to change the goals, e.g., to drainage, fenestration, and coagulation.

Endoscopic removal requires adequate room. The absence of ventriculomegaly makes cannulation of the ventricles more difficult and reduces the available working space. In addition, the fornices are more at risk during manipulation of the colloid cyst since the foramina of Monro are usually not enlarged in these cases. When the ventricles are small, a better working space can be obtained by not using a peel-away sheath and attaching a fluid management system that will both irrigate and gently distend the ventricular space (▶ Fig. 17.1). Thus, although endoscopic removal in normal-sized (nondilated) ventricles is technically feasible in highly experienced hands, open removal should be favored in these cases.[3]

With respect to location, an important feature to look for on imaging is location of the colloid cyst in the sagittal and in the coronal plane. A colloid cyst posterior to the foramen of Monro (corresponding to zones II and III according to Beaumont et al) or extending superiorly up between the fornices will be more difficult to remove endoscopically since its attachment point cannot be seen and controlled (▶ Fig. 17.2).[4] It is usually preferable for the approach side to be the nondominant side since the entry point is very lateral and often too close to where Broca's area would be on the dominant side. However, this can also be influenced somewhat by preferring to approach from where the colloid cyst seems to be the most attached.

In summary, the ideal cyst and patient for the endoscopic approach is a small-to-medium size colloid cyst presenting at the foramen of Monro, without extension between the fornices and not posterior to the foramen of Monro, preferably presenting to the nondominant side, where the fornices do not appear excessively thin, in patients with ventriculomegaly (▶ Fig. 17.3).

## 17.3 Technique (▶ Video 17.1)

When surgery is indicated and an endoscopic approach is chosen, appropriate equipment is mandatory. This includes a multichannel neuroendoscope (this technique uses the MINOP endoscope, Aesculap, Tuttlingen, Germany), associated endoscopic instruments, and the use of a neuronavigation system. Instruments that are essential include a suction cannula that fits down the working channel, a bipolar and/or monopolar cautery, endoscopic scissors and graspers, and a small flexible grasper, the last of these to be deployed down a side port on the side anterior to the cyst and with a small bend near the tip that allows it to exit the endoscope at a converging angle.

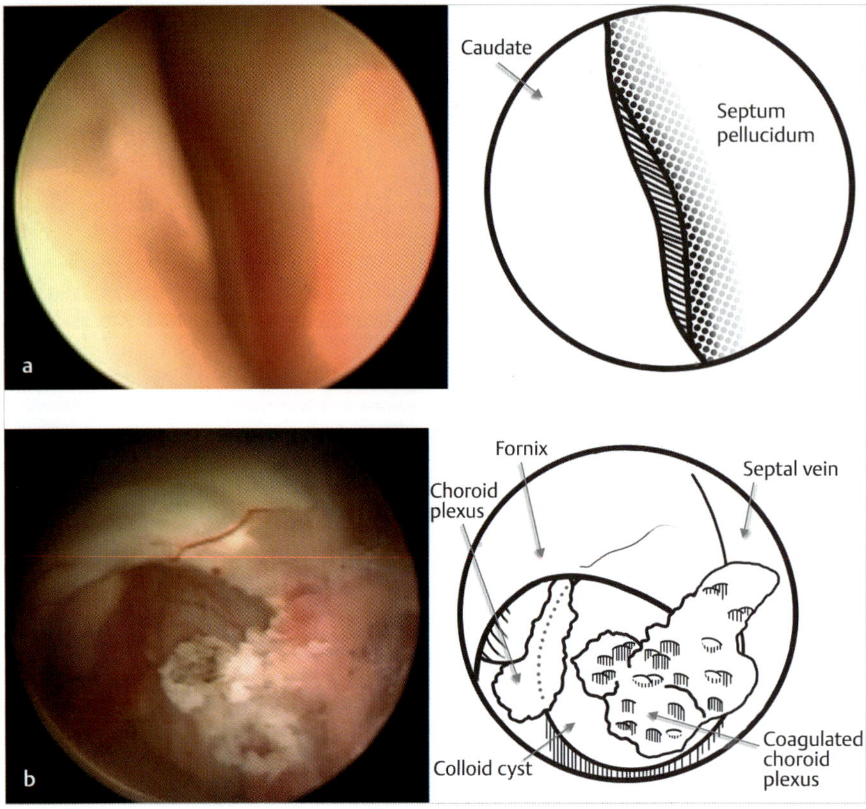


**Fig. 17.1** The effect of using or not using a peel-away sheath in a patient with small ventricles; left-sided approach. **(a)** The ventricle with the peel-away sheath in is collapsed. **(b)** With the peel-away sheath removed, the ventricles distend under mild irrigation; the coagulated choroid plexus, fornix, and cyst can be seen.

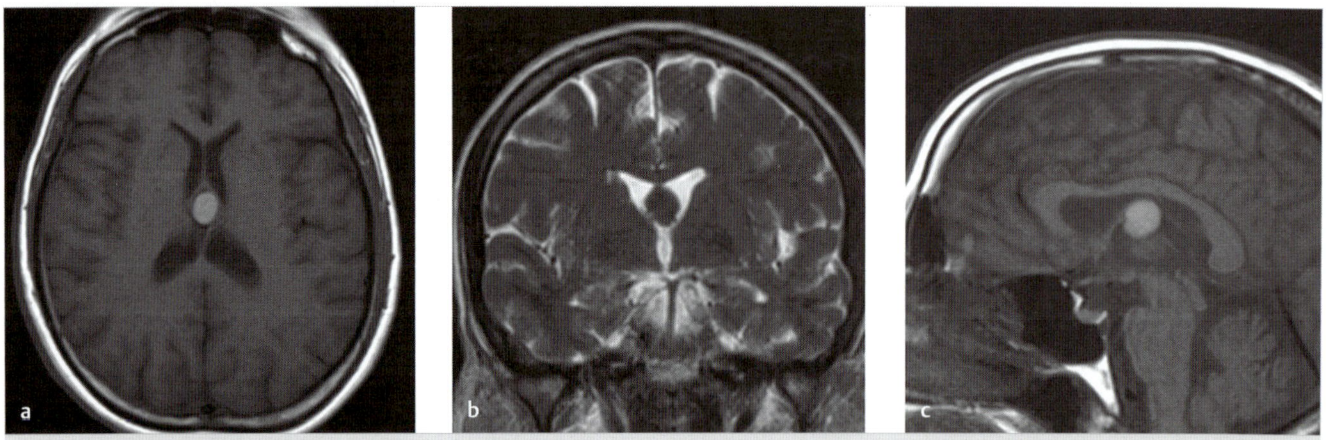


**Fig. 17.2** A colloid cyst anatomically unfavorable for an endoscopic approach. **(a)** Axial T1 magnetic resonance imaging (MRI) showing a colloid cyst with the fornices bowing around it. **(b)** Coronal T2 MRI showing that the cyst is located almost entirely above the foramen of Monro. **(c)** Sagittal T1 MRI showing the cyst is also posterior to the foramen on Monro in zone II.

Everything, including the video chain and the optics of the endoscope, should be confirmed to be in good working order before beginning the procedure.

The patient is positioned supine with the head flexed and fixed in a rigid head clamp so that the sagittal suture is perpendicular to the floor. The head should be raised above the heart to lower the venous pressure, which reduces brain fullness and helps with hemostasis. The surgeon is also positioned so as to be in the same trajectory as the endoscope; thus, the screen is across the head from the patient instead of at the foot (▶ Fig. 17.4).

A cylindrical burr hole 8 mm in diameter is placed about 5 cm anterior to the coronal suture and 5 to 7 cm lateral to the midline on the side that the cyst presents the most, preferably on the nondominant side as previously noted. This more anterolateral

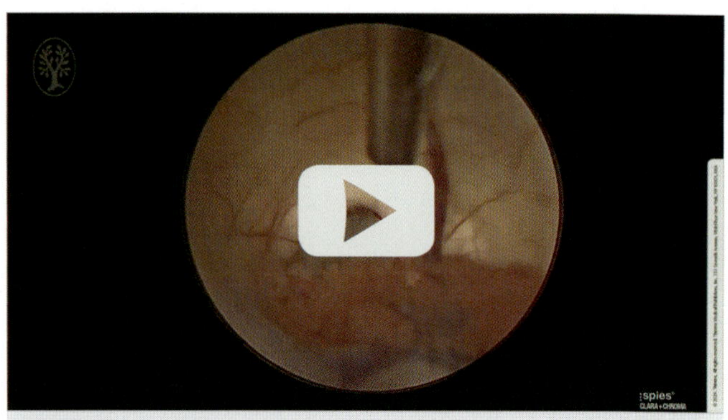

**Video 17.1** Bimanual endoscopic technique using an anterolateral approach for the resection of colloid cysts.

approach allows the endoscope to see up under the arch of the fornix to the attachment point on the roof of the third ventricle. The trajectory is modified according to sidedness (i.e., less lateral on the left to avoid Broca's area) and according to the specific anatomy of the frontal horn and the presence of ventriculomegaly; usually the larger the ventricles the more anterolateral the approach that can be achieved. It should avoid the head of the caudate nucleus and be aimed directly at the colloid cyst and its attachment point in order to reduce the need to sweep the endoscope during surgery which can damage the brain parenchyma and cause bleeding. Neuronavigation is an invaluable tool to confirm the best entry point using these criteria.

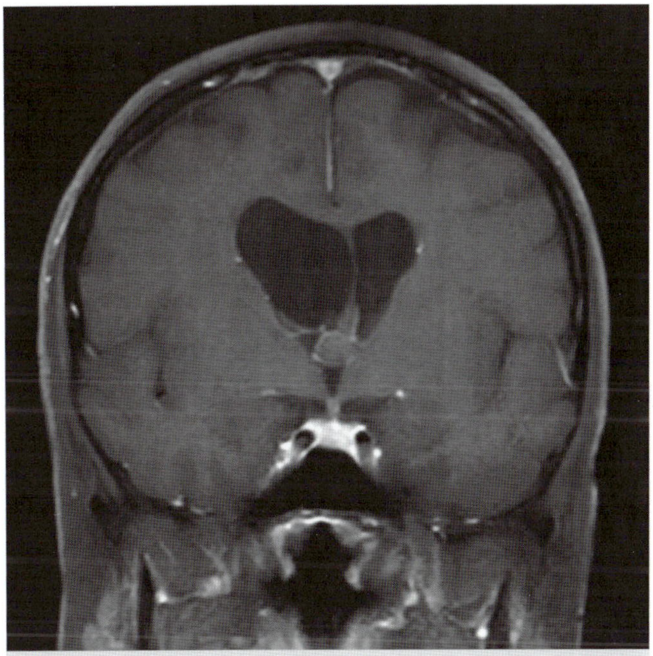

**Fig. 17.3** Coronal T1 magnetic resonance imaging (MRI) with gadolinium showing a 9-mm colloid cyst in a patient in whom the ventricle is dilated on the nondominant side where the cyst is present. This constellation of findings constitutes good conditions for a right-sided endoscopic approach.

A working peel-away sheath is optional but preferred by many surgeons, as it allows easy egress of fluid, preventing increased intracranial pressure from over-irrigation. The disadvantage of the peel-away sheath is that the cerebrospinal fluid (CSF) pressure is low, which may lend to more venous bleeding, and drainage of spinal fluid may cause the ventricles to collapse; removal of the sheath and direct placement of the endoscope can reverse these conditions when they present a problem.[3] The neuroendoscope is advanced under stereotactic guidance into the lateral ventricle. The 30-degree endoscope is used since it keeps the instruments in sight from the moment they leave the trocar and allows to work close to the endoscope. The procedure is done under intermittent irrigation using body temperature lactated Ringer's solution. This fluid is chosen since it resembles CSF more than normal saline and causes less ionic shift in the CSF.

When the cyst is visualized, its capsule is coagulated with bipolar cautery, taking care to avoid the fornix. The capsule is punctured, and the cyst contents are aspirated using a trimmed pediatric endotracheal suction catheter.[5] Then a two-instrument technique is used to dissect the cyst wall from the surrounding neurovascular structures.[2]

The two-instrument technique is carried out as follows: an assistant holds the endoscope which permits the primary surgeon to use a bimanual technique to create tension on the wall of the colloid cyst. This is made possible using several tricks. First, a flexible grasping forceps, which is bent very slightly 1.5 cm from the tip, is brought in through the side channel so that it is anterior to the foramen (left channel for a left approach, right channel for a right approach). The flexible forceps grasps the cyst wall and pulls it anteriorly away from the roof of the third ventricle, across the path of the main channel, allowing the main channel instruments to access the cyst wall at the attachment point (▶ Fig. 17.5). By drawing the flexible forceps into the trocar, tension is maintained, and the attachment point is revealed. A combination of coagulation and sharp dissection can be used to remove the cyst wall

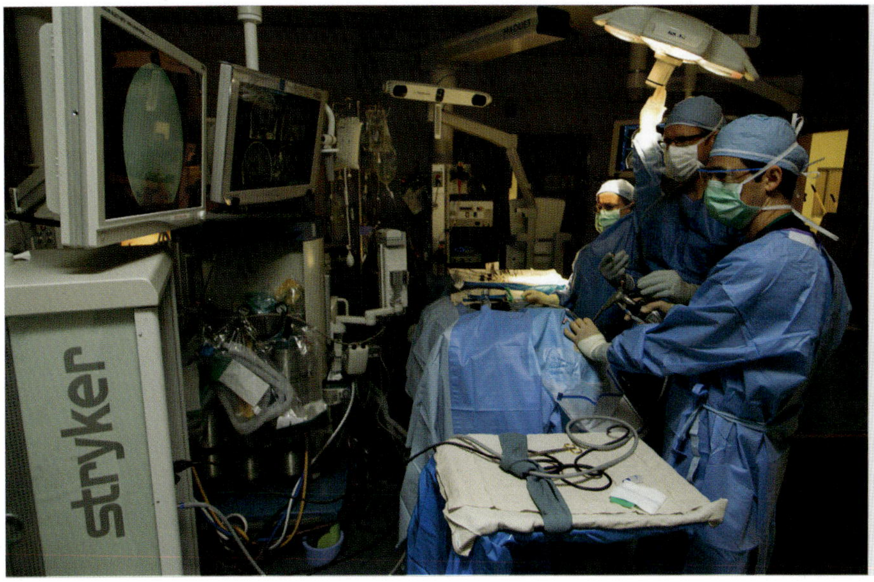


**Fig. 17.4** Room setup for endoscopic colloid cyst removal. The screen is across the head from the surgeon and assistant.

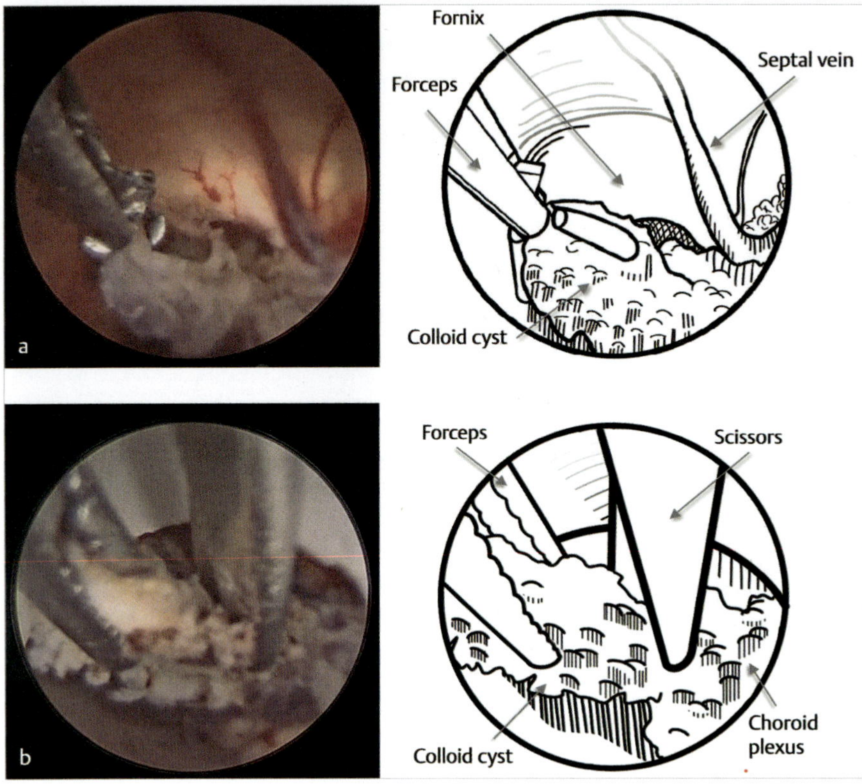


**Fig. 17.5** The small grasping forceps has a small bend in it, so that even coming through a side channel, it can be rotated back to the middle of the exposure, and by rotating it back, **(a)** drag the grasped cyst past the main working channel where **(b)** it can be coagulated and cut.

under tension. By rotating the flexible instrument, the cyst wall can be placed under tension and drawn up and pulled to expose the plane between the cyst and normal tissue, so that another instrument can be used to dissect the cyst further. Lastly, the endoscope itself can be rotated, which again creates tension and can expose the desired dissection plane, with the advantage that there is no need to swing the endoscope shaft within the brain parenchyma. With the tension on the cyst dome provided by the small flexible grasper, the bipolar is used to coagulate the attachment, followed by scissors which separates the colloid cyst from the roof of the third ventricle. It is helpful to have one person hold the grasping forceps and the other hold the endoscope and work the main channel. After detachment from the roof of the third ventricle, the cyst and the endoscope are all drawn together from the brain through the peel-away sheath. Hemostasis is obtained and the roof of the third ventricle is inspected for residue. A septum pellucidotomy is performed if there is any concern about the patency of the foramen of Monro.

Using these techniques, excellent removal can be obtained, in the order of 86.7% removal with low morbidity.[2,3]

## 17.4 Conclusion

Key elements of the definition of an optimal outcome in endoscopic colloid cyst surgery include complete cyst removal without a residue that results in recurrence. For this to be achieved, careful microdissection under tension is essential, which is most easily achieved in microsurgery with two instruments. Although true bimanual dissection is not possible with a single-entry point, a reasonable functional facsimile can be achieved by using two instruments of proper configuration through the same endoscope trocar.

## References

[1] Sethi A, Cavalcante D, Ormond DR. Endoscopic versus microscopic transcallosal excision of colloid cysts: a systematic review in the era of complete endoscopic excision. World Neurosurg. 2019; 132:e53–e58

[2] Wilson DA, Fusco DJ, Wait SD, Nakaji P. Endoscopic resection of colloid cysts: use of a dual-instrument technique and an anterolateral approach. World Neurosurg. 2013; 80(5):576–583

[3] Wait SD, Gazzeri R, Wilson DA, Abla AA, Nakaji P, Teo C. Endoscopic colloid cyst resection in the absence of ventriculomegaly. Neurosurgery. 2013; 73(1) Suppl Operative:ons39–ons46, ons46–ons47

[4] Beaumont TL, Limbrick DD, Jr, Rich KM, Wippold FJ, II, Dacey RG, Jr. Natural history of colloid cysts of the third ventricle. J Neurosurg. 2016; 125(6):1420–1430

[5] Souweidane MM, Luther N. Endoscopic resection of solid intraventricular brain tumors. J Neurosurg. 2006; 105(2):271–278

# 18 Resection of Colloid Cysts Using Flexible Endoscopy: How I Do It?

*Islas-Aguilar Mario Alberto and Jaime Gerardo Torres-Corzo*

**Abstract**

Colloid cysts are benign intracranial lesions that make up a significant fraction of intraventricular tumors, with symptoms often including headaches, hydrocephalus, and cognitive disturbances. Flexible neuroendoscopy has proven to be an effective surgical approach due to its minimal invasiveness and versatility, particularly noted for its single burr hole technique for lesion inspection, coagulation, and extraction. This method is especially beneficial for pediatric cases due to its smaller diameter compared to rigid endoscopes. The ability to access and treat both lateral ventricles via septostomy, along with its low complication rates such as fistula and infection, underscores its advantages. Despite limitations in instrument variety, leading to challenges in achieving total cyst resection, the technique's efficacy is supported by a low recurrence rate, indicating that cyst wall retraction and extraction are generally sufficient for positive clinical outcomes.

The surgical procedure requires careful planning based on imaging studies, and specific patient positioning to optimize access and minimize risks. The technique involves a single burr hole, avoiding the need for repositioning during septostomy and contralateral ventricle exploration. Key steps include ventricular puncture, cerebrospinal fluid exchange, and the use of peel-away catheters and fiberscopes for tissue protection and precise intraventricular pressure control. The use of holmium laser for cyst wall coagulation and the strategic approach to cyst content drainage underscore the procedure's sophistication. Despite the challenges of not always achieving total gross resection, the method's emphasis on minimizing postoperative complications and leveraging neuronavigation for complex cases.

*Keywords:* flexible endoscopy, cyst resection, neuroendoscopy, holmium laser, hydrocephalus

## 18.1 Introduction

Colloid cysts are benign intracranial lesions, with an incidence ranging from 0.5 to 2.0% of all intracranial tumors, representing 15% of all intraventricular lesions.[1,2] Commonly, the patient presents with headache, altered level of consciousness, ataxia, and memory difficulties; hydrocephalus might be unilateral or bilateral according to the Monro level of obstruction.[3,4]

Flexible neuroendoscopy is a surgical technique that over the years has shown good results because of the versatility it offers.

Removal of colloid cysts of the third ventricle with flexible neuroendoscopy has several advantages. A single burr hole is used to perform all the procedures (inspection of the lesion, wall coagulation using monopolar or laser when needed and content extraction); also the average diameter is smaller than a rigid endoscope. This is especially relevant when treating pediatric patients.[5,6]

The contralateral ventricle can be reached through a septostomy, allowing to work in both Monro foramina and releasing both lateral ventricles. Flexible neuroendoscopy has a low incidence of fistula, infection, hygroma, and subdural hematoma; therefore, it allows to perform a "second look" in a quick and simple way for reexamination.

Among the disadvantages of this technique is the low number of instruments to facilitate a total resection of the cyst because of the single working channel. However, colloid cysts are not neoplastic lesions. We believe that extraction and retraction of the cyst wall are enough to achieve good clinical results in most cases. In our experience, no single case has recurred. We do not perform a total resection because of the high risk of the deep venous system bleeding that arises posteriorly causing complications such as hydrocephalus, cerebral aqueduct stenosis, post-hemorrhagic arachnoiditis, etc.[1,7,8]

## 18.2 Surgical Technique

Flexible neuroendoscopy requires surgical planning based on imaging studies analysis, either magnetic resonance image or computed tomography, topography, surgical approaching site, lateral ventricle morphology, septum pellucidum characteristics, size of the third ventricle and characteristics of the convexity, and subarachnoid space of the skull base.

General anesthesia is used with an armed single-lumen endotracheal tube. The patient is placed supine with the head in neutral position fixed on a doughnut pillow or in a three-pin fixation Mayfield head holder with the head flexed at 30 degrees when a neuronavigation system is needed. A neuronavigation system is used. The head is flexed at 30 degrees. We place the endoscope on a special holder to improve the handling of the device (▶ Fig. 18.1).

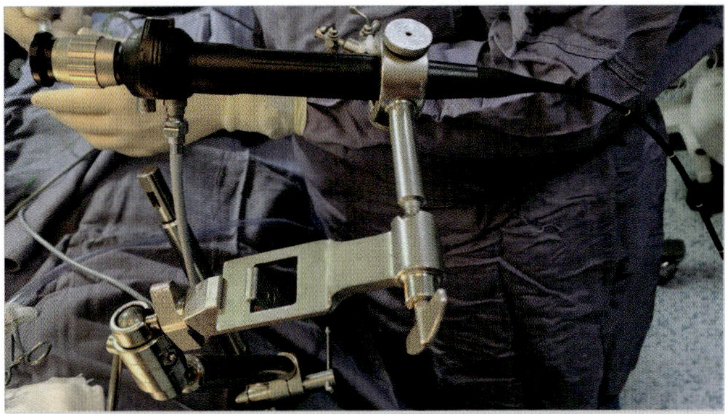

**Fig. 18.1** Flexible neuroendoscope holder.

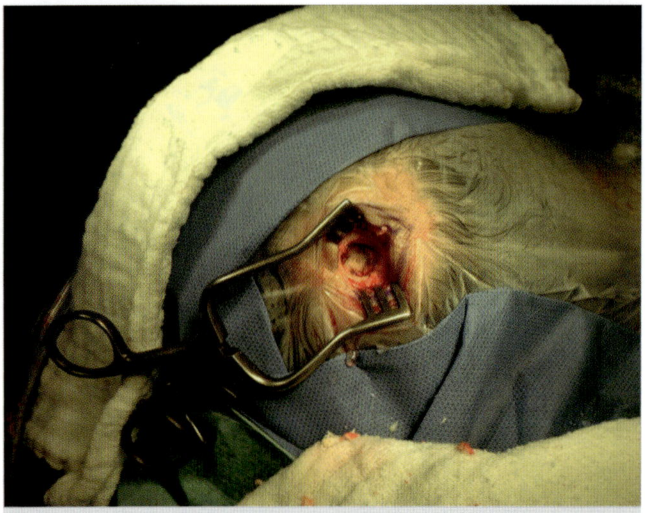

Fig. 18.2 Burr hole prior to dural incision.

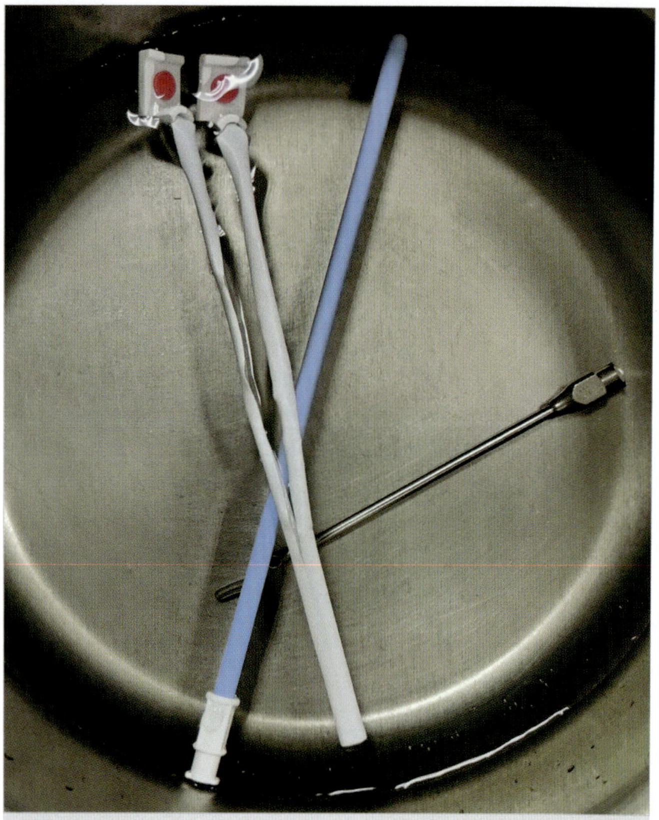

Fig. 18.3 Peel-away catheter introducer and ventricular needle.

Partial pressure of carbon dioxide is kept close to 35 mmHg (1,850 MASL) to prevent position changes of the brain parenchyma. It is important to remember that suggested $CO_2$ partial pressure varies according to the height above the sea level of the region.

Shaving and linear skin incision parallel to the sagittal suture in Kocher point are performed. A single burr hole is used in flexible neuroendoscopy. No change in position is needed to perform the septostomy and exploration of contralateral ventricle. The burr hole is made 1 cm in front of the coronal suture and 3 cm lateral to the midline (▶ Fig. 18.2). A dural cruciate incision is made. The borders are coagulated where the puncture is made to reduce the risk of hygroma or subdural hematoma. Ventricular puncture using a rigid ventricular needle is performed. Then 5 mL of cerebrospinal fluid is collected for analysis and the same amount of liquid is replaced with Ringer lactate solution to keep intraventricular pressure, especially when neuronavigation system is used.[9]

A peel-away catheter introducer (▶ Fig. 18.3) (Codman Neuro, Rayham, Massachusetts, USA) is used in every procedure to protect brain tissue and control intraventricular pressure. The fiberscope (Karl Storz Gmbh, Tuttlingen, Germany) is inserted through the peel-away sheath into the right lateral ventricle. Before the resection is performed, primary anatomic landmarks are visualized. Colloid cyst wall is coagulated. Next, the lesion is punctured with forceps and intracystic content is drained with a semiflexible 2-French epidural catheter inserted in the working channel. Sometimes the intracystic content is highly viscous and the use of forceps or laser is necessary. We have used holmium laser for resection and wall coagulation with good results. Foramen of Monro is opened as the cyst retraction and removal are achieved. Third ventricle colloid cysts always require a septum pellucidum fenestration to achieve contralateral removal of the cyst where the same technique is performed. This way both Monro foramina are free. When possible, total gross resection is achieved but in most cases the wall is attached to the third ventricle roof. In our experience, there is no growth of the remnant wall. A third ventriculostomy is not necessary. We conclude the procedure with ventricular lavage, then the fiberscope is removed from the cortex, and the surgical tract is filled with a rolled Gelfoam sponge (Pfizer Inc., New York, New York, USA). Measure of the ventricular pressure is done at the end of surgery with a rigid ventricular needle.

We use a 1-mm coagulating electrode with 5 to 8 joules. The holmium YAG (Ho:YAG) laser is used with a 200-µm fiber, 1.5 joules, 12 watts, and 8 Hz. This configuration might be changed according to the size of the cyst and wall thickness. When ventriculomegaly is absent or anatomical relationships might complicate the procedure, we use neuronavigation-assisted flexible neuroendoscopy (▶ Fig. 18.4) (Fiagon Gmbh, Henningsdorf, Berlin, Germany). In our experience, it has proven useful and beneficial in these cases (▶ Fig. 18.5).[10]

## 18.3 Clinical Case

A 45-year-old female patient presented with ataxia, tremor, dysdiadochokinesia, dysmetria, and cephalgia, lasting 1 year; no sensitive or motor alterations were observed.

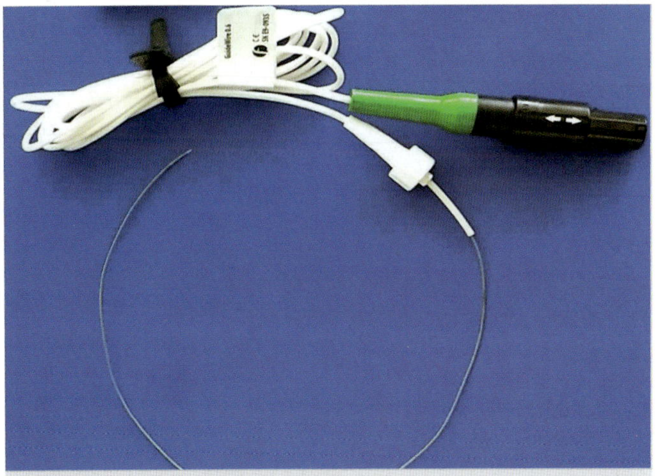

Fig. 18.4 Guidewire system.

Sagittal and axial magnetic resonance imaging (MRI) showed a hyperintense lesion in T1 occupying the third ventricle and obstructing both Monro foramina producing hydrocephalus (▶ Fig. 18.6).

### 18.3.1 Preoperative Plan

MRIs are evaluated prior to surgery, measuring ventricular diameter and analyzing anatomical variants to plan the procedure. Ventricular diameter and anatomical variants are observed. We positioned the patient in neutral position on a doughnut pillow and flexed the head at 30 degrees. Surgery is started using the previously described technique.

### 18.3.2 Endoscopic Findings

A precoronal burr hole in Kocher point was used to introduce the fiberscope through a peel-away sheath (▶ Fig. 18.7).

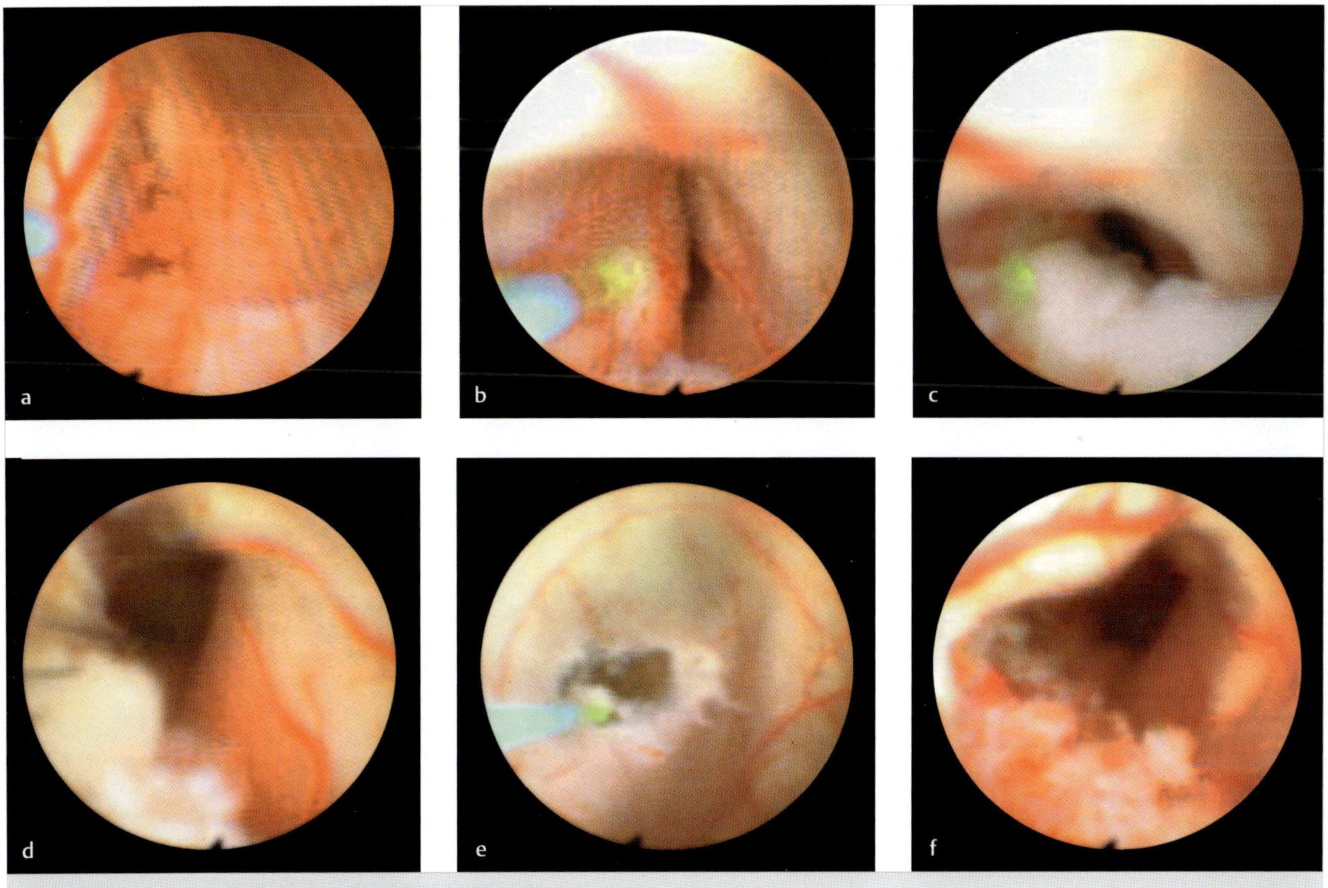



**Fig. 18.5** **(a)** A mass displacing the lateral wall and roof of the third ventricle is observed above the choroid plexus. **(b)** A holmium YAG laser is used to fenestrate the cyst wall; thereafter, small veins are coagulated using this device. **(c)** The inner cyst content is released. **(d)** The inner cyst content is drained using an epidural catheter. **(e)** After complete drainage and wall coagulation are achieved, a septostomy is performed to work on the contralateral Monro foramen using laser. **(f)** Image showing a complete aperture of the right Monro foramen.

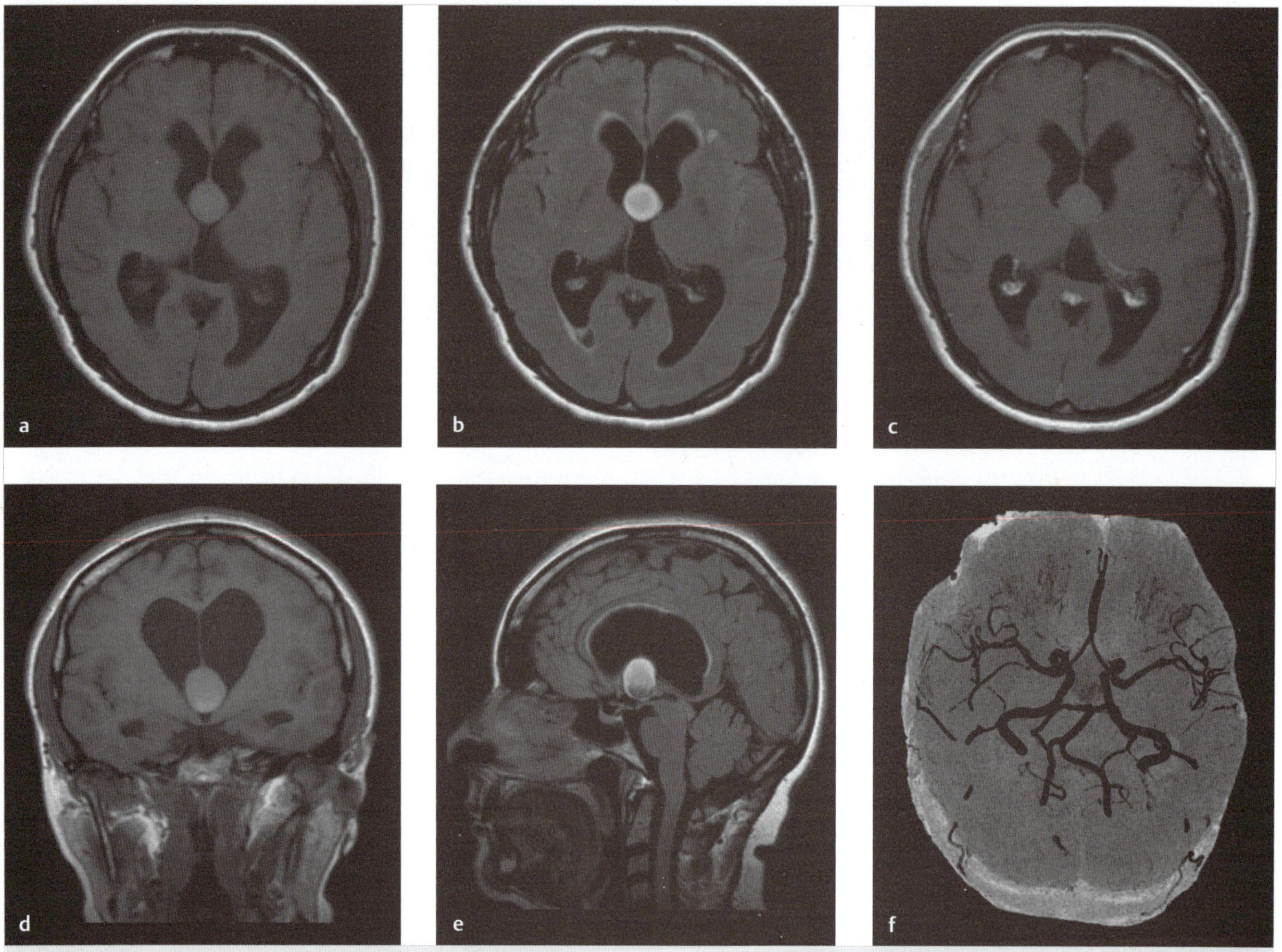

Fig. 18.6 (a) Axial T1-weighted magnetic resonance imaging showing a solid, isointense image occupying the third ventricle. Ventricular enlargement is observed suggesting a bilateral obstruction of Monro foramina. (b) Axial T2-weighted magnetic resonance imaging showing a hyperintense change on the lesion, and transependymal edema is evident. (c) Axial T1-weighted magnetic resonance imaging with contrast showing no reinforcement of the lesion. (d) Coronal T1-weighted magnetic resonance imaging showing a bilateral obstruction of Monro foramina and a slight difference in the ventricular enlargement of the left lateral horn. (e) Sagittal T2-weighted magnetic resonance imaging showing a lesion occupying the third ventricle and displacing the third ventricle walls. (f) Three-dimensional reconstruction showing no relevant vascular involvement by the lesion.

Anatomic landmarks were visualized. Right caudate and fornix, thalamostriate, and septal and caudate veins were visualized as well as the choroid plexus to locate the right foramen of Monro. A complete obstruction at this level by a mass was observed, displacing the medial wall and roof of the third ventricle. The wall and adjacent vascular structures were coagulated using Ho:YAG laser. Then the wall was opened using the same device. White cottoned material was drained using an epidural 18-gauge catheter inserted through the working channel. This procedure was repeated until the foramen of Monro was wide open. A septostomy was performed and contralateral foramen of Monro was observed. The same steps were done on the contralateral foramen of Monro. Ventricular lavage and closure were performed (▶ Fig. 18.8; ▶ Video 18.1).

### 18.3.3 Results

The hydrocephalus was solved, and symptoms disappeared. In a 4-year follow-up, the patient remains free of hydrocephalus, and there has been no cyst enlargement.

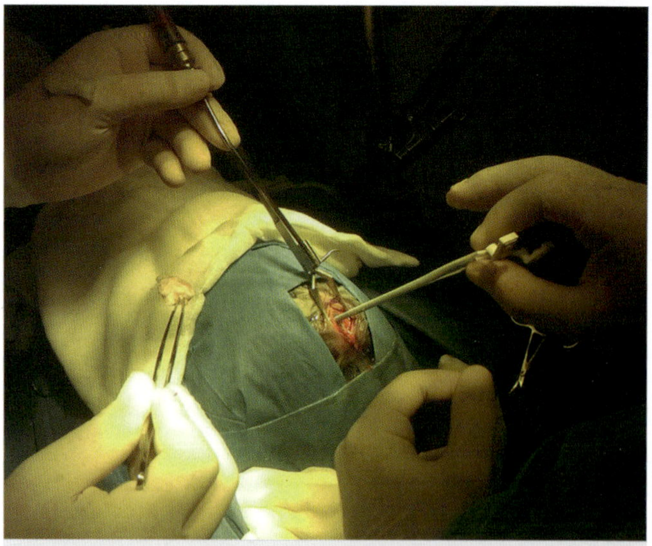

Fig. 18.7 Peel-away catheter is introduced after ventricular puncture.

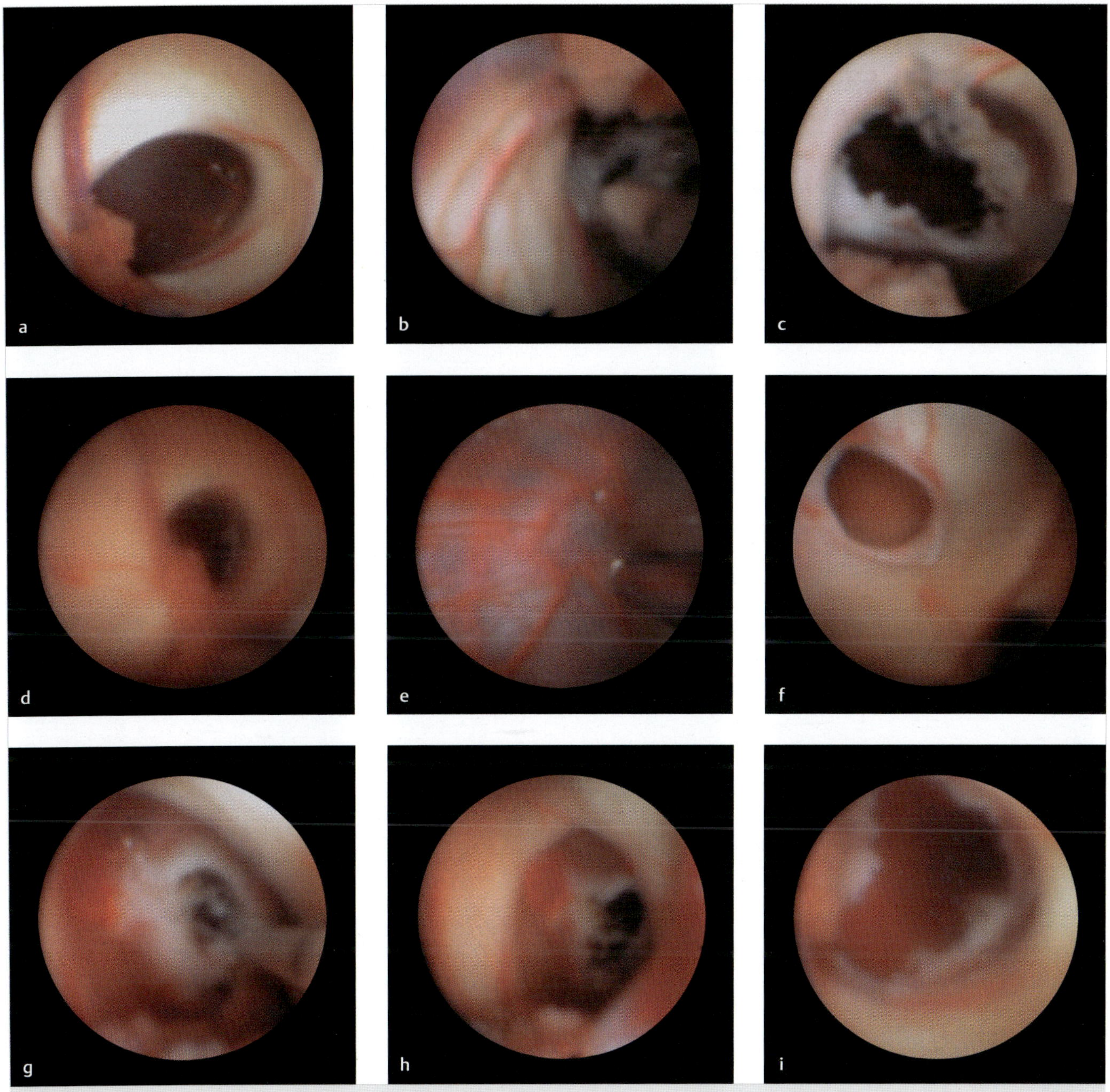


**Fig. 18.8 (a)** Right foramen of Monro is occluded by a colloid cyst. The membrane is visualized, and the clamp is introduced for cyst puncture and drainage. **(b, c)** The wall is coagulated using a 2-French coagulating electrode. **(d)** Right foramen of Monro is released. **(e)** The wall of the cyst next to the floor of the third ventricle is opened using anatomical landmarks as reference. **(f)** A septostomy is performed to work on the contralateral foramen of Monro. **(g, h)** The wall of the cyst occupying the left Monro foramen is opened and coagulated. **(i)** Left foramen of Monro is permeable.

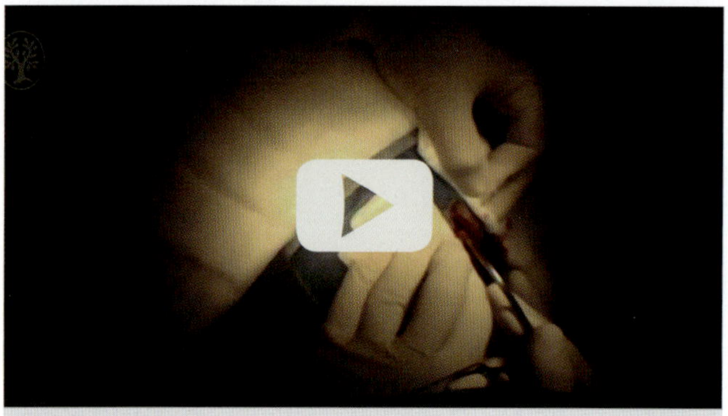

**Video 18.1** Colloid cyst resection technique.

# References


[1] Torres-Corzo JG, Rangel-Castilla L, Nakaji P, eds. Neuroendoscopic Surgery. Stuttgart: Georg Thieme Verlag; 2016

[2] Sheikh AB, Mendelson ZS, Liu JK. Endoscopic versus microsurgical resection of colloid cysts: a systematic review and meta-analysis of 1,278 patients. World Neurosurg. 2014; 82(6):1187–1197

[3] Brostigen CS, Meling TR, Marthinsen PB, Scheie D, Aarhus M, Helseth E. Surgical management of colloid cyst of the third ventricle. Acta Neurol Scand. 2017; 135(4):484–487

[4] Sabanci PA, Aras Y, Ali A, et al. Transcortical removal of third ventricular colloid cysts: comparison of conventional, guided microsurgical and endoscopic approaches and review of the literature. Turk Neurosurg. 2017; 27(4):546–557

[5] Torres-Corzo J, Rangel-Castilla L. Flexible neuroendoscopy: Part III—Basic endoscopic procedures and advantages of flexible neuroendoscopy. Contemp Neurosurg. 2013; 35(5):1–6

[6] Rangel-Castilla L, Torres-Corzo J. Flexible neuroendoscopy: Part II—Clinical and diagnostic indications. Contemp Neurosurg. 2013; 35(4):1–5

[7] Torres-Corzo J, Rangel-Castilla L. Flexible neuroendoscopy: Part IV—Advanced endoscopic procedures and complications of flexible neuroendoscopy. Contemp Neurosurg. 2013; 35(6):1–5

[8] Longatti P, Godano U, Gangemi M, et al. Italian neuroendoscopy group. Cooperative study by the Italian neuroendoscopy group on the treatment of 61 colloid cysts. Childs Nerv Syst. 2006; 22(10):1263–1267

[9] Torres-Corzo JG, Islas-Aguilar MA, Cerecedo-López CD. Flexible neuroendoscopic diagnosis and management of ventricular tumors: a retrospective cohort study. World Neurosurg. 2018; 118:e707–e712

[10] Torres-Corzo JG, Rangel-Castilla L, Islas-Aguilar MA, Vecchia RR-D. A novel approach of navigation-assisted flexible neuroendoscopy. Oper Neurosurg (Hagerstown). 2018; 14(3):E33–E37

# Index

*Note:* Page numbers set **bold** or *italic* indicate headings or figures, respectively.